Total Hip Arthroplasty: A Comprehensive Clinical Guide

Total Hip Arthroplasty: A Comprehensive Clinical Guide

Edited by Jasper Max

AMERICAN
MEDICAL PUBLISHERS
www.americanmedicalpublishers.com

American Medical Publishers,
41 Flatbush Avenue,
1st Floor, New York,
NY 11217, USA

Visit us on the World Wide Web at:
www.americanmedicalpublishers.com

ISBN: 978-1-63927-404-8

Cataloging-in-Publication Data

Total hip arthroplasty : a comprehensive clinical guide / edited by Jasper Max.
p. cm.
Includes bibliographical references and index.
ISBN 978-1-63927-404-8
1. Total hip replacement. 2. Orthopedics. 3. Orthopedic surgery. I. Max, Jasper.
RD549 .T68 2022
617.581 059 2--dc23

Table of Contents

Preface

This book was inspired by the evolution of our times; to answer the curiosity of inquisitive minds. Many developments have occurred across the globe in the recent past which has transformed the progress in the field.

Total hip arthroplasty is a surgical procedure in which a damaged or worn out hip joint is replaced with a prosthetic implant. This surgery is usually performed to resolve a hip fracture or a severe case of arthritis. Rheumatoid arthritis, osteoarthritis and traumatic arthritis commonly affect the hip joint. Other conditions that can cause joint failure of the hips include benign and malignant bone tumors, avascular necrosis, protrusio acetabuli, etc. A total hip replacement involves the replacement of the acetabulum and the femoral heal. This is a very common orthopedic procedure. Certain complications may occur after total hip arthroplasty. Dislocation is the chief complication in such surgeries. It may occur due to relaxed soft tissues and incomplete scar formation. Other complications include intraoperative fractures, vein thrombosis, loosening of the prosthesis, osteolysis, metal sensitivity and toxicity, etc. Most of these complications are however infrequent and largely preventable. Employing strategies such as using antibiotics routinely, using improved prosthetic materials and surfaces, etc. can prevent complications from arising. This book explores all the important aspects of total hip arthroplasty in the present day scenario. It strives to provide a fair idea about this operative procedure and to help develop a better understanding of the latest advances in its execution. With state-of-the-art inputs by acclaimed experts of orthopedics, this book targets students and professionals.

This book was developed from a mere concept to drafts to chapters and finally compiled together as a complete text to benefit the readers across all nations. To ensure the quality of the content we instilled two significant steps in our procedure. The first was to appoint an editorial team that would verify the data and statistics provided in the book and also select the most appropriate and valuable contributions from the plentiful contributions we received from authors worldwide. The next step was to appoint an expert of the topic as the Editor-in-Chief, who would head the project and finally make the necessary amendments and modifications to make the text reader-friendly. I was then commissioned to examine all the material to present the topics in the most comprehensible and productive format.

I would like to take this opportunity to thank all the contributing authors who were supportive enough to contribute their time and knowledge to this project. I also wish to convey my regards to my family who have been extremely supportive during the entire project.

Editor

1

Subtrochanteric shortening osteotomy during cementless total hip arthroplasty in young patients with severe developmental dysplasia of the hip

Duan Wang[1†], De-Hua Li[2,3†], Qi Li[1†], Hao-Yang Wang[1†], Ze-Yu Luo[1], Yang Yang[4], Fu-Xing Pei[1] and Zong-Ke Zhou[1*]

Abstract

Background: This retrospective study was designed to determine complications, functional and radiographic results of transverse subtrochanteric osteotomy during cementless, modular total hip arthroplasty (THA) in a series of active patients younger than 45 years with Crowe Type-III or IV developmental dysplasia of the hip (DDH).

Methods: We followed 49 patients (56 hips) with DDH who were treated with cementless THA, where the acetabular cup was positioned in the anatomic hip center and where a simultaneous transverse femoral osteotomy was performed. Complication rate evaluation and clinical outcomes were measured by validated clinical scores and radiographic evaluation were performed at a mean follow up of 10 years (range, 4.8–14.3 years).

Results: The mean limb-length discrepancy was reduced from 4.2 cm to 1.1 cm ($P < 0.01$). The mean Harris hip score (HSS) significantly improved from 40.6 points to 87.4 points ($P < 0.01$). Similarly, severity of low back pain, modified MAP, HOOS, and SF-12 also showed significant improvement ($P < 0.01$). There were 3 cases of postoperative dislocation, 3 cases of transient nerve palsy, 2 cases of nonunion, and 4 cases of intraoperative fracture. At 10 years follow-up, the estimated survival rate with any component revision as end points was 92%.

Conclusion: The cementless THA combined with transverse subtrochanteric osteotomy is a reliable technique with restoration of a more normal limb, satisfactory clinical outcomes, and mid-term survival of components.

Background

Characterized by anatomical abnormalities, biomechanical alterations, femoral deformities and severe soft tissue contractures, severe developmental dysplasia of the hip (DDH) increases the complexity of performing total hip arthroplasty (THA) [1, 2]. In most patients with Crowe Type-III or IV DDH, the true acetabulum is the best position for supporting cup due to sufficient bone stock and good biomechanics [3]. Therefore, placement of the acetabular cup in the true acetabulum has proved to obtain durable clinical and favorable biomechanical results of THA in such patients [4–6]. However, the limb may be lengthened by more than 4 cm during restoration of the anatomical hip rotation center, which resulted in overstretching of neurovascular structures and difficulty in reducing the hip. In addition, overstretching of peri-articular structures, including muscles and tendons, may lead to the dysfunction of the abductor muscles, hip stiffness, and early loosening of the components [7].

To address these concerns during THA for severe dysplasia, femoral shortening is sometimes necessary and an effective in most cases to correct femoral malrotation, facilitate the reduction, and equalize limb lengths without tension forces and increased risk of neurological traction injury [5, 7, 8]. Shortening osteotomy at different anatomic levels, including greater trochanter,

* Correspondence: zongke@126.com
†Equal contributors
1Department of Orthopedics, West China Hospital/West China School of Medicine, Sichuan University, 37# Wuhou Guoxue road, Chengdu 610041, People's Republic of China
Full list of author information is available at the end of the article

subtrochanteric region,, and distal femur, has been described previously. Subtrochanteric osteotomies can be performed with various techniques, such as transverse, oblique, Z-shaped, and chevron-shaped, each of which has their own advantages and disadvantages [2, 9–11]. The main disadvantage of the osteotomy is the risk of fracture and nonunion. The transverse type of bone cutting is a simpler and effective technique with similar rotational stability compared with other types of osteotomy in young patients [10]. Compared with a non-modular standard stem, a modular stem may be desirable to provide good fit and fill in the femoral canal and to obtain torsional stability at the osteotomy site [12]. In our center, we have performed cementless THA combined with transverse subtrochanteric osteotomy with use of modular stem in most patients with severe dysplasia [13].

Several prior reports have described short- to mid-term results of cementless THA combined femoral osteotomy shortening using modular stem in limited number of patients with severe dysplasia. However, these reports have included mixed groups of cemented and cementless femoral and acetabular components, different types of femoral osteotomy techniques, or even no femoral osteotomy in patients with large age span [9, 11, 14–16]. Moreover, many patients with severe DDH have complained not only of hip pain but also of low back pain and needed intensive treatment for such pain [17]. Lumbar spine and hip arthritis often coexist. Some studies demonstrated that THA could relieve the low back pain in patients with hip arthritis [18]. Nevertheless, no previous studies evaluated the low back pain after THA combined with femoral shorting osteotomy in active young patients who present severe hip dysplasia.

The purpose of the present study was to evaluated (1) mid-term clinical outcomes, (2) radiographic evaluation, (3) complications, and (4) mid-term survival of components in a group of active young patients with Crowe type-III and IV DDH who underwent cementless THA with transverse simultaneous subtrochanteric shortening osteotomy. We hypothesized that the cementless THA combined with transverse subtrochanteric shortening osteotomy is a reliable method in restoration of a more normal limb and satisfactory clinical outcomes, with mid-term survival of components for young patients with Crowe type-III and IV DDH.

Methods

Ethics statement

The study protocol was approved by the local institutional review board of West China Hospital, Sichuan University. Informed consent (including patients' details, images, or videos) was obtained from all participants. All experiments were performed in accordance with relevant guidelines and regulations.

Patients

We retrospectively reviewed 53 consecutive patients (62 hips) in whom cementless THA combined with transverse subtrochanteric shortening osteotomies was performed for Type-III or IV DDH according to Crowe classification from 2002 to 2012 in joint registry. One patient (1 hip) did not attend due to health issues unrelated to the THA, and one patient (2 hips) did not attend owing to no longer being interested. Two patients (3 hips) were lost to follow up after surgery and could not be contacted by phone or email at least 5 attempts. In the remaining 49 patients (56 hips), the hip dislocation was presented unilaterally in 42 patients and bilaterally in 7 patients. In bilateral high dislocations, 5 patients had Crowe type-IV, and 2 patients had Crowe type-IV dislocation of one hip and Type-III of the other. Therefore, 8 hips (14.3%) were Crowe Type III, while the other 48 hips (85.7%) were Crowe Type IV.

Severe pain unresponsive to non-operative management, pelvic obliquity, and functional impairment with limp in daily activities were the indication for surgery. There were 9 males and 40 females with mean age of 36.9 years (range, 19–45 years) at the time of index THA. Previous Schanz osteotomy was performed in two patients. Modular femoral stem (S-ROM®, DePuy Orthopadics, Marsaw IN.) with porous-coated acetabular component (PINNACLE®, POROCOAT®, DePuy Orthopadics, Marsaw IN.) was identical in all hips. The mean postoperative follow-up period was 10.2 years (range, 4.8–14.3 years). The pre-, peri- and post-operative data and surgical data were prospectively collected onto a predefined data collection form for patients with DDH. Table 1 showed the demographics of our study group.

Surgical planning and procedures

All operations were planned with transparencies and performed with use of cementless femoral and acetabular components. An acetabular template was placed at anatomical hip center, and a femoral template was correspondingly interiorized. The amount of femoral shortening was calculated to improve leg length discrepancy and lengthen the leg by no more than 3–4 cm to avoid nerve injury. Three-dimensional computed tomography (CT) scans was utilized to evaluate the acetabular bone stock.

All patients were operated on using a posterolateral approach in the lateral decubitus position. After resection of the femoral head and total capsulectomy were conducted, the position of the true acetabulum was reached and exposed through removal of fibrous scar tissue and osteophyte covering the true acetabulum. Soft-tissue release was applied in all hips. Transverse and round ligament was good indicator for recognizing true acetabulum. If the true acetabulum was not reachable

Table 1 Demographics and clinical results

Indicator	Pre-op clinical features		Overall (Pre-op)	Overall (Post-op)	*P* Value[a]
	Crowe Type-III	Crowe Type-IV			
No. of hips	8	48	56	56	
Gender (No. of pts)					
Male	0	9	9	–	
Female	8	34	40	–	
Affected side (No. of hips)					
Left	3	21	24	–	
Right	5	17	22	–	
Bilateral	0	10	10	–	
Harris Hip Score					
Mean in points (range)	54.6 (48–59)	38.2 (23–57)	40.6 (23–59)	87.4 (77–98)	<0.01
Rating (no. of hips)					
Excellent (90–100 points)	0	0	0	15	
Good (80–89 points)	0	0	0	39	
Fair (70–79 points)	0	0	0	2	
Poor (<70)	8	48	56	0	
PMA					
Mean in points (range)	7.6 (6–9)	6.5 (4–9)	6.6 (4–12)	16 (14–18)	<0.01
Pain	2.5 (2–3)	2.1 (1–4)	2.2 (1–4)	5.5 (5–6)	<0.01
Motion	2.4 (2–3)	2.3 (1–3)	2.3 (1–3)	5.2 (5–6)	<0.01
Function	2.6 (2–3)	2.0 (1–3)	2.1 (1–3)	5.3 (4–6)	<0.01
Rating (no. of hips)					
Excellent (18 points)	0	0	0	6	
Good (15–18 points)	0	0	0	43	
Fair (12–15 points)	0	0	0	7	
Poor (<12 points)	8	48	56	0	
Limp (no. of Pts.)					
Severe	3	28	31	0	
Moderate	4	15	19	3	
Slight	1	5	6	11	
None	0	0	0	42	
Limb-length discrepancy					
Mean in mm (range)	2.8 (2.1–3.7)	4.4 (2.3–6.5)	4.2 (2.1–6.5)	1.1 (0.6–1.4)	<0.01
< 1 cm (no. of hips)	0	0	0	24	
1–2 cm (no. of hips)	0	0	0	32	
2–3 cm (no. of hips)	5	4	9	0	
3–4 cm (no. of hips)	3	13	16	0	
4–5 cm (no. of hips)	0	18	18	0	
5–6 cm (no. of hips)	0	10	10	0	
> 6 cm (no. of hips)	0	3	3	0	
HOOS subscale scores					
Symptoms	10.8 (8–12)	8.8 (4–12)	9.1 (4–12)	16.6 (14–19)	<0.01
Pain	20.6 (17–24)	15.9 (6–23)	16.6 (6–24)	36.5 (34–40)	<0.01
Activities of daily living	34.1 (32–37)	28.7 (19–36)	29.4 (19–37)	60.9 (57–67)	<0.01

Table 1 Demographics and clinical results *(Continued)*

Indicator	Pre-op clinical features		Overall (Pre-op)	Overall (Post-op)	*P* Value[a]
	Crowe Type-III	Crowe Type-IV			
Sports and recreation	7.4 (5–8)	5.5 (3–8)	5.8 (3–8)	12.8 (10–16)	<0.01
Quality of life	6.9 (5–8)	5 (3–8)	5.3 (3–8)	13.7 (12–16)	<0.01
Trendelenburg sign (no. of hips)					
Yes	6	47	53	1	
No	2	1	3	55	
SF-12					
PCS	15.5 (12–17)	10.9 (6–16)	11.6 (6–17)	22.7 (19–25)	<0.01
MCS	18.3 (15–20)	13.8 (9–19)	14.4 (9–20)	25.6 (22–29)	<0.01

Values are expressed as mean with range
MAP Merle d'Aubigne and Postel, *PCS* Physical component summary, *MCS* Mental component summary, *ROM* range of motion, *HOOS* Hip dysfunction and Osteoarthritis Outcome Score
[a]$P < 0.05$ is significant

due to the obstruction of the proximal part of the femur, a transverse femoral osteotomy approximately 1–2 cm distal to the lesser trochanter was performed. If there was proximal femoral canal deformity, an osteotomy was conducted at the level of the deformity. Elevation or split of a short section of the vastus lateralis was performed to approach the subtrochanteric area. Next, the proximal femoral fragment was translated anteriorly to reach the true acetabulum after the performance of transverse osteotomy. The acetabulum was widened and deepened with use of hemispherical reamers at a designated angle of antevertion and abduction to obtain bleeding cancellous, which indicated an interference fit between the anterior and posterior columns (Fig. 1a). As for insufficient coverage or severe acetabular bone defects, augmentation of the acetabulum was conducted by a structural autograft or titanium alloy (Ti-alloy) mesh combined with bulk bone grafting from the resected femoral head. Femoral head structural bone autografts fixed with screws were used in thirty-eight hips to improve coverage of the cup due to insufficient coverage, whereas Ti-alloy mesh and impaction bone grafting were used in nine hips owing to severe acetabular bone defects according to the three-dimensional CT. Implantation of the acetabular cup was conducted using press-fit technique (Fig. 1b). The median diameter of the acetabular cup was 48 mm (range, 44 to 52 mm). The 28-mm femoral head was used in twenty-six hips, 32-mm head in twenty-two hips, and 36-mm head in eight hips. Ceramic-on-ceramic wear bearing was applied in forty-eight hips, and metal-on-poly in eight hips.

After the acetabular component was inserted, attention was then directed to the more distal femur. A second transverse subtrochanteric osteotomy was conducted to shorten the femur by the planned amount. If proximal femoral canal deformity existed, correction of rotational deformity of the proximal femur was conducted before axial reaming through subtrochanteric osteotomy. Four cases (4 hips) with such femoral canal deformity were corrected in our series. The straight axial intramedullary reaming process was conducted in the distal femur, and the proximal part of the femur was then prepared for the cementless implant (Fig.1c-d). Then, sequential rasping was performed until the appropriate femoral component size was achieved. The proximal and distal bone fragments were then aligned, and they were properly rotated on the trial component. If a trial reduction of the hip could not be achieved following the first cut of the osteotomy, the additional osteotomy was gradually performed in sequence also with a transverse design to archive satisfactory hip reduction. The average amount of femoral shorting was 2.7 cm (range, 1.9–4.5 cm). After the proximal sleeve was implanted, the straight stem was then inserted into the femur across the osteotomy site when the rotational alignment of the 2 fragments was adjusted to allow approximately 15°-20°of anteversion of the femoral component (Fig. 1e). If necessary, prophylactic cable fixation could be used to prevent femoral fracture. After the insertion of femoral component, the gap at the osteotomy site was grafted with autogenous morselized bone and stabilized by cable fixation to enhance biologic healing in forty-six cases (Fig. 1f). In most cases, cortical autograft struts cut from the resected femoral bone fragment was applied for additional stabilization of the osteotomy site. After the insertion of femoral and acetabular components, C-arm X ray was used in most patients to ensure the position of the cup and stem (Fig. 1g).

Postoperative rehabilitation

All patients were encouraged to conduct isometric exercises and active motion on a bed immediately after surgery. The patients walked with partial weight bearing under the protection of crutches for approximately 2 weeks. Then, gradually progressive full weight bearing

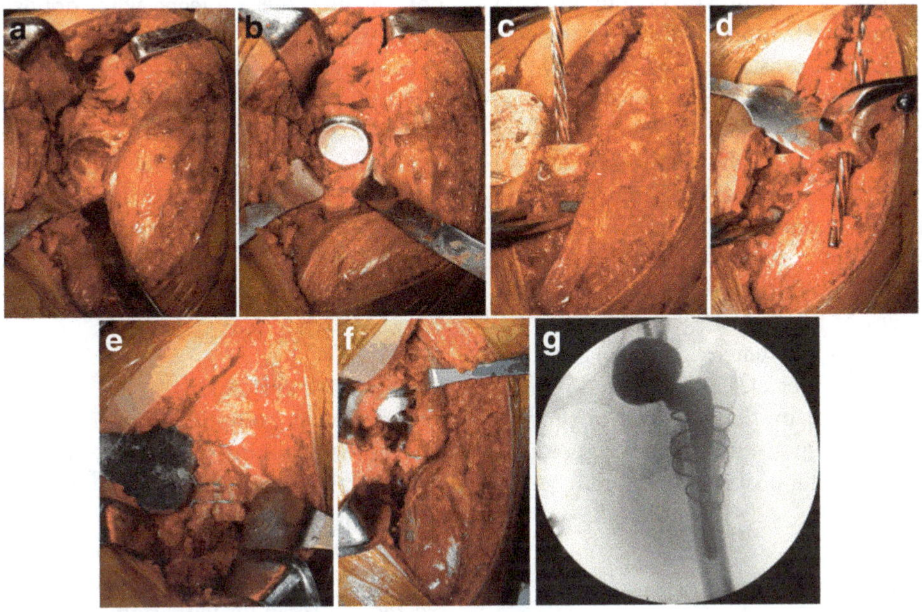

Fig. 1 Intraoperative photographs of THA in a thirty-one-year-old woman with Crowe type-IV DDH. (**a**) Acetabulum was widened and deepened to obtain bleeding cancellous and femoral head autograft was applied. (**b**) The insertion of acetabular cup. (**c**) The straight axial intramedullary reaming process was conducted in the distal femur. (**d**) The proximal part of the femur was then prepared for the cementless implant. (**e-f**) The straight stem was then inserted into the femur across the osteotomy site, at which the gap was grafted with autogenous morselized bone and stabilized by cable fixation. (**g**) C-arm X ray was used to ensure the position of the cup and stem

was allowed 4–6 weeks depending on stability of the femoral stem and positively osseous healing at osteotomy site. The mean hospital stay was 7.2 days (range, 6–15 days).

Clinical analysis

Clinical evaluation was conducted at 3 weeks, 6 weeks, 12 weeks, and 6 months after the surgery and annually thereafter until the last follow-up. A informative, concise follow-up data correction form was designed by the senior author (Z.K.Z.) for the patients with DDH [13]. The form included Hip dysfunction and Osteoarthritis Outcome Score (HOOS) (covering pain, symptoms, daily living, Sports, and quality of life), which is a validated and highly reproducible tool for evaluation of patient's opinion about their hips, assessment of symptoms and functional limitations related to DDH, and description of their hip disability [19]. In addition, 12-item short-form health survey questionnaire (SF-12) is more sensitive than HOOS regarding the hip-related quality of life in younger active patients [13]. We decided to use HOOS and SF-12 as accurate measure of life quality and hip disability. In our center, the Harris Hip Score (HHS) and modified Merle d'Aubigne and Postel (MAP) hip score (including pain, motion, and gait function) are collected routinely to evaluate the function of the hip [13, 20, 21]. In addition to the validated patient-reported outcomes, all pre- and post-operative evaluations regarding the severity of limp and Trendelenburg test status were also achieved. The limb-length discrepancy (LLD) was also recorded in pre- and post-operative periods, which was measured from the anterior superior iliac spine to the medial malleolus suggesting the length discrepancy of lower extremities. At each visit, a specific questionnaire about the presence of low back pain and details of such pain was completed. We also asked the back-pain location and evaluated the intensity of the pain with use of the visual analogue scale (VAS). All complications were reviewed.

Radiographic analysis

At each visit, all patients had standard anteroposterior and lateral radiographs of the hip, full-length view of the lower extremities. All radiographic measurements were adjusted for magnification. Radiographs were evaluated by authors who were not involved in the surgery. The amount of limb length was calculated by subtracting the amount of intraoperative femoral shortening from the amount of difference between the pre- and post-operative tip of the greater trochanter [22]. Bone union of the osteotomy site was evaluated on serial radiographs with the following radiographic criteria, including the presence of callus, cortical continuity, and no progressive gapping at the osteotomy site [23]. In addition, we also evaluated whether and when bone union occurred at the osteotomy site. Serial radiographs were also examined with respect to peri-prosthetic radiolucency, component migration, heterotopic ossification, osteolysis, and subsidence. Peri-prosthetic radiolucency was documented in acetabulum and femoral components according Delee and Charnley [24]. Heterotopic ossification was classified according to the method of Brooker et al. [25]. The seven zones around the femoral component on radiographs were described by Gruen et al. [26]. The mode of fixation of the femoral component was classified as bone ingrown, fibrous stable or unstable according to the system of Engh et al. [27]. Subsidence of femoral stem was also evaluated according to the method described by Engh et al. [27]. The loosening of acetabular cup was defined by the presence of progressive radiolucent lines >2 mm around the inserted cup, or migration, or a change in the position of the cup.

Statistical analysis

Two-sided paired Student t test was used to analyze preoperative and postoperative continuous variables. Statistical significance was set at $P < 0.05$. The χ^2 test was performed to analyze categorical variables. These data are presented as mean values with ranges. Kaplan-Meier was used to conduct analysis of cumulative survival rate of acetabular and femoral components. The end points for survival were defined as revision for any reason (including radiographic signs of loosening at the latest follow-up). Statistical analysis was performed with the use of SPSS Statistics software version 19.0 (IBM, Armonk, NY).

Results

Clinical outcomes

The mean HHS improved significantly from 40.6 points (range, 23–59 points) preoperatively to 87.4 points (range, 77–98 points) by the final follow-up ($P < 0.01$). Similarly, the mean modified MAP hip score improved from 6.6 points (range, 4 to 12 points) preoperatively to 16 points (range, 14 to 18 points) at the time of the latest follow-up, and the difference revealed significance ($P < 0.01$). For patient-reported outcomes, the mean HOOS and SF-12 scores significantly improved at the final follow-up ($P < 0.01$) (Table 1). Two of our patients were lost to follow-up.

Pre-operatively, the mean clinically measured LLD for unilateral THA was 4.2 cm (range, 2.1–6.5 cm) and it significantly improved to 1.1 cm (range, 0.6–1.4 cm) at the latest follow-up ($P < 0.01$), and no patients had >2 cm LLD postoperatively. At the final follow-up time, limp was moderate in three hips (5.4%), slight in eleven (19.6%), and none in 42 (75%) in the whole patient cohort. Moreover, positive Trendelenburg sign was presented in one patient (one hip) postoperatively. We did not include the subjects with opposite side DDH or other contralateral hip deformity.

The preoperative VAS score for low back pain was rated as severe in 10 patients (23.8%), moderate in 28 patients (66.7%), and mild in 4 patients (9.5%). At the final follow-up, the low back pain was moderate in 3 patients (7.1%), mild in 12 patients (28.6%), and none in 27 patients (64.3%). The low back pain improved over time, and the improvement was significant at every follow-up time point ($P < 0.01$) (Table 1, Fig. 2).

Radiographic evaluation

All acetabular components were placed in the position of true acetabulum (Fig. 3). Bone union of osteotomy site was archived in fifty-four hips with no complication, and the mean time to bone union was 6 months (range, 4–9 months). Serial radiographs showed two cases (4.1%) of nonunion at osteotomy site. One patient was treated successfully with bone grafting and medication, and showed bone union of the osteotomy site within 8 months without any complication at last follow-up time; the other one showed progressive stem subsidence and then the signs of radiographic loosening through the postoperative period, and it was revised with fully porous-coated stem at postoperatively 3.4 years and the new femoral component was stable at last follow-up time. Femoral stem that remained in situ after THA on radiographs indicated bone ingrowth in fifty hips (89.3%) at final follow-up time. Radiographic analyses of the femoral stem revealed radiolucency in three patients (6.1%) (three hips). However, no signs of progressive subsidence or loosening of femoral component were observed at the last follow-up in any hip. One patient (2.0%) (one hip) suffered from peri-prosthetic fracture around the femoral stem at 4.2 years, which was stabilized with a longer stem and cerclage wires, and fully healed without further complication. One patient (2.0%) (one hip) sustained peri-prosthetic fracture of distal femur at 5 years, and cerclage wires and bone graft were applied successfully for fixation. In addition, two patients (4.1%) (two hips) sustained acetabular fracture and loosening of the acetabular cup at postoperative five and seven years, respectively. They have been successfully treated by cup revision and bone grafting with no further complication (Table 2). Asymptomatic Brooker class-I and II heterotopic ossification were observed in three and two hips, respectively (Fig. 4). In addition, focal osteolysis was observed in five hips (Zone I in one hip, Zone II in two hips, and Zone 3 in two hips) on follow-up radiographs, but the cups showed bony incorporation and no surgery was required (Fig. 4).

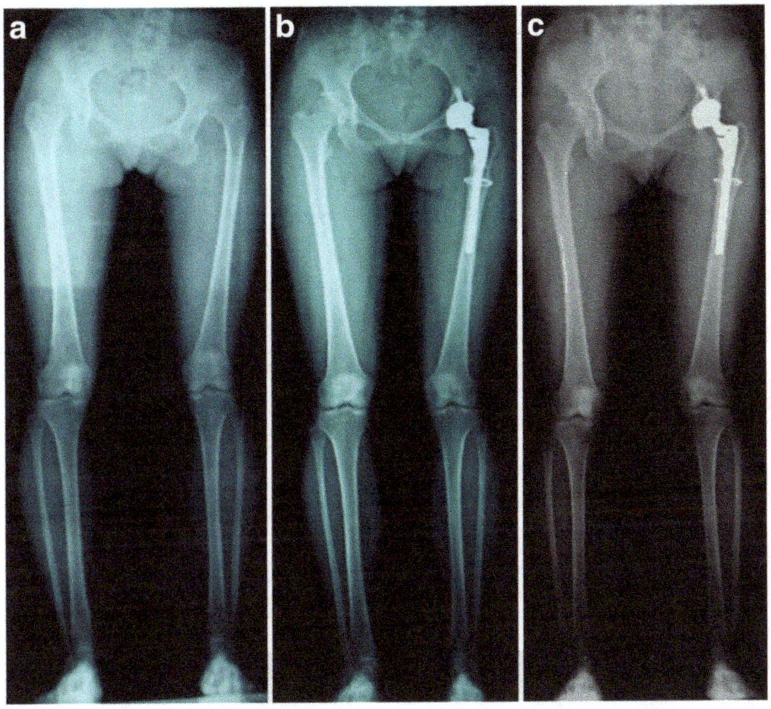

Fig. 2 Full-length radiographs of a twenty-five-year-old woman with unilateral Crowe type-IV DDH. The serial post-operative radiographic image showed that pelvic inclination was normalized over time. (**a**) Pre-operative radiographic image; (**b**) Radiographic image after four years follow-up; (**c**) Radiographic image after nine years follow-up

Complications

According to the Clavien-Dindo classification, the classification of surgical complications was grade I in 33 patients (67.3%), grade II in 9 patients (18.4%), and grade III in 7 patients (14.3%), respectively [28]. At the beginning of the series, an intraoperative nondisplaced fracture occurred in proximal femur in two hips and in distal femur in two hips, which were successfully treated with internal fixation with cerclage bands without further complication. Three patients (6.1%) (three hips) experienced transient nerve injury with weaknesses of ankle extension and dropfoot, who were treated with medication and physical therapy and fully recovered within 1 year without functional defects. Three patients (6.1%) (three hips) had dislocation postoperatively. In two cases, dislocation was treated successfully with closed reduction without further sequelae (Fig. 4). In one case, dislocation recurred two

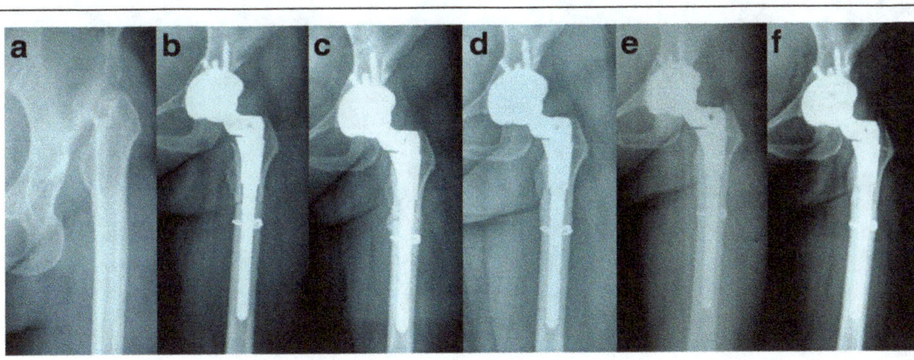

Fig. 3 Radiographs of a twenty-nine-year-old woman with unilateral Crowe type-IV DDH. (**a**) Preoperative anteroposterior view. (**b**) Post-operative radiographic image at four months follow-up. Total hip arthroplasty was combined with simultaneous transverse osteotomy. Cerclage wires were placed at osteotomy site, and the acetabulum was reconstructed with screws. (**c**) Post-operative radiographic image at one year follow-up. (**d**) At four years follow-up, bone union was detected at the osteotomy site without radiolucent lines around the stem. (**e**) At eight years follow-up, the femoral and acetabular components showed no radiographic signs of loosening. (**f**) Post-operative radiographic image at eleven years follow-up. The femoral and acetabular components were stable

Table 2 Complications

Case	Complication	Treatment	Results
5	Dislocation at 7 days	Closed reduction	No recurred dislocation
13	Dislocation at 2 years	Open reduction	No recurred dislocation
16	Dislocation at 2 weeks	Closed reduction	No recurred dislocation
9	Intraoperative femoral proximal fracture	Cerclage wires for fixation	No further complications
12	Intraoperative femoral proximal fracture	Cerclage wires for fixation	No further complications
19	Intraoperative femoral distal fracture	Cerclage wires for fixation	No further complications
24	Intraoperative femoral distal fracture	Cerclage wires for fixation	No further complications
14	Transient nerve injury	Medication and physical therapy	Full recovery
15	Transient nerve injury	Medication and physical therapy	Full recovery
21	Transient nerve injury	Medication and physical therapy	Full recovery
20	Nonunion of the osteotomy site, aseptic loosening of femoral component	Fully coated femoral component used in revision, bone graft at 3.4 years	Bone ingrowth and stable
35	Nonunion of the osteotomy site	Bone grafting and medication	Satisfactory clinical results
36	Peri-prosthetic fracture around the femoral stem	A longer stem and cerclage wires used in revision at 4.2 years	Bone ingrowth and stable
40	Peri-prosthetic fracture of distal femur	Cerclage wires and bone graft used in surgery at 5 years	Full healed
31	Acetabular fracture and thereby loosening of the acetabular cup	Cup revision and bone grafting at 5 years	No further complication
17	Acetabular and greater trochanter fracture, and screw breakage, and thereby loosening of the acetabular cup	Cup revision and bone grafting at 7 years	No further complication

years after indexed THA and could not be resolved with closed reduction, and required open reduction. Moreover, four patients (8.2%) complained of longer or shorter contralateral limb length. But no limbs were longer or shorter based on the result of radiographic measurement. No vascular complications, infection and deep venous thrombosis was recorded (Table 2). In summary, three (6.1%) and four patients (8.2%) required reoperation and revision surgery in the follow-up period, respectively.

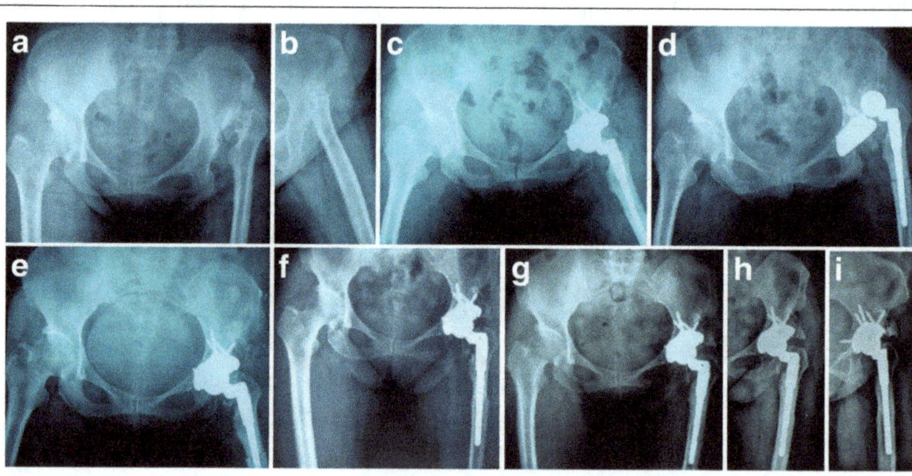

Fig. 4 Radiographs of a forty-two-year-old woman with unilateral Crowe type-IV DDH. (**a**-**b**) Pre-operative anteroposterior view. (**c**) Radiographic image at postoperative 1 day. Total hip arthroplasty was performed combined with transverse osteotomy in left hip. (**d**-**e**) Postoperative anteroposterior view showed dislocation at 1-week follow-up, which was treated successfully through closed relocation. (**f**) Radiographic image after five years follow-up showed that no radiolucent lines around the femoral and acetabular components were identified. But osteolysis around the stem at the distal tip and heterotopic ossification were identified. (**g**-**i**) At eleven years follow-up, the postoperative Harris hip score was 97, and the femoral stem was judged to be stable with bone ingrowth

Survivorship analysis

Kaplan-Meier survivorship with an end point of any component revision was 92% (95% confidence interval 84–99) at postoperative 10 years. Kaplan-Meier survivorship with an end point of aseptic loosening of the stem was 96% (95% confidence interval 87–99) at 10 years (Fig. 5).

Discussion

Crowe Type-III or IV developmental dysplasia is technically demanding for cementless THA in young patients, such as anatomical and biomechanical abnormalities, soft tissue contractures, and femoral deformities. In THA for severe DDH, satisfactory clinical and radiographic results have been reported with placement of the acetabular component in the true acetabulum and a femoral shortening osteotomy. However, the majority of studies reported series of a small number of patients who treated with THA combined with a subtrochanteric shortening osteotomy have included different surgical techniques with mixed groups of cemented and cementless implants or combinations of other osteotomy techniques, and the results are not consistent [5, 6, 8, 23, 29–39] (Table 3). To our knowledge, this is the largest reported series of young patients with Crowe Type-III and IV DDH, in which the clinical and radiographic outcomes and related complications of exclusively THA combined with simultaneous transverse femoral subtrochanteric shortening osteotomy were evaluated. The major finding of this study was that the cementless THA combined with transverse subtrochanteric shortening osteotomy could improve function, resort a more normal limb, and provide stable fixation in hips with Crowe Type-III and IV DDH.

We noted some limitations of the current study. First, the number of patients was relatively small. Second, there was a retrospective study with no control group. Third, there was no evaluation of inter-observer reliability, and all operations were performed by five senior surgeons. Forth, low back pain was measured with VAS scale and lacks objective evidence in this study.

Previous studies reported that superior placement of the acetabular component could result in improper components orientation, unfavorable biomechanical environment and even higher rates of components loosening, especially in young patients with severe DDH [40, 41]. Therefore, we placed all acetabular cups in true acetabulum and restored the anatomical center of hip rotation in our series. In addition, considering the young age of our series and the risk of the need for potential revision surgery, structural acetabular autograft was conducted in most cases. Linde et al. found that the rate of mechanical loosening of the acetabular cup was 13% in the group with the anatomical position of acetabular components compared with 42% in the group with superior placement of the acetabular cups at 15 years follow-up, and the difference revealed significance [40]. In our

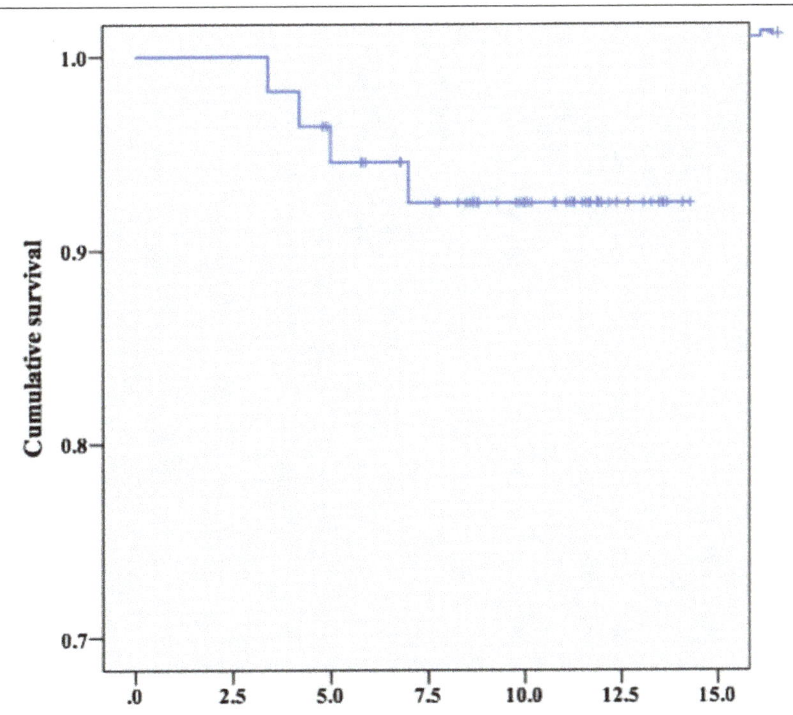

Fig. 5 Kaplan-Meier survivorship curve with revision for any component as the end points

Table 3 Overview of relevant literature in the treatment of Crowe III or IV dysplasia combined with subtrochanteric femoral shortening osteotomy

Study	Year	Hips (n)	DDH type	Femoral osteotomy	Mean age (Yrs)	Stem Type	Acetabular Type	Clinical results		Revision	Nonunion	Aseptic Loosening		Introp fracture		Heterotopic ossification	Nerve injury	Dislocation	Survival (end points)	FU (Yrs)
								Pre-operation	Post-operation			Act AL	Fem AL	Introp AF	Introp FF					
Ozan et al.	2016	32 (25)	III&IV	Transverse	51 (35–70)	Cementless	Cementless	HHS: 49 (25–72)	HHS: 87 (74–94)	2 (6.2%)	0 (0%)	2 (6.2%)	0 (0%)	0 (0%)	0 (0%)	0 (0%)	0 (0%)	3 (9.3%)	93% (Loosening)	5.1
Verettas et al.	2015	66 (62)	III&IV	Transverse	46 (24–74)	Cementless	Cementless	NA	NA	4 (6%)	0 (0%)	0 (0%)	0 (0%)	0 (0%)	0 (0%)	0 (0%)	1 (1.5%)	2 (3%)	94% (Revision)	9
Sofu et al.	2015	73 (68)	III&IV	Transverse	47 (31–69)	Cementless (Stryker)	Cementless (Stryker)	HHS: 38.6 ± 2.9 Pain: 16 ± 3.7	HHS: 83.7 ± 6.8 Pain: 40 ± 4.6	6 (8.2%)	4 (5.5%)	0 (0%)	4 (5.5%)	0 (0%)	0 (0%)	2 (2.7%)	0 (0%)	1 (1.3%)	87% (Femoral loosening; nonunion)	5
Desteli et al.	2015	60 (52)	III&IV	Transverse	51 ± 13	Cementless (HA)	Cementless (HA)	HHS: 39(25–60) Pain: 3 (1–5) Function: 3(1–5) Motion: 2 (1–4)	HHS:93(80–100) Pain: 5.4 (3–6) Function: 4(3–5) Motion: 5 (4–6)	0 (0%)	0 (0%)	0 (0%)	0 (0%)	0 (0%)	0 (0%)	0 (0%)	0 (0%)	0 (0%)	NA	6.5
Ogawa et al.	2011	6 (6)	III&IV	Transverse	58 ± 7.2	Cementless (S-ROM)	Cementless (Stryker; Depuy)	JOA: 35.5 ± 5.7 Pain: 7.0 ± 3.4 Function:9.3 ± 1.3 Motion:11.2 ± 1.3	JOA: 72.3 ± 2.1 Pain: 35.8 ± 1.5 Function:14 ± 0.8 Motion: 16 ± 0.5	0 (0%)	0 (0%)	0 (0%)	0 (0%)	0 (0%)	0 (0%)	0 (0%)	0 (0%)	2 (33.3%)	100% (Loosening)	8.1
Akiyama et al.	2011	15 (11)	III&IV	Transverse	59 (42–77)	Cemented	Cemented	MAP: 8.1 ± 2.5	MAP: 15.1 ± 1.3	3 (20%)	3 (20%)	0 (0%)	0 (0%)	0 (0%)	0 (0%)	0 (0%)	0 (0%)	2 (13.3%)	80% (Revision)	3–10
Togrul et al.	2010	21 (14)	III&IV	Transverse	42 (33–52)	Cementless	Cementless	Pain: 2.9 (1–5) Motion: 4.4(3–5) Walking:3.7(2–5)	Pain: 5.2 (4–6) Motion:5.4(5–6) Walking:5.5(5–6)	1 (4 .8%)	0 (0%)	0 (0%)	0 (0%)	0 (0%)	0 (0%)	0 (0%)	0 (0%)	2 (9.5%)	95% (Revision)	3.4
Howie et al.	2010	35 (28)	III&IV	Transverse	47 (26–75)	Cemented	Cemented	OHS: 40.2 SF12: 79.6	OHS: 26.7 SF12: 103.3	7 (20%)	2 (3%)	2 (3%)	0 (0%)	0 (0%)	0 (0%)	0 (0%)	2 (6%)	3 (9%)	80% (Revision)	5.6
Biant et al.	2009	28 (22)	III&IV	Transverse	45 (23–74)	Cementless (S-ROM)	Cementless	HHS: 37 (19–69) SF12: NA WOMAC: 27	HHS:83(44–100) SF12: 95.6 WOMAC: 23	4 (14%)	0 (0%)	2 (7.1%)	0 (0%)	0 (0%)	2 (7.1%)	0 (0%)	1 (3.6%)	0 (0%)	NA	10
Park et al.	2007	24 (23)	III&IV	Transverse	49 (20–66)	Cementless	Cementless	HHS: 35.6	HHS: 81.7	4 (17%)	3 (12%)	1 (4%)	3 (13%)	0 (0%)	3 (13%)	0 (0%)	0 (0%)	1 (4%)	83% (Revision)	4.7
Gotze et al	2007	7 (7)	III&IV	Transverse	42 (29–64)	Cementless	Cementless	HHS: 43 (29–61)	HHS: 77 (66–90)	1 (14%)	0 (0%)	0 (0%)	1 (14%)	0 (0%)	0 (0%)	0 (0%)	0 (0%)	0 (0%)	86% (Revision)	1.5
Onodera et al.	2006	14 (13)	III&IV	Transverse	55 (44–69)	Cementless	Cementless	HHS: 38 (15–55)	HHS: 82 (35–93)	1 (7%)	1 (7%)	0 (0%)	1 (7%)	0 (0%)	6 (43%)	0 (0%)	NA	1 (7%)	93% (Revision)	5
Erdemli et al.	2005	25 (22)	III&IV	Transverse	44 (28–61)	Cementless	Cementless	HHS: 37 Pain: 2.3 Function: 2.3 Motion: 2.3	HHS: 95 Pain: 5.7 Function: 4.5 Motion: 4.4	4 (16%)	1 (4%)	0 (0%)	2 (8%)	1 (4%)	2 (8%)	1 (4%)	1 (4%)	1 (4%)	84% (Revision)	6
Masonis et al..	2003	11	III&IV	Transverse	49 (21–70)	Cementless	Cementless	HHS: 33 (22–45)	HHS:74(42–100)	5 (24%)	1 (9%)	0 (0%)	0 (0%)	0 (0%)	0 (0%)	0 (0%)	0 (0%)	0 (0%)	76% (Revision)	5.8
		10	III&IV	Transverse	49 (21–70)	Cemented	Cemented				1 (10%)	0 (0%)	0 (0%)	0 (0%)	0 (0%)	0 (0%)	0 (0%)	3 (30%)		5.8
Bruce et al.	2000	9	III&IV	Transverse	53 (26–77)	Cementless (S-ROM)	Cementless	HHS: 31 (20–25)	HHS: 81 (60–98)	2 (22%)	0 (0%)	0 (0%)	1 (11%)	0 (0%)	2 (22%)	0 (0%)	0 (0%)	1 (11%)	78% (Revision)	4.7
Present study	2016	56 (49)	III&IV	Transverse	36 (19–45)	Cementless (S-ROM)	Cementless (S-ROM)	HHS: 40 (23–59) Pain: 2.2 (1–4) Function: 2 (1–3) Motion: 2.3(1–3) PCS: 11.6 (6–17) MCS: 14.4(9–20)	HHS: 87 (77–98) Pain: 5.5 (5–6) Function: 5 (4–6) Motion: 5.2(5–6) PCS: 22 (19–25) MCS: 25 (22–29)	1 (1.8%)	1 (1.8%)	1 (1.8%)	0 (0%)	0 (0%)	3 (5.4%)	2 (3.6%)	3 (5.4%)	3 (5.4%)	98% (Revision)	10.1

LLD length discrepancy, *Introop AF* intraoperative acetabular fracture, *Introop FF* intraoperative femoral fracture, *Acet AL* acetabulum aseptic loosening, *Fem AL* femoral component aseptic loosening, *PW* polyethylene wear, *FNI* femoral nerve injury, *SNI* sciatic nerve injury, *OHS* oxford hip scores, *DVT* deep vein thrombosis, *PE* pulmonary embolism, *HHS* harris Hip Score, *MAP* Merle d'Aubigne and Postel, *JOA* Japanese Orthopaedic Association hip score

series, only two patients (two hips) showed acetabular component loosening (3.5%) due to acetabular fracture and screw breakage.

Femoral shortening osteotomy is sometimes necessary to assist anatomic placement of acetabular cup without sciatic nerve compromise and excessive soft tissue tension [6, 31]. Subtrochanteric osteotomies can be performed at different anatomic levels with various surgical techniques, including Z-shaped, transverse, oblique, and double Chevron [2, 10, 11]. A biomechanical study by Muratli et al. compared four different subtrochanteric osteotomies techniques, and demonstrated that there was no single inherent feature increasing the stability of the osteotomy designs [10]. Li et al. performed a meta-analysis comparing transverse and modified osteotomy regarding complications and survivorship and no difference was found [42]. And, transverse osteotomy may be recommended compared with other techniques due to technical simplicity, convenience of adjusting the anteversion angle, correction of the rotational deformity, preservation of the proximal femoral metaphysis, relatively short learning curve for precise performance and minimal damage of the periosteum in patients with severe DDH [5, 42]. Therefore, transverse subtrochanteric osteotomy was utilized in all hips. Common complications in femoral shortening osteotomy were intraoperative femoral fracture with rates from 5 to 24% [6, 8, 23] and nonunion at the osteotomy site with rates from 7 to 22% [31, 32, 35]. Great attention should be paid to narrow and straight femoral canals, which are so vulnerable to fracture during broaching or insertion of femoral stem. Our union rate of osteotomy site was 96.4%. In our series, several methods were available to prevent nonunion. First, the interface between the osteotomy fragments should be cut as smoothly as possible. Second, autologous morselized bone grafts were used to augment the osteotomy gap, and the resected bone from femoral head was wrapped around osteotomy site. Third, great care was taken to minimize the damage of periosteum circumferentially during preparation of osteotomy sites and prophylactic cerclage wiring to keep the osteoblastic activity of periosteum. At the beginning of our series, no precautions were taken to decrease the risk of intraoperative femoral fracture, three cases of fracture were recorded that was successfully treated with cerclage bands and healed with no further complications. To obtain a strong fixation and minimize the risk of fracture, we subsequently paid more attention to fracture signs (e.g. sudden much more subsidence of the implant, rotational instability of stem at final insertion) during broaching and performed prophylactic cable fixation before the insertion of implant. The risk of intraoperative fracture decreased after prevention of fracture.

In this study, we consider dislocation as an important complication, which may compromise the press-fit between femoral component and femoral fragment and result in disengagement and early loosening of stem [43]. Total dislocation rates were 5.3% in our series that compared favorably with dislocation rates in other studies [8, 34, 36, 38]. The relatively low incidence of dislocation can be interpreted by the stronger muscle strength in younger and more active patients, proper cup orientation, and restoration of abductor muscles lever arm and center of hip rotation [3, 6, 7, 31]. Another important complication was transient nerve injury in three patients, which were recovered with no weakness or numbness in the limb by the latest follow-up evaluation. Some researchers reported that femoral lengthening increase the incidence of nerve palsy, and thereby they recommended lengthening the femur by <3 cm, < 4 cm, or <5 cm to avoid this complication [3, 12]. The transient nerve injuries occurred in our series due to relatively large amount of leg lengthening and less experience, and time-consumption at the beginning. We estimated the bone shortening based on preoperative templating, and believed that the leg lengthening of <3.5 cm may decrease the risk of nerve injury [13].

The function outcomes, including HSS, HOOS, and SF-12, improved significantly in our study group comparable to the results reported in the literature, which may be attributed to the relief of preoperative pain, improvement of LLD, and restoration of abductor muscles lever arm and femoral offset [5, 34, 35, 38]. In addition, we should pay more attention to chronic complications of the lumber spine and concomitant back pain, which was due to the compensation of lumber scoliosis and pelvic inclination for LLD. The results showed the significant improvement of patient's low back pain in this study, which can be explained by the two reasons: (1) LLD was decreased, and (2) thereby pelvic inclination and excess scoliosis or lordosis was normalized over time after this procedure.

It is generally accepted that the rates of implant failure were higher in young and more active patients due to a high grade of physical activity and functional demand, compared with elderly and inactive patients. As a result of high failure rate of components in cemented THA, cementless THA with ceramic on ceramic can provide long-term stable fixation and became the gold standard in younger cases. In addition, modular standard stem is very suitable in cases with severe DDH with a need for femoral osteotomy, which provides good fit and fill in dysplastic narrow femoral canal and stable fixation of the metaphyseal and diaphyseal fragments, and thereby obtains torsional stability [12, 31]. With regards to the long-term survival, overall failure rate was 7.1% in our series, which was is comparable to other published studies recording a failure rate of 0–10% [31, 44].

Conclusion

For young patients with Crowe Type-III or IV DDH, THA is very difficult due to the abnormal anatomy of the proximal femur and acetabular structure. The mid-term clinical and radiographic results of THA for these patients were good in our study. Thus, we demonstrated that cementless THA combined transverse subtrochanteric femoral shortening osteotomy in hips with Crowe Type-III or IV DDH is a reliable technique, which provides satisfactory outcomes, including acceptable rate of major lengthening-related complications, stable fixation of cementless implant, and significant improvement of function and relief of back pain.

Abbreviations

DDH: developmental dysplasia of the hip; THA: Total hip arthroplasty; HOOS: Hip dysfunction and Osteoarthritis Outcome Score; HHS: Harris Hip Score; SF-12: 12-item short-form health survey questionnaire; MAP: Merle d'Aubigne and Postel; LLD: Limb-length discrepancy; VAS: Visual analogue scale

Funding

None

Acknowledgements

We would like to thank the relevant staff for guidance and assistance for their support and collaboration in our hospital.

Authors' contributions

ZKZ. and FXP. conceived and designed this study; DW, DHL, and QL collected the data; DW, HYW, YY and ZYL performed the statistical analysis; HYW, YY and ZYL prepared Tables 1–3; DW, HYW, YY and ZYL prepared Figs. 1–5; DW, QL and HYW wrote the manuscript; DW, DHL, and ZKZ revised this manuscript. All authors reviewed the final manuscript. All authors agree to be accountable for all aspects of the work.

Consent for publication

Not applicable.

Competing interests

The authors declare that they have no competing interests.

Author details

[1]Department of Orthopedics, West China Hospital/West China School of Medicine, Sichuan University, 37# Wuhou Guoxue road, Chengdu 610041, People's Republic of China. [2]Key Laboratory of Birth Defects and Related Diseases of Women and Children, Ministry of Education, Sichuan University, Chengdu 610041, People's Republic of China. [3]Department of Nursing, West China Second University Hospital/West China Women's and Children's Hospital, Chengdu 610041, China. [4]State Key Laboratory of Oral Diseases, West China Hospital of Stomatology, Sichuan University, Chengdu 610041, People's Republic of China.

References

1. Noble PC, Kamaric E, Sugano N, Matsubara M, Harada Y, Ohzono K, Paravic V. Three-dimensional shape of the dysplastic femur: implications for THR. Clin Orthop Relat Res. 2003;417:27–40.
2. Bao N, Meng J, Zhou L, Guo T, Zeng X, Zhao J. Lesser trochanteric osteotomy in total hip arthroplasty for treating CROWE type IV developmental dysplasia of hip. Int Orthop. 2013;37(3):385–90.
3. Ahmed E. Ibrahim el G, Ayman B: Total hip arthroplasty with subtrochanteric osteotomy in neglected dysplastic hip. Int Orthop. 2015;39(1):27–33.
4. Eskelinen A, Helenius I, Remes V, Ylinen P, Tallroth K, Paavilainen T. Cementless total hip arthroplasty in patients with high congenital hip dislocation. J Bone Joint Surg Am. 2006;88(1):80–91.
5. Sofu H, Kockara N, Gursu S, Issin A, Oner A, Sahin V. Transverse subtrochanteric shortening osteotomy during Cementless Total hip arthroplasty in Crowe type-III or IV developmental dysplasia. J Arthroplast. 2015;30(6):1019–23.
6. Howie CR, Ohly NE, Miller B. Cemented total hip arthroplasty with subtrochanteric osteotomy in dysplastic hips. Clin Orthop Relat Res. 2010;468(12):3240–7.
7. Zagra L, Bianchi L, Mondini A, Ceroni RG. Oblique femoral shortening osteotomy in total hip arthroplasty for high dislocation in patients with hip dysplasia. Int Orthop. 2015;39(9):1797–802.
8. Togrul E, Ozkan C, Kalaci A, Gulsen M. A new technique of subtrochanteric shortening in total hip replacement for Crowe type 3 to 4 dysplasia of the hip. J Arthroplast. 2010;25(3):465–70.
9. Mu W, Yang D, Xu B, Mamtimin A, Guo W, Cao L. Midterm outcome of Cementless Total hip arthroplasty in Crowe IV-Hartofilakidis type III developmental dysplasia of the hip. J Arthroplast. 2016;31(3):668–75.
10. Muratli KS, Karatosun V, Uzun B, Celik S. Subtrochanteric shortening in total hip arthroplasty: biomechanical comparison of four techniques. J Arthroplast. 2014;29(4):836–42.
11. Yalcin N, Kilicarslan K, Karatas F, Mutlu T, Yildirim H. Cementless total hip arthroplasty with subtrochanteric transverse shortening osteotomy for severely dysplastic or dislocated hips. Hip Int. 2010;20(1):87–93.
12. Takao M, Ohzono K, Nishii T, Miki H, Nakamura N, Sugano N. Cementless modular total hip arthroplasty with subtrochanteric shortening osteotomy for hips with developmental dysplasia. J Bone Joint Surg Am. 2011;93(6): 548–55.
13. Wang D, Li LL, Wang HY, Pei FX, Zhou ZK. Long-term results of Cementless Total hip arthroplasty with subtrochanteric shortening osteotomy in Crowe type IV developmental dysplasia. J Arthroplast. 2016;32(4):1211–19.
14. Krych AJ, Howard JL, Trousdale RT, Cabanela ME, Berry DJ. Total hip arthroplasty with shortening subtrochanteric osteotomy in Crowe type-IV developmental dysplasia. J Bone Joint Surg Am. 2009;91(9):2213–21.
15. Charity JA, Tsiridis E, Sheeraz A, Howell JR, Hubble MJ, Timperley AJ, Gie GA. Treatment of Crowe IV high hip dysplasia with total hip replacement using the Exeter stem and shortening derotational subtrochanteric osteotomy. J Bone Joint Surg Br. 2011;93(1):34–8.
16. Imam MA, Fathalla I, Holton J, Nabil M, Kashif F. Cementless Total hip replacement for the Management of Severe Developmental Dysplasia of the hip in the middle eastern population: a prospective analysis. Front Surg. 2016;3:31.
17. Hasegawa Y, Iwase T, Kanoh T, Seki T, Matsuoka A. Total hip arthroplasty for Crowe type developmental dysplasia. J Arthroplast. 2012;27(9):1629–35.
18. Parvizi J, Pour AE, Hillibrand A, Goldberg G, Sharkey PF, Rothman RH. Back pain and total hip arthroplasty: a prospective natural history study. Clin Orthop Relat Res. 2010;468(5):1325–30.
19. Swarup I, Marshall AC, Lee YY, Figgie MP. Implant survival and patient-reported outcomes after total hip arthroplasty in young patients with developmental dysplasia of the hip. Hip Int. 2016;26(4):367–73.
20. Zeng WN, Wang FY, Chen C, Zhang Y, Gong XY, Zhou K, Chen Z, Wang D, Zhou ZK, Yang L. Investigation of association between hip morphology and prevalence of osteoarthritis. Sci Rep. 2016;6:23477.
21. Zeng WN, Zhou K, Zhou ZK, Shen B, Yang J, Kang PD, Pei FX. Comparison between drainage and non-drainage after total hip arthroplasty in Chinese subjects. Orthop Surg. 2014;6(1):28–32.
22. Li W, Zhang W, Bai G, Huang Z, Shen R. Total hip arthroplasty for treatment of Crowe type IV congenital dysplasia of hip with dislocation in adults. Zhongguo Xiu Fu Chong Jian Wai Ke Za Zhi. 2013;27(10):1153–6.
23. Masonis JL, Patel JV, Miu A, Bourne RB, McCalden R, Macdonald SJ, Rorabeck CH. Subtrochanteric shortening and derotational osteotomy in primary total hip arthroplasty for patients with severe hip dysplasia: 5-year follow-up. J Arthroplast. 2003;18(3 Suppl 1):68–73.
24. DeLee JG, Charnley J. Radiological demarcation of cemented sockets in total hip replacement. Clin Orthop Relat Res. 1976;121:20–32.
25. Brooker AF, Bowerman JW, Robinson RA, Riley LH, Jr.: Ectopic ossification

following total hip replacement. Incidence and a method of classification. J Bone Joint Surg Am 1973, 55(8):1629–1632.

26. Gruen TA, McNeice GM, Amstutz HC. "modes of failure" of cemented stem-type femoral components: a radiographic analysis of loosening. Clin Orthop Relat Res. 1979;141:17–27.
27. Engh CA, Massin P, Suthers KE. Roentgenographic assessment of the biologic fixation of porous-surfaced femoral components. Clin Orthop Relat Res. 1990; 257:107–28.
28. Dindo D. The Clavien–Dindo classification of surgical complications. Springer London. 2014;250:187–96.
29. Desteli EE, Imren Y, Tan E, Erdogan M, Ozcan H. Clinical results of cementless total hip arthroplasty with shortening osteotomy for high dislocation with developmental dysplasia. Acta Orthop Belg. 2015;81(1):30–5.
30. Verettas DA, Chloropoulou P, Xarchas K, Drosos G, Ververidis A, Kazakos K. Small diameter acetabulum and femoral head in total hip arthroplasty for developmental dysplasia of the hip, with no femoral osteotomy. Hip Int. 2015;25(3):209–14.
31. Biant LC, Bruce WJ, Assini JB, Walker PM, Walsh WR. Primary total hip arthroplasty in severe developmental dysplasia of the hip. Ten-year results using a cementless modular stem. J Arthroplast. 2009;24(1):27–32.
32. Bruce WJ, Rizkallah SM, Kwon YM, Goldberg JA, Walsh WR. A new technique of subtrochanteric shortening in total hip arthroplasty: surgical technique and results of 9 cases. J Arthroplast. 2000;15(5):617–26.
33. Erdemli B, Yilmaz C, Atalar H, Guzel B, Cetin I. Total hip arthroplasty in developmental high dislocation of the hip. J Arthroplast. 2005;20(8):1021–8.
34. Onodera S, Majima T, Ito H, Matsuno T, Kishimoto T, Minami A. Cementless total hip arthroplasty using the modular S-ROM prosthesis combined with corrective proximal femoral osteotomy. J Arthroplast. 2006;21(5):664–9.
35. Park MS, Kim KH, Jeong WC. Transverse subtrochanteric shortening osteotomy in primary total hip arthroplasty for patients with severe hip developmental dysplasia. J Arthroplast. 2007;22(7):1031–6.
36. Ozan F, Uzun E, Gurbuz K, Koyuncu S, Altay T, Kayali C. Total hip arthroplasty in the developmental dysplasia of the hip using transverse subtrochanteric osteotomy. J Orthop. 2016;13(4):259–63.
37. Akiyama H, Kawanabe K, Yamamoto K, Kuroda Y. So K, Goto K, Nakamura T: cemented total hip arthroplasty with subtrochanteric femoral shortening transverse osteotomy for severely dislocated hips: outcome with a 3- to 10-year follow-up period. J Orthop Sci. 2011;16(3):270–7.
38. Ogawa H, Ito Y, Shinozaki M, Matsumoto K, Shimizu K. Subtrochanteric transverse shortening osteotomy in cementless total hip arthroplasty achieved using a modular stem. Orthopedics. 2011;34(3):170.
39. Gotze C, Winkelmann W, Gosheger G, Rodl R. Is there a need of an additional extramedullary fixation in transverse subtrochanteric shortening in primary total hip arthroplasty for patients with severe hip dysplasia? Short-term experience in seven patients with congenital dislocation. Z Orthop Unfall. 2007;145(5):568–73.
40. Linde F, Jensen J, Pilgaard S. Charnley arthroplasty in osteoarthritis secondary to congenital dislocation or subluxation of the hip. Clin Orthop Relat Res. 1988; 227:164–71.
41. Makita H, Inaba Y, Hirakawa K, Saito T. Results on total hip arthroplasties with femoral shortening for Crowe's group IV dislocated hips. J Arthroplast. 2007;22(1):32–8.
42. Li C, Zhang C, Zhang M, Ding Y. Comparison of transverse and modified subtrochanteric femoral shortening osteotomy in total hip arthroplasty for developmental dysplasia of hip: a meta-analysis. BMC Musculoskelet Disord. 2014;15:331.
43. Zhu J, Shen C, Chen X, Cui Y, Peng J, Cai G. Total hip arthroplasty with a non-modular conical stem and transverse subtrochanteric osteotomy in treatment of high dislocated hips. J Arthroplast. 2015;30(4):611–4.
44. Vermersch T, Viste A, Desmarchelier R, Fessy MH. Prospective longitudinal study of one hundred patients with total hip arthroplasty using a second-generation cementless dual-mobility cup. Int Orthop. 2015;39(11):2097–101.

2

Surgical accuracy, function, and quality of life of simultaneous versus staged bilateral total hip arthroplasty in patients with osteonecrosis of the femoral head

Seung-Chan Kim, Young-Wook Lim, Woo-Lam Jo, Dong-Chul Park, Jin-Woo Lee, Won-Woo Kang and Yong-Sik Kim*

Abstract

Background: The optimal surgical option for patients requiring bilateral hip replacement remains controversial. The purpose of this study was to compare surgical accuracy; functional outcome and health-related quality of life; and prosthetic-related complications and revision surgery of a simultaneous bilateral total hip arthroplasty (THA) with those of a staged bilateral THA with an interval between procedures <12 months.

Methods: A total of 123 unselected consecutive patients (mean age, 43.3 years) who underwent bilateral THAs for osteonecrosis of the femoral head (ONFH) with a minimum follow-up of two years (mean, 60.2 months) were studied retrospectively; 63 simultaneous procedures served as a test group and 60 staged procedures served as a control group.

Results: The mean postoperative leg-length discrepancy (LLD) and the percentage of patients who had an LLD >3 mm were significantly lower in the simultaneous group ($P < 0.001$ and $P = 0.001$, respectively). A higher number of cups within the safe zones, a higher correction rate, and a lower failure rate for the cup placement in the second-operated hip were also identified in the simultaneous group. The mean Harris hip score, EuroQol-5D index, and EuroQol-visual analogue scale score were all better in the simultaneous group at the latest follow-up ($P < 0.001$, in all comparisons). We found that the simultaneous procedure was associated with a lower incidence of postoperative prosthetic-related complications and revision surgery.

Conclusions: We suggest that bilateral ONFH could be treated with a simultaneous THA rather than a staged THA to achieve a better surgical outcome.

Keywords: Total hip arthroplasty, Bilateral, Simultaneous, Staged, Accuracy, Osteonecrosis of the femoral head

Background

It has been estimated that approximately 15–25% of patients being considered for primary total hip arthroplasty (THA) require a second contralateral procedure within five years [1–3]. Specifically, non-traumatic osteonecrosis of the femoral head (ONFH) is a progressive disease primarily affecting bilateral hip joints of young adults [4, 5]. Once ONFH begins, 80% of femoral heads may collapse if no treatment is administered, thus, it frequently may result in the need for THA [6]. However, the optimal timing of surgery in patients requiring bilateral hip replacement still remains controversial, and the surgeon and patient must decide whether to perform simultaneous bilateral THA (BTHA) or staged BTHA with an interval between procedures.

Simultaneous BTHA has several potential benefits over a staged procedure, including a decrease in cost and overall length of hospital stay, use of a single anesthetic, better functional recovery, and earlier return

* Correspondence: yongsik@korea.com
Department of Orthopaedic Surgery, Seoul St. Mary's Hospital, College of Medicine, The Catholic University of Korea, Banpodae-ro 222, Seocho-gu, Seoul 137-701, South Korea

to daily activities [7, 8]. Simultaneous BTHA, however, also poses a potential increased risk of venous thromboembolic events, heterotopic ossification, higher blood transfusion requirement, and increased need for transfer to a rehabilitation facility [2, 3, 8–13]. Nevertheless, there is a recent consensus that there is no significant difference in the safety of the simultaneous BTHA and the staged BTHA in regard to complication rate and mortality [8, 9, 14, 15]. However, some studies have not supported this practice [2].

Although the literature contains a number of studies regarding perioperative and socioeconomic implications of simultaneous BTHA vs. staged BTHA, to the best of our knowledge, only a few studies have compared accuracy in surgical procedures, radiographic outcome, functional outcome, and quality of life. We hypothesized that patients who underwent a simultaneous BTHA would have superior surgical accuracy, better functional outcome, and quality of life. We secondarily hypothesized that there would be no difference in surgical outcome of the first-operated hip of a BTHA between the two procedures.

Therefore, we sought to (1) compare the postoperative leg-length discrepancy (LLD) and the accuracy of acetabular cup placement (in particular, of the second-operated hip) based on the safe zones proposed by Lewinnek et al. [16] and Callanan et al. [17]; (2) compare the functional outcome and quality of life in patients with simultaneous BTHA versus those in patients with staged BTHA; and (3) determine whether differences in the incidence of perioperative prosthetic-related complications and revision surgery were present between the two groups.

Methods

After institutional review board approval, we retrospectively reviewed a consecutive series of 177 patients (354 hips) who underwent bilateral cementless THAs from October 2007 through October 2013 with either a simultaneous or staged procedure. All patients with a preoperative diagnosis of bilateral ONFH and known clinical outcomes through regular follow-up (minimum follow-up period: two years) were considered for inclusion. Patients with primary or secondary osteoarthritis, inflammatory arthritis, bony ankylosis, neurologic diseases, previous hip surgery, and significant involvement of the knee, ankle and/or spine were excluded. Ultimately, a total of 123 patients (246 hips), consisting of 71 male (142 hips) and 52 female patients (104 hips), were included in the study. Mean patient age at the time of surgery was 43.3 years (range, 17 to 77) and mean follow-up duration was 60.2 months (range, 24 to 101).

The patients were divided into two groups according to type of surgery; 63 patients who underwent simultaneous BTHA, comprised the test group; the control group comprised 60 patients whose operations were performed as a staged procedure with an interval < 12 months (mean, 4.8 months; range, 2 weeks to 12 months). The procedure was selected primarily based on symptoms and patient preference. A simultaneous procedure was chosen if the patient presented with bilateral intractable hip pain, while a staged procedure was planned when the patient presented with one-sided intractable pain or preferred to undergo a two-stage procedure. A summary of the demographics and clinical data of the patients of the two groups is shown in Table 1. No significant differences were found between the two groups in regard to age, sex, body mass index (BMI), American Society of

Table 1 Patient demographics and clinical data

Data	Simultaneous BTHA	Staged BTHA	*P* value
Number of patients (hips)	63 (126)	60 (120)	
Mean age (years; range)	43.1 (20 to 69)	43.5 (17 to 77)	0.871#
Sex (n; %)			0.336†
Male	39 (62)	32 (53)	
Female	24 (38)	28 (47)	
Mean BMI (kg/m^2; range)	22.9 (15.8 to 30.9)	23.3 (16.4 to 37.9)	0.568#
ASA grade (n; %)			0.404†
1	19 (30)	18 (30)	
2	38 (60)	40 (67)	
3	6 (10)	2 (3)	
4/5	0	0	
ARCO stage in ONFH (hips; %)			0.638†
III	89 (71)	88 (73)	
IV	37 (29)	32 (27)	
Ceramic head (n; %)			0.817†
28 mm	18 (14)	14 (12)	
32 mm	40 (32)	38 (31)	
36 mm	68 (54)	68 (57)	
Mean follow-up (months; range)	57.8 (24 to 98)	62.7 (24 to 101)	0.767‡
Mean length of hospital stay (days; range)	10.5 (4 to 28)	18.7 (8 to 45)	< 0.001‡
Mean hospital charge ($; range)	12,608 (9645 to 21,469)	14,910 (11,428 to 27,146)	< 0.001‡
Mean operative time (min; range)	172 (108 to 245)	162 (104 to 275)	0.058#
Mean intraoperative blood loss (mL; range)	1037 (550 to 2000)	1145 (600 to 2700)	0.098‡

BTHA bilateral total hip arthroplasty, *ASA* American Society of Anesthesiologists, *ONFH* osteonecrosis of the femoral head, *ARCO* Association Research Circulation Osseous
#Independent *t*-test
†Chi-square test
‡Mann-Whitney test

Anesthesiologists (ASA) grade, disease stage, ceramic head diameter implanted, follow-up duration, operative time, and intraoperative blood loss; however, a shorter length of hospital stay and a smaller amount of hospital charge were noted in the simultaneous BTHA group.

In all patients, preoperative planning with digital templating on standardized radiographs of the pelvis was performed. Preoperative templating was performed to determine the hip center of rotation, femoral offset, and preoperative LLD, as well as to estimate the optimal size and position of the acetabular and femoral component. The radiographs comprised an anteroposterior (AP) view of the pelvis centered over the pubic symphysis with the pelvis and legs in a neutral position and at 15° of internal rotation to control for femoral anteversion, and lateral views of both hips. Each template radiograph included a standard calibration marker positioned as close to the coronal plane of the hip joint as possible; thus, facilitating the adjustment of the magnification. The head-to-lesser-trochanter distance (HLD) was measured as described in our previous study and recorded preoperatively as a reference standard for minimizing the occurrence of LLD in all cases [18]. In our unit, all radiographs are digitized using the Picture Archiving and Communication System (PACS; Marosis, Infinite, Seoul, Korea).

Six months postoperatively, standardized pelvic radiographs were taken on the radiographic coronal plane to evaluate the postoperative LLD, radiographic cup inclination and anteversion angle the same as the protocol for preoperative AP pelvic radiographs (Fig. 1). When taking standardized plain radiographs, effort was made to decrease an anterior or posterior pelvic tilt throughout the study. The LLD on radiographs was defined as the difference in perpendicular distance in millimeters between the inter-teardrop-line to the corresponding tip of the lesser trochanter [19]. The actual value of the LLD was obtained using a known size of the prosthetic head implanted. The orientation of acetabular components was measured with the use of digital measurement tools on PACS workstations. The cup inclination angle was directly measured as the angle between the long axis of the opening ellipse and the inter-teardrop line. The anteversion angle was computed using the method described by Lewinnek et al. (= arcsin (short axis/long axis)) [20, 21]. Thus, the angles measured on a plain AP radiographs by this method were radiographic anteversion and inclination since the radiographic definition and radiographic coronal plane (functional coronal plane) were consistently used in this study; Lu et al. [22] demonstrated that measurement of the orientation of acetabular components on radiographic coronal plane using Lewinnek's method is reliable and accurate compared with measurement on CT scans. To test a cup alignment, two safe zones for inclination and anteversion (the safe zone of Lewinnek et al. [16] (inclination, 30° to 50°; anteversion, 5° to 25°) and the modified safe zone of Callanan et al. [17] (inclination, 30° to 45°; anteversion, 5° to 25°)) were used as standard references in this study. Calculation of the number of hips that were in those safe zones regarding inclination, anteversion, and a combination of both were done for both groups. For the analyses of surgical accuracy in positioning of the acetabular component, the cup placement of the second hip of the BTHA was determined as 'correction' if the cup of the second-operated hip was within the safe zone while the cup of the first-operated hip was outside the safe zone. In contrast, the cup placement of the second hip was determined as 'failure' if the cup of the second hip was outside the safe zone while the cup of the first hip was within the safe zone. One independent investigator (one of the authors) who was not involved in any of the operations and blinded to the study groups, evaluated all radiographs.

All surgeries were performed by a single surgeon (the senior author) at our institution under general anesthesia in a standard fashion. A posterolateral approach with a short external rotator preservation procedure was used to enhance joint stability with the patient in the lateral decubitus position for all procedures [23]. All patients received a cementless hemispheric porous-coated acetabular component (BENCOX®; Corentec, Cheonan, Korea) and a cementless double-tapered wedge femoral component (BENCOX®; Corentec) with ceramic-on-ceramic bearing couples (BIOLOX®; CeramTec AG, Polchingen, Germany). The surgeon positioned the cup using its aligning guide with the goal of cup position at 40° of abduction and 15° of anteversion. All THAs were performed with the use of the HLD method to minimize the occurrence of LLD [18]. Additionally, the legs were palpated on the table intraoperatively to confirm the leg length. In cases of simultaneous BTHA, the surgical team strove to reduce the time for repositioning the patient and preparing the skin of the second hip. Nevertheless, the average time from the skin closure of the first hip to the skin incision of the second hip was approximately 15 min (mean, 15.3 min). The operative time, intraoperative blood loss, and any intraoperative complications were recorded in the operative notes immediately after surgery.

Clinical and radiologic evaluations were performed at 6 weeks, 3, 6, 12 months, and yearly thereafter postoperatively. The patients were assessed with the Harris Hip Score (HHS) at each follow-up visit to evaluate functional outcome and completed the self-administered EuroQol-5 dimension (EQ-5D) questionnaires and the EuroQol-visual analogue scale (EQ-VAS) measurement

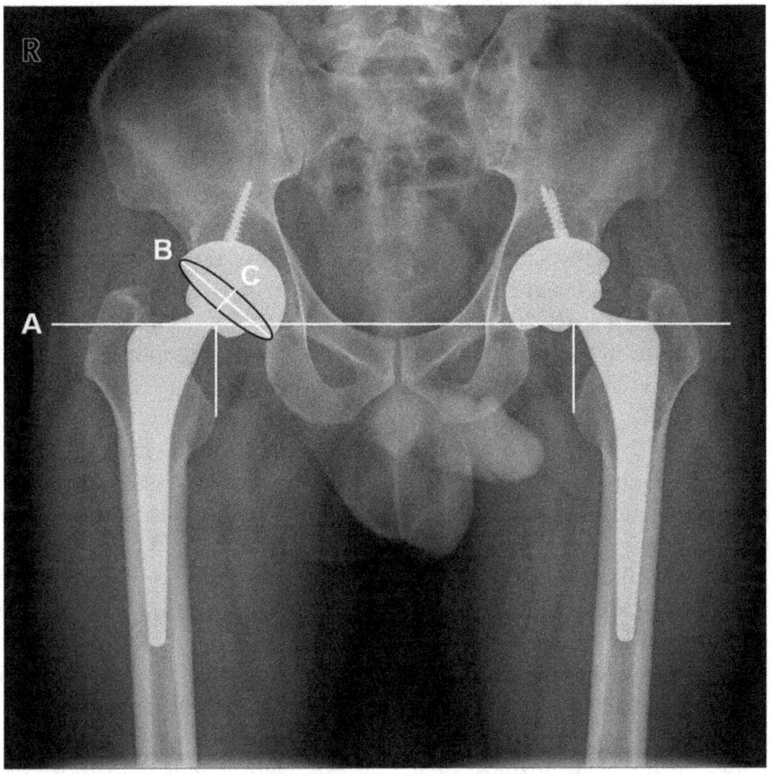

Fig. 1 A standardized anteroposterior pelvic radiograph of a 39-year-old male patient with bilateral osteonecrosis of the femoral head at 6 months after simultaneous bilateral total hip arthroplasty showing the radiographic measurement of leg-length discrepancy and acetabular cup orientation. The line A indicates the inter-teardrop line as a reference line. The line B is the long axis and the line C is the short axis of the opening ellipse of the acetabular component, respectively

at the time of the latest follow-up to evaluate health-related quality of life and health status [24]. The EQ-5D has five dimensions (mobility, self-care, usual activities, pain/discomfort, and anxiety/depression) and each item has three levels (no problem, some problem, or major problem); an EQ-5D index score of 1 represents the best possible health status, and a score of 0 represents the worst possible health status. The EQ-VAS is a vertical visual analogue scale ranging from 0 (indicating the worst imaginable health status) to 100 (indicating the best imaginable health status). The incidence and details of any postoperative prosthetic-related complications and revisions at any time point during follow-up were noted. Postoperative systemic complications were not addressed in this study except for death since those have been evaluated in several previous studies [2, 8, 9, 14, 15, 25–27]. All clinical information was collected by a research assistant (one of the authors) using medical records.

A post hoc power analysis was performed using a G*Power software [28] (version 3.1; Düsseldorf University, Düsseldorf, Germany) for each sample size of the cohorts and the means (and standard deviations) of the outcome measure LLD of each group, resulting in a power value of 0.98. Statistical analysis was performed using SPSS for Windows (version 21; SPSS, Chicago, Illinois, USA). The distribution of variables was tested for normality using the Kolmogorov-Smirnov test. The independent *t*-test was used for comparison of normally distributed continuous variables and the Mann-Whitney U test was used for nonparametric continuous variables in independent groups. The Pearson chi-square test or Fisher's exact test was used for categorical variables. $P < 0.05$ was considered statistically significant.

Results

Among 246 hips with ONFH, no significant difference was found between the simultaneous and staged BTHA groups in stage of the disease based on the Association Research Circulation Osseous (ARCO) classification system [29]. At the time of each surgery, there were 89 stage-III hips and 37 stage-IV hips in the simultaneous BTHA group, and 88 stage-III hips and 32 stage-IV hips in the staged BTHA group ($P = 0.638$). The independent comparison of the second-operated hips also showed no significant difference in stage between the two groups: 49 stage-III hips and 14 stage-IV hips in the simultaneous group, and 45 stage-III hips and 15 stage-IV hips in the staged group ($P = 0.717$).

The mean postoperative LLD was significantly lower in the simultaneous BTHA group (2.1 mm) compared to the staged BTHA group (4.3 mm; $P < 0.001$). A percentage of patients who had an LLD < 3 mm postoperatively in the simultaneous group was significantly higher than that of the staged group (75% vs. 42%; $P = 0.001$). We still found a higher percentage of patients in the simultaneous group who had an LLD < 5 mm, although significance of the difference disappeared (92% vs. 73%; $P = 0.068$). No patient (0%) had an LLD of >10 mm in the simultaneous group, whereas 2 patients (3.3%) had an LLD of >10 mm in the staged group (one with an LLD of 14.1 mm, and the other with an LLD of 10.8 mm).

There were no significant differences between groups in the mean radiographic cup inclination angle or anteversion angle for the first-operated hip as well as the second-operated hip of the BTHA (Table 2). When comparing the first-operated hip of the simultaneous group to that of the staged group independently, no significant differences in the number of cups within each safe zone for inclination and anteversion were found. However, the comparison of the second-operated hip showed significant differences between the two groups. The number of cups within each safe zone for inclination was found to be higher in the simultaneous group: 95% vs. 85% for Lewinnek ($P = 0.056$), and 81% vs. 65% for Callanan ($P = 0.046$). The number of cups within the safe zone for anteversion was also significantly higher in the simultaneous group: 95% vs. 77% ($P = 0.003$).

In the analyses of accuracy of acetabular cup placement of the second-operated hip, the simultaneous group showed a higher correction rate and a lower failure rate for both inclination and anteversion (Table 3). The failure rate for anteversion in the simultaneous group, in particular, was significantly lower: 2% vs. 23% ($P = 0.001$).

The mean postoperative HHS, EQ-5D index, and EQ-VAS score at the time of the latest follow-up in the simultaneous group were all significantly higher than those of the staged group (Table 4).

The results of perioperative prosthetic-related complications and revision surgery in the two groups are summarized in Table 5. No dislocations occurred in either group and there were no significant differences in the overall incidence of intraoperative fracture, dislocation, aseptic loosening, wound infection, periprosthetic fracture, or revision between the two groups. However, both the number of occurrences in the second hip and the proportion of second hip occurrences in the staged group were higher than those in the simultaneous group for all events except dislocation and periprosthetic fracture. On the contrary, the proportion of second hip

Table 2 Comparison of accuracy in acetabular cup placement according to type of surgery

Parameter	Simultaneous BTHA (*N* = 63)	Staged BTHA (*N* = 60)	*P* value
Mean inclination (°; mean ± SD; range)			
First-operated hip	42.0 ± 6.2 (29.3 to 55.7)	40.8 ± 7.3 (24.5 to 61.6)	0.333[#]
Second-operated hip	40.7 ± 5.4 (22.8 to 52.4)	41.7 ± 7.2 (25.8 to 63.5)	0.401[#]
Mean anteversion (°; mean ± SD; range)			
First-operated hip	16.7 ± 6.9 (2.7 to 30.5)	17.3 ± 7.5 (4.7 to 36.3)	0.639[#]
Second-operated hip	17.9 ± 5.2 (7.8 to 30.8)	17.5 ± 7.7 (3.8 to 34.6)	0.706[#]
Cups within safe zone for inclination (n; %)			
First-operated hip			
Lewinnek (30° to 50°)	56 (89)	51 (85)	0.522[†]
Callanan (30° to 45°)	42 (67)	45 (75)	0.310[†]
Second-operated hip			
Lewinnek (30° to 50°)	60 (95)	51 (85)	0.056[†]
Callanan (30° to 45°)	51 (81)	39 (65)	0.046[†]
Cups within safe zone for anteversion (n; %)			
First-operated hip			
Lewinnek, or Callanan (5° to 25°)	50 (79)	47 (78)	0.889[†]
Second-operated hip			
Lewinnek, or Callanan (5° to 25°)	60 (95)	46 (77)	0.003[†]

BTHA bilateral total hip arthroplasty, *SD* standard deviation
[#]Independent *t*-test
[†]Chi-square test.

Table 3 Comparison of correction rate and failure rate in acetabular cup placement during second THA according to type of surgery

Parameter	Simultaneous BTHA (N = 63)	Staged BTHA (N = 60)	P value
Correction rate for inclination (n; %)			
Lewinnek (30° to 50°)	7/7 (100)	7/9 (78)	0.475‡
Callanan (30° to 45°)	16/21 (76)	9/15 (60)	0.465‡
Failure rate for inclination (n; %)			
Lewinnek (30° to 50°)	3/56 (5)	7/51 (14)	0.188‡
Callanan (30° to 45°)	7/42 (17)	15/45 (33)	0.074†
Correction rate for anteversion (n; %)			
Lewinnek, or Callanan (5° to 25°)	11/13 (85)	10/13 (77)	1.000‡
Failure rate for anteversion (n; %)			
Lewinnek, or Callanan (5° to 25°)	1/50 (2)	11/47 (23)	0.001†

BTHA bilateral total hip arthroplasty
†Chi-square test
‡Fisher's exact test.

occurrences in the simultaneous group did not exceed 50% for all events. In the simultaneous group, there were 2 revisions (1.6%; 1 of 2 performed on the second hip) for aseptic loosening of the femoral component during the entire follow-up period. Four revisions (3.3%; 4 of 4 performed on the second hip) were required in the staged group; these included 1 femoral component revision and 1 acetabular component revision for aseptic loosening, and 2 two-stage revisions for septic loosening (one was on the acetabular component and the other on the femoral component). Mortality did not differ significantly between the two groups at any time point (Table 5).

Discussion

Patients often present with bilateral hip disease, and the patient and surgeon must decide whether to perform simultaneous bilateral THA or unilateral THA, with replacement of the other hip in the future. Since the introduction of the simultaneous procedure in 1967 [30], the two procedures have been repeatedly evaluated in regard to safety and socioeconomic factors [2, 8, 25–27]. However, the literature contains only a limited amount of studies that assess the accuracy of the surgical procedure, radiographic outcome, functional outcome, and quality of life in regard to simultaneous versus staged BTHA. In patients with bilateral ONFH, the present study showed that simultaneous BTHA resulted in a superior surgical accuracy, better functional outcome, higher quality of life, and fewer prosthetic-related complications, compared to a staged BTHA. In particular, there has been a remarkable difference regarding accuracy of cup placement when comparing the second-operated hip independently between the two groups.

The restoration of normal anatomy and biomechanics after THA, such as leg-length and acetabular orientation, are thought to be important factors in achieving pain-free and well-functioning hip joint, as well as ensuring the stability of the prosthetic hip and patient satisfaction [18, 19, 31, 32]. There currently is no defined limit of acceptable LLD in terms of hip function and patient satisfaction. Nevertheless, there is a general consensus among hip surgeons that most patients can tolerate a discrepancy of <10 mm [33, 34]. We have found a significantly lower LLD after a simultaneous BTHA than that after a staged procedure. In the simultaneous group, no patient had an LLD of >10 mm, whereas 2 patients had an LLD of >10 mm in the staged group and had much lower clinical scores than the other patients (one with an LLD of 14.1 mm, HHS of 70, EQ-5D index of 0.757, EQ-VAS of 60; and one with an LLD of 10.8 mm, HHS of 65, EQ-5D index of 0.766, EQ-VAS of 50). Our findings do not agree with a previous study reporting no significant difference in the postoperative LLD (4.5 mm vs. 5.3 mm; P = 0.239) [9]. In their study, however, a lower LLD was also identified in the simultaneous group.

Our findings indicate that a simultaneous BTHA is associated with a superior surgical outcome. In this study, the second-operated hips in the simultaneous group showed better results in regard to the number of cups within the safe zones and the correction rate/failure rate for the acetabular cup placement, compared to those of the staged group. In a previous randomized controlled trial, Bhan et al. [9] found no significant difference in the mean abduction angle of the acetabular component between the two groups. However, unlike the present study, they merely assessed the mean value of the inclination angle of all cups implanted on bilateral hips. We suggest that the reason for this difference in surgical accuracy between the two groups may be due to

Table 4 Comparison of postoperative Harris hip score, EQ-5D and EQ-VAS score at the time of the latest follow-up after THA according to type of surgery

Parameter	Simultaneous BTHA (N = 63)	Staged BTHA (N = 60)	P value
Harris hip score (mean ± SD; range)	95.9 ± 4.8 (73 to 100)	90.7 ± 8.2 (64 to 100)	< 0.001†
EQ-5D$_{index}$ (mean ± SD; range)	0.94 ± 0.08 (0.72 to 1.00)	0.87 ± 0.09 (0.68 to 1.00)	< 0.001†
EQ-VAS (mean ± SD; range)	86.0 ± 10.6 (50 to 100)	74.1 ± 15.6 (30 to 100)	< 0.001†

BTHA bilateral total hip arthroplasty, *SD* standard deviation
†Mann-Whitney test.

Table 5 Prosthetic-related complications and mortality of simultaneous and staged BTHA during entire follow-up period

Complication	Simultaneous BTHA (126 hips)		Staged BTHA (120 hips)		*P* value
	Overall incidence	Proportion of second hip given occurrence (n; %)	Overall incidence	Proportion of second hip given occurrence (n; %)	
Intraoperative fracture (n; %)[a]	10 (8)	3/10 (30)	7 (6)	5/7 (71)	0.516[†]
Dislocation (n; %)[a]	0 (0)	0/0 (0)	0 (0)	0/0 (0)	1.000[‡]
Aseptic loosening (n; %)[a]					
Acetabular component	0 (0)	0/0 (0)	1 (1)	1/1 (100)	0.488[‡]
Femoral component	2 (2)	1/2 (50)	1 (1)	1/1 (100)	1.000[‡]
Superficial or deep wound infection (n; %)[a]	0 (0)	0/0 (0)	2 (2)	2/2 (100)	0.237[‡]
Periprosthetic fracture (n; %)[a]	0 (0)	0/0 (0)	0 (0)	0/0 (0)	1.000[‡]
Revision surgery (n; %)[a]	2 (2)	1/2 (50)	4 (3)	4/4 (100)	0.437[‡]
Mortality (n; %)[b]					
6 weeks	0 (0)	-	0 (0)	-	1.000[‡]
1 year	1 (2)	-	0 (0)	-	1.000[‡]
2 year	1 (2)	-	1 (2)	-	1.000[‡]

BTHA bilateral total hip arthroplasty
† Chi-square test
‡ Fisher's exact test
[a] Data are presented as number of joints affected
[b] Data are presented as number of patients affected

immediate positive feedback from a vivid memory of the first-operated hip in a simultaneous procedure.

The influence of type of surgery on the functional outcome, quality of life, and health status in the present study appears to be significant. We demonstrated that the mean postoperative HHS, EQ-5D index, and EQ-VAS score in the simultaneous group were all significantly better than those of the staged group. Our findings do not agree with previous studies that have reported similar HHS postoperatively in the groups [2, 9, 25]. The reasons for this are unclear, but this could be caused by more accurate surgical procedures, no delayed rehabilitation time for the first-operated hip and reduced time lost from work in a simultaneous procedure.

With a mean follow-up of more than 60 months, we found the staged procedure resulted in an increase in postoperative prosthetic-related complications and revision surgery, especially for the second-operated hip compared to the simultaneous procedure. The reported arthroplasty-related complication rates and revision rates between the two procedures appear to vary [9, 25–27]. Berend et al. [2] reported a higher revision rate (3.9% vs. 0.5%; $P = 0.010$) and a higher dislocation rate in the simultaneous group. However, Rasouli et al. [8] demonstrated that local complications occurred significantly more frequently in a staged BTHA compared to a simultaneous BTHA (4.05% vs. 6.20%; $P < 0.001$). A possible explanation for the result in our study could be the superiority of surgical accuracy in simultaneous BTHA over staged BTHA.

The study has several limitations. First, this was a retrospective cohort study. Second, the study population was relatively small. A higher number would be more appropriate to generalize our findings. Third, preoperative clinical scores in regard to functional outcome and quality of life were not evaluated. Thus, perioperative improvements in each score could not be addressed. Fourth, we did not examine hip diseases other than ONFH, and the results of the current study may not be applicable to patients with other conditions such as primary or secondary osteoarthritis. The above limitations are offset by the strengths of the study, which was an analysis of a single-surgeon case series with the same approach. Accordingly, a potential bias related to the surgical technique may not be considered. In addition, in order to objectively assess the surgical accuracy, only ONFH was included in this study because, compared to other conditions, non-traumatic ONFH usually has relatively little radiographic evidence of acetabular abnormality and infrequent bilateral asymmetry of the acetabulum at the time of surgery [35].

Conclusion

With greater surgical accuracy, better functional outcome, and higher quality of life, simultaneous BTHA has been shown to be superior to staged BTHA in patients with bilateral ONFH. This may be attributed to immediate feedback from a more recent surgery. Our results suggest that for medically operable patients, bilateral hip disease could be treated with a simultaneous procedure rather than a staged procedure to achieve a better surgical outcome.

Abbreviations

ARCO: Association Research Circulation Osseous; ASA: American Society of Anesthesiologists; BMI: Body mass index; BTHA: Bilateral total hip arthroplasty; EQ-5D: EuroQol-5 dimension; EQ-VAS: EuroQol-visual analogue scale; HHS: Harris hip score; HLD: Head-to-lesser-trochanter distance; LLD: Leg length discrepancy; ONFH: Osteonecrosis of the femoral head; PACS: Picture archiving and communication system; SD: Standard deviation; THA: Total hip arthroplasty

Acknowledgement

We thank all the patients involved in the study.

Funding

This study is an independent study, not supported by any funding.

Authors' contributions

YSK supervised the study design and data analysis, revised the manuscript and acted as the corresponding author. SCK participated in designing the study, drafted the manuscript, and was responsible for the analysis and interpretation of the data as the first author. YWL, WLJ performed the radiographic measurements and the interpretation of the data, and helped draft the manuscript. DCP performed the statistical analysis. JWL, WWK contributed to data acquisition and study coordination. All authors read and approved the final manuscript.

Competing interests

The authors declare that they have no competing interests.

Consent for publication

Written informed consent was obtained from the patient shown in Fig. 1 for the publication of the image.

References

1. Lazansky MG. A method for grading hips. J. Bone Joint Surg. Br. 1967;49: 644–51.
2. Berend KR, Lombardi AV, Adams JB. Simultaneous vs staged Cementless bilateral Total hip Arthroplasty. J Arthroplast. 2007;22:111–5.
3. Parcells BW, Macknet DM, Kayiaros ST. The Direct Anterior Approach for 1-Stage Bilateral Total Hip Arthroplasty: Early Outcome Analysis of a Single-Surgeon Case Series. J. Arthroplasty [Internet]. 2015 [cited 2015 Dec 6]; Available from: http://linkinghub.elsevier.com/retrieve/pii/S0883540315007950.
4. Papanagiotou M, Malizos KN, Vlychou M, Dailiana ZH. Autologous (non-vascularised) fibular grafting with recombinant bone morphogenetic protein-7 for the treatment of femoral head osteonecrosis. Bone Jt J. 2014;96:31–5.
5. Zeng Y, Qi X, Feng W, Li J, Li F, Zeng J, et al. One-sided hip-preserving and concurrent contralateral total hip arthroplasty for the treatment of bilateral osteonecrosis of the femoral head in different stages: short-medium term outcomes. BMC Musculoskelet. Disord. [Internet]. 2015 [cited 2016 Apr 10];16. Available from: http://www.ncbi.nlm.nih.gov/pmc/articles/PMC4455936/.
6. Zhu H, Cai X, Lin T, Shi Z, Yan S. Low-intensity pulsed ultrasound enhances Bone repair in a rabbit model of steroid-associated Osteonecrosis. Clin Orthop Relat res. 2015;473:1830–9.
7. Reuben JD, Meyers SJ, Cox DD, Elliott M, Watson M, Shim SD. Cost comparison between bilateral simultaneous, staged, and unilateral total joint arthroplasty. J Arthroplast. 1998;13:172–9.
8. Rasouli MR, Maltenfort MG, Ross D, Hozack WJ, Memtsoudis SG, Parvizi J. Perioperative morbidity and mortality following bilateral Total hip Arthroplasty. J Arthroplast. 2014;29:142–8.
9. Bhan S, Pankaj A, Malhotra R. One- or two-stage bilateral total hip arthroplasty a PROSPECTIVE, RANDOMISED, CONTROLLED STUDY IN AN ASIAN POPULATION. J Bone Joint Surg Br. 2006;88–B: 298–303.
10. Parvizi J, Pour AE, Peak EL, Sharkey PF, Hozack WJ, Rothman RH. One-stage bilateral total hip arthroplasty compared with unilateral total hip arthroplasty: a prospective study. J Arthroplast. 2006;21:26–31.
11. Stavrakis AI, SooHoo NF, Lieberman JR. Bilateral Total hip Arthroplasty has similar complication rates to unilateral Total hip Arthroplasty. J Arthroplast. 2015;30:1211–4.
12. Glait SA, Khatib ON, Bansal A, Hochfelder JP, Slover JD. Comparing the incidence and clinical data for simultaneous bilateral versus unilateral Total hip Arthroplasty in New York state between 1990 and 2010. J Arthroplast. 2015;30:1887–91.
13. Romagnoli S, Zacchetti S, Perazzo P, Verde F, Banfi G, Viganò M. Simultaneous bilateral total hip arthroplasties do not lead to higher complication or allogeneic transfusion rates compared to unilateral procedures. Int Orthop. 2013;37:2125–30.
14. Lindberg-Larsen M, Joergensen CC, Husted H, Kehlet H. Simultaneous and staged bilateral total hip arthroplasty: a Danish nationwide study. Arch Orthop Trauma Surg. 2013;133:1601–5.
15. Garland A, Rolfson O, Garellick G, Kärrholm J, Hailer NP. Early postoperative mortality after simultaneous or staged bilateral primary total hip arthroplasty: an observational register study from the swedish Hip arthroplasty register. BMC Musculoskelet. Disord. [Internet]. 2015 [cited 2015 Dec 1];16. Available from: http://www.biomedcentral.com/1471-2474/16/77.
16. Lewinnek GE, Lewis JL, Tarr R, Compere CL, Zimmerman JR. Dislocations after total hip-replacement arthroplasties. J. Bone Jt. Surg. 1978;60:217–20.
17. Callanan MC, Jarrett B, Bragdon CR, Zurakowski D, Rubash HE, Freiberg AA, et al. The John Charnley award: risk factors for cup Malpositioning: quality improvement through a joint registry at a tertiary hospital. Clin Orthop Relat res. 2010;469:319–29.
18. Lim YW, Chang YJ, Kwon SY, Kim YS. A simple method using a PACS to minimize leg length discrepancy in primary THA. J Arthroplast. 2013;28: 1791–5.
19. Mahmood SS, Mukka SS, Crnalic S, Sayed-Noor AS. The Influence of Leg Length Discrepancy after Total Hip Arthroplasty on Function and Quality of Life: A Prospective Cohort Study. J. Arthroplasty [Internet]. [cited 2015 May 6]; Available from: http://www.sciencedirect.com/science/article/pii/S0883540315002776.
20. Widmer K-H. A simplified method to determine acetabular cup anteversion from plain radiographs. J Arthroplast. 2004;19:387–90.
21. Shin WC, Lee SM, Lee KW, Cho HJ, Lee JS, Suh KT. The reliability and accuracy of measuring anteversion of the acetabular component on plain anteroposterior and lateral radiographs after total hip arthroplasty. Bone Jt J. 2015;97–B:611–6.
22. Lu M, Zhou Y-X, Du H, Zhang J, Liu J. Reliability and validity of measuring Acetabular component orientation by plain Anteroposterior radiographs. Clin Orthop Relat res. 2013;471:2987–94.
23. Kim YS, Kwon SY, Sun DH, Han SK, Maloney WJ. Modified posterior approach to Total hip Arthroplasty to enhance joint stability. Clin. Orthop. 2008;466:294–9.
24. Dawson J, Fitzpatrick R, Frost S, Gundle R, McLardy-Smith P, Murray D. Evidence for the validity of a patient-based instrument for assessment of outcome after revision hip replacement. J Bone Joint Surg Br. 2001; 83:1125–9.
25. Parvizi J, Tarity TD, Sheikh E, Sharkey PF, Hozack WJ, Rothman RH. Bilateral total hip arthroplasty: one-stage versus two-stage procedures. Clin Orthop. 2006;453:137–41.
26. Alfaro-Adrián J, Bayona F, Rech JA, Murray DW. One- or two-stage bilateral total hip replacement. J Arthroplast. 1999;14:439–45.
27. Salvati EA, Hughes P, Lachiewicz P. Bilateral total hip-replacement arthroplasty in one stage. J Bone Joint Surg am. 1978;60:640–4.
28. Faul F, Erdfelder E, Buchner A, Lang A-G. Statistical power analyses using G*power 3.1: tests for correlation and regression analyses. Behav. Res. Methods. 2009;41:1149–60.
29. Mont MA, Cherian JJ, Sierra RJ, Jones LC, Lieberman JR. Nontraumatic Osteonecrosis of the femoral head: where do we stand today?: a ten-year update. J Bone Jt Surg. 2015;97:1604–27.

30. Jaffe WL, Charnley J. Bilateral Charnley low-friction arthroplasty as a single operative procedure. A report of fifty cases. Bull. Hosp. Joint Dis. 1971;32: 198–214.
31. D'Lima DD, Urquhart AG, Buehler KO, Walker RH, Colwell CW. The effect of the orientation of the acetabular and femoral components on the range of motion of the hip at different head-neck ratios. J Bone Joint Surg am. 2000; 82:315–21.
32. Biedermann R, Tonin A, Krismer M, Rachbauer F, Eibl G, Stöckl B. Reducing THE risk of dislocation after total hip arthroplasty THE EFFECT OF ORIENTATION OF THE ACETABULAR COMPONENT. J. Bone Joint Surg. Br. 2005;87-B:762–9.
33. Ranawat CS, Rodriguez JA. Functional leg-length inequality following total hip arthroplasty. J Arthroplast. 1997;12:359–64.
34. Halai M, Gupta S, Gilmour A, Bharadwaj R, Khan A, Holt G. The Exeter technique can lead to a lower incidence of leg-length discrepancy after total hip arthroplasty. Bone Jt. J. 2015;97-B:154–9.
35. Steinberg ME, Corces A, Fallon M. Acetabular involvement in Osteonecrosis of the femoral head*. J Bone Jt Surg am. 1999;81:60–5.

3

Direct anterior approach for total hip arthroplasty with a novel mobile traction table

Junichi Nakamura[1*], Shigeo Hagiwara[1], Sumihisa Orita[1], Ryuichiro Akagi[1], Takane Suzuki[2], Masahiko Suzuki[3], Kazuhisa Takahashi[1] and Seiji Ohtori[1]

Abstract

Background: The purpose of this prospective cohort study was to clarify the safety and efficacy of total hip arthroplasty via the direct anterior approach in the supine position with a novel mobile traction table.

Methods: The first experience of consecutive surgeries by a single surgeon using the direct anterior approach with a traction table is described with a two-year follow-up period. Of 121 patients, 100 patients without previous hip surgeries, severe deformity, or cemented implants were divided into two groups comprising the first 50 patients and the second 50 patients.

Results: The implant survival rate was 99% at the two-year follow-up. Revision surgery was required for periprosthetic femoral fracture in one patient. The complication rate possibly related to the traction table was 5% (5 patients): three anterior dislocations, one periprosthetic femoral fracture, and one intraoperative perforation caused by femoral rasping. The complication rate tended to decrease in the second group compared to the first group (4% versus 6%). Mean surgical time (72.0 minutes versus 82.5 min, $p = 0.027$), rate of allogeneic blood transfusion (2% versus 24%, $p = 0.001$), and cup alignment in the safe zone (100% versus 88%, $p = 0.027$) were significantly improved in the second group compared to the first group.

Conclusion: The direct anterior approach with a novel mobile traction table showed a positive learning curve for surgical time, rate of allogeneic blood transfusion, and cup alignment in the safe zone.

Keywords: Mobile traction table, Total hip arthroplasty, Direct anterior approach in supine position

Background

Total hip arthroplasty (THA) is a successful treatment for painful hip disorders. The direct anterior approach (DAA) for this surgery has become of great interest because of its quicker recovery and lower dislocation rate over the last decade [1–3]. DAA is a muscle sparing approach that separates both the true inter-muscular and inter-nervous planes to reach the hip joint using the distal part of the Smith-Petersen approach (Hueter approach) [4, 5]. Theoretically, DAA is the most minimally invasive technique for hip surgery and is gaining in popularity [6]. On the other hand, DAA is technically demanding. The traction table, initially proposed by Judet et al. [7], assists the surgery by providing efficient exposure of the hip joint [8–11]. Fluoroscopy also guides implant position and insertion [12, 13]. However, Steiger RN et al. indicated that only 20% of orthopedic surgeons in Australia have mastered DAA with a traction table (traction DAA) [14]. Moreover, an earlier fixed-type special traction table is large and expensive for those just starting to use DAA. An alternative technique for DAA is manual leg control using a standard surgical table [15–18]. Homma et al. [18] suggested that manual leg control with a standard surgical table was sufficient for DAA, although the rate at which surgeons have discontinued the procedure is unknown. Besides, the direction of a surgical table is structurally opposite (180°) for the traction table, and for manual leg control. Because of the

* Correspondence: njonedr@chiba-u.jp
[1]Department of Orthopaedic Surgery, Graduate School of Medicine, Chiba University, 1-8-1 Inohana, Chuo-ku, Chiba City, Chiba 260-8677, Japan
Full list of author information is available at the end of the article

different direction, an incorrect table setting could cause a serious problem with femoral exposure using the manual leg control approach as this procedure uses a bending function of the surgical table to extend the hip joints around the buttocks. Thirdly, the fixed type traction table is large and expensive for a surgeon inexperienced with DAA. Therefore, we developed a novel mobile traction table to facilitate traction DAA. The table is less expensive and saves operating room space. The purpose of this prospective cohort study was to clarify the safety and efficacy of THA via DAA in the supine position with a novel mobile traction table.

Methods

The research protocol of this prospective cohort study was in compliance with the Helsinki Declaration, approved by the Institutional Review Boards, and registered with the University Hospital Medical Information Network. Written informed consent was obtained from all study participants. The inclusion criterion was primary THA; all THAs for which the first author was not the surgeon were excluded. From May 2012 to April 2014, 121 primary THAs were performed on consecutive patients in our institute using traction DAA. The first author operated on 114 patients, and less experienced surgeons operated on seven patients who were not included in this study. Fourteen patients were regarded as the refractory group: five patients with previous hip surgeries, five patients with severe osteoporosis requiring cemented implants, and four patients with severe deformity requiring special stems. The remaining 100 patients (18 male and 82 female, 61 right and 39 left) were regarded as the standard group without previous hip surgeries, severe deformity, or cemented implants. The standard group of 100 patients was divided into two groups consisting of the first 50 patients and the second 50 patients to undergo surgery. Baseline patient characteristics of the standard group and the refractory group are shown in Table 1. Characteristics of the two groups within the standard group are shown in Table 2. One or more comorbidities were noted in 67 of 114 patients (59%). Physical status was classified using the American Society of Anesthesiologists classification [19]. In the standard group, cementless, rectangular cross section type, straight-stems were used, with a highly cross-linked polyethylene cementless cup, and cobalt-chrome femoral head. In the refractory group, 4 patients used this same combination, but 5 patients used cementless, cylindrical modular type, straight-stems to adjust for excessive anteversion. The other 5 patients used cemented, polished, double tapered, rectangular straight-stems, with a cementless cup in two patients and a cemented cup in three patients.

Table 1 Comparison of the standard group and the refractory group

	Standard group (n = 100)	Refractory group (n = 14)	p values
Gender (Male: Female)	18:82	5:9	0.154
Age	62.3 ± 13.7	66.8 ± 7.7	0.231
Diagnosis (OA:ION:RA)	62:32:6	10:1:3	0.039[b]
ASA-PS (I:II:III)	37:44:19	2:5:7	0.027[b]
BMI	23.6 ± 3.8	23.7 ± 4.1	0.903
Preoperative Hb	12.6 ± 1.5	12.3 ± 1.4	0.411
Preoperative JOA hip score	38.8 ± 13.4	38.1 ± 17.6	0.864
Surgical time (minutes)	77.3 ± 23.7	115.1 ± 40.7	0.001[a]
Intraoperative blood loss (ml)	256 ± 186	506 ± 558	0.001[a]
Estimated total blood loss (ml)	835 ± 340	1084 ± 649	0.026[a]
Allogeneic blood transfusion	13 (13%)	5 (36%)	0.045[b]
Cup abduction angle (degrees)	41.0 ± 4.1	42.2 ± 7.9	0.388
Cup anteversion (degrees)	16.8 ± 5.1	18.5 ± 6.9	0.254
Cup safe zone	94 (94%)	11 (79%)	0.080
Stem varus angle (degrees)	0.1 ± 0.5	0.0 ± 0.0	0.494
Stem flexion angle (degrees)	0.6 ± 1.0	0.3 ± 0.7	0.262
Stem safe zone	94 (94%)	14 (100%)	1.000
Leg length discrepancy (mm)	6.4 ± 9.0	5.4 ± 7.4	0.673
Postoperative JOA hip score			
At three months	84.4 ± 9.4	77.9 ± 7.6	0.014[a]
At two years	87.8 ± 8.2	83.6 ± 6.1	0.066
Surgical complication (category 2 and 3)	5 (5%)	0 (0%)	1.000
Revision	1 (1%)	0 (0%)	1.000

OA osteoarthritis, *ION* idiopathic osteonecrosis, *RA* rheumatoid arthritis, *ASA-PS* American Society of Anesthesiologists-Physical status, *BMI* body mass index, *Hb* hemoglobin, *JOA* Japanese Orthopedic Association.
Mean ± standard deviation
[a]Student's t-tests and [b]Pearson χ^2 tests

The first author had 8 years of surgical experience as an adult hip surgeon. He used the direct lateral approach in the lateral decubitus position in 61 patients for the first 2 years, the anterolateral (modified Watson-Jones) approach in the lateral decubitus position in 53 patients the following year and a half, and then used the direct anterior approach in the supine position without a traction table in 6 patients. He learned the direct anterior approach from Dr. Oinuma at Funabashi Orthopedic Hospital (Japan). After that, he introduced the traction table for this approach. Therefore, the first author had

Table 2 Comparison of the first 50 cases and the second 50 cases in the standard group

	First 50 cases	Second 50 cases	*p* values
Gender (Male:Female)	7:43	11:39	0.436
Age	64.5 ± 13.4	60.1 ± 13.7	0.110
Diagnosis (OA:ION:RA)	30:16:4	32:16:2	0.694
ASA-PS (I:II:III)	17:20:13	20:24:6	0.203
BMI	23.8 ± 3.8	23.4 ± 3.8	0.674
Preoperative Hb	12.3 ± 1.4	13.0 ± 1.5	0.020[a]
Preoperative JOA hip score	34.9 ± 12.2	42.8 ± 13.5	0.003[a]
Surgical time (minutes)	82.5 ± 27.1	72.0 ± 18.6	0.027[a]
Intraoperative blood loss (ml)	263 ± 172	249 ± 201	0.704
Estimated total blood loss (ml)	866 ± 361	803 ± 318	0.359
Allogeneic blood transfusion	12 (24%)	1 (2%)	0.001[b]
Cup abduction angle (degrees)	41.9 ± 4.5	40.1 ± 3.6	0.032[a]
Cup anteversion (degrees)	17.7 ± 6.0	15.8 ± 3.9	0.070
Cup safe zone	44 (88%)	50 (100%)	0.027[b]
Stem varus angle (degrees)	0.1 ± 0.8	0.1 ± 0.6	0.888
Stem flexion angle (degrees)	0.5 ± 1.1	0.7 ± 0.9	0.165
Stem safe zone	47 (94%)	47 (94%)	1.000
Leg length discrepancy (mm)	5.0 ± 5.7	7.9 ± 11.2	0.109
Postoperative JOA hip score			
At three months	85.1 ± 10.4	83.7 ± 8.3	0.478
At two years	89.0 ± 8.0	86.7 ± 8.3	0.176
Surgical complication (category 2 and 3)	3 (6%)	2 (4%)	1.000
Revision	1 (2%)	0 (0%)	0.999

OA osteoarthritis, *ION* idiopathic osteonecrosis, *RA* rheumatoid arthritis, *ASA-PS* American Society of Anesthesiologists-Physical status, *BMI* body mass index, *Hb* hemoglobin, *JOA* Japanese Orthopedic Association.
Mean ± standard deviation
[a]Student's t-tests and [b]Pearson χ^2 tests

previous experience with 120 total hip arthroplasties at the beginning of the study.

Surgical procedure

Preoperative planning was based on computed tomography-assisted, three dimensional software (ZedHip, LEXI, Tokyo, Japan). After induction of general anesthesia, 1 g of tranexamic acid was intravenously injected before skin incision. Traction DAA for THA was performed with the patient in a supine position, lying on a novel mobile traction table, ~As You Walk~ LECURE ® (Surgical Alliance, Tokyo, Japan) (Fig. 1). This table can be set up with a standard orthopedic surgical table, and can hold the leg in hip flexion/extension, internal/external rotation, adduction/abduction, or traction, distraction, or compression (Fig. 2). A non-scrubbed and non-sterile assistant handled the traction table. The table provides wide exposure of the proximal femur and the acetabulum both with direct visualization and fluoroscopy. The leather boot is designed to fit the foot and ankle snugly with a double locking bandage mechanism to avoid slipping off the foot. From the superior anterior iliac spine, Heuter's interval between the tensor fascia lata and sartorius muscle is palpated. The skin incision runs along the mid-line of the tensor fascia lata. This line links the anterior superior iliac spine and the lateral femoral condyle and is more than one finger's breadth from Heuter's interval, avoiding injury of the lateral femoral cutaneous nerve. The incision begins 3 cm proximal from the tip of the greater trochanter and 9 cm distal to the trochanter (12 cm long in total). With fluoroscopy, a vertical line passing though the tip of the greater trochanter is identified and the pelvic tilt is adjusted by symmetry of the obturator foramina, centering the coccyx with the symphysis.

The sheath of the tensor fascia lata is incised longitudinally in the direction of the muscle fibers. The muscle fibers of the tensor fascia lata are intentionally pulled laterally within the sheath by the surgeon's index finger and relaxed by exposing the intermuscular space toward the anterior superior iliac spine. The deep fascia of the rectus femoris is identified by white tendinous fibers, muscle fibers as red, and fat tissue as yellow (tricolor sign). A wound retractor is utilized without a surgical arm or a sinker to hold the retractor. After hemostasis of the arteriole branch, the deep fascia is incised longitudinally at the boundary of the fat tissue to spare the rectus femoris within the sheath. The femoral head is outlined by two narrow Homann retractors, one at the piriformis fossa and the other at the medial aspect of the femoral neck. The triangle of the anterior capsule is visualized; the medial line is the inferior iliofemoral ligament, the lateral line is the insertion of the vastus lateralis muscle and the capsule, and the superior line is the superior iliofemoral ligament. After capsulectomy, the upper outline of the cervicotrochanteric junction is visualized, then 45° of external rotation makes the lower outline clear, and mild traction causes subluxation. The osteotomy is performed in situ, perpendicular to the anterior intertrochanteric plane. With traction, the osteotomy site is spontaneously opened and the femoral head can be easily removed. The posterior capsule between the acetabulum and the greater trochanter (ischiofemoral ligament and superior iliofemoral ligament) is resected. A blunt forked retractor is placed at the recess of the posterior wall of the acetabulum.

Femoral preparation is recommended before acetabular reaming (femoral first technique). Elevating the calcar femorale with a blunt hook, a sharp fork retractor is inserted into the posterolateral aspect of the greater trochanter. To avoid a hinge phenomenon of the greater trochanter at the posterior wall of the acetabulum, it is useful to apply internal rotation in the neutral position first, and then to apply elevation and external rotation to 90° to

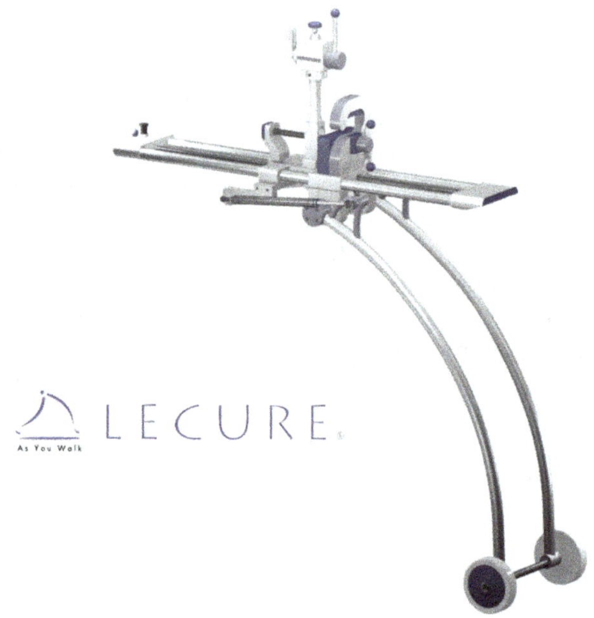

Fig. 1 ~As You Walk~ LECURE ®, a novel mobile traction table

visualize the calcar. The ischiofemoral ligament and the superior iliofemoral ligament need to be detached until sufficient anterior mobilization of the greater trochanter is obtained. The pubofemoral ligament also needs to be detached to obtain sufficient lateral mobilization of the calcar. Hyperextension of 35°, relaxation and compression, and adduction of 10° are applied with the traction table. This relaxation technique prevents excessive stretch of the femoral nerve and also assists femoral exposure. A Z-shaped canal finder (Tanaka Ika, Tokyo, Japan) is an essential tool to identify the axis of the medullary canal and anteversion of the calcar. The entry point of the canal finder is the piriformis fossa, avoiding flexion insertion or perforation of the femur. Varus insertion can be avoided by removing the cancellous bone of the lateral femoral canal with the shoulder of this canal finder. Femoral rasps are inserted sequentially.

Acetabular reaming is performed with a straight holder, avoiding excessive reaming of the anterior and posterior walls of the acetabulum. Fluoroscopy intermittently monitors the height and the depth of the reaming, and the cup position. In severely dysplastic hips, the outline for the reaming is prepared with a round chisel. Cup fixation is press-fit and screw fixation uses two 20 mm screws. Reduction is performed by internal rotation and traction. Alignment of the implant and leg length discrepancy are confirmed with fluoroscopy. Anterior stability is examined by external rotation of 90° with mild traction. The acetabular bone defect is reconstructed with morselized autograft. At closure, no suction drains are applied, the fascia of the tensor is sutured continuously but the skin is not sutured, rather it is coated with an adhesive agent (Dermabond, Ethicon, NJ). A water-proof wound dressing is wrapped with a compressive bandage for a few days to prevent hematoma. Postoperative rehabilitation begins on postoperative day one and the patients are allowed full weight bearing.

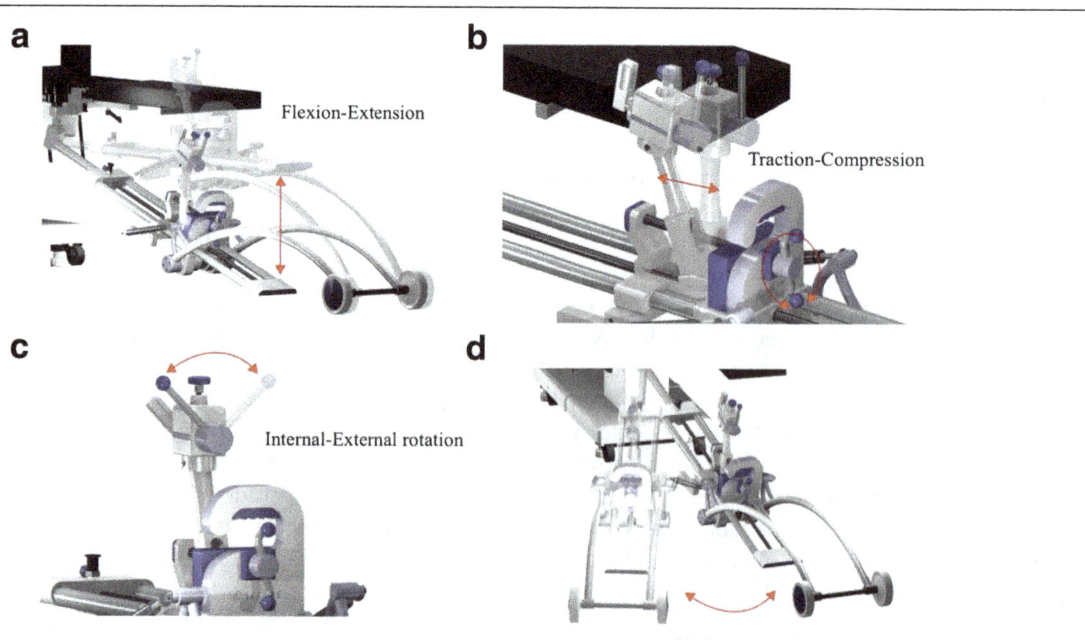

Fig. 2 Movement of the mobile traction table. This table can hold the leg in hip flexion/extension (**a**), traction, distraction, or compression (**b**), internal/external rotation (**c**), or adduction/abduction (**d**)

Measurements and outcomes

The primary outcome was implant survival at the end point of conversion to revision surgery. The secondary outcomes were surgical complications, surgical time, and blood loss. Surgical complications were categorized as (1) complications definitely not related to the traction table, (2) complications that may be related to the traction table, and (3) complications related to the traction table. Stem sinking was defined as more than 3 mm of stem subsidence compared to an X-ray taken immediately after surgery; subsidence was evaluated by two authors. Excessive acetabular reaming was defined as an iatrogenic bone defect of the acetabular wall created by reaming and was evaluated by the surgeon intraoperatively. Cup migration was defined as more than 5° of change of cup alignment on adjusted pelvic tilt compared to an X-ray taken immediately after surgery; migration was evaluated by two authors. Blood loss consisted of intraoperative blood loss recorded by the anesthesiologists, blood transfusion, and estimated total blood loss [20]; Estimated total blood loss = Estimated blood volume × (preoperative hemoglobin - post operative-day one hemoglobin) / preoperative hemoglobin + autologous blood transfusion volume + allogeneic blood transfusion volume. Other outcomes were the safe zone for implant alignment [21], and the preoperative and postoperative Japanese Orthopedic Association (JOA) hip scores [22] at three months and two years. Lateral inclination of 40 +/- 10° and anteversion of 15 +/- 10° measured from an anteroposterior X-ray of the pelvis in the supine position were regarded as the safe zone for cup alignment by Lewinnek et al. [4]. Cup anteversion was calculated by measurement of the short diameter and long diameter of the ellipse as follows:

Cup anteversion = $\sin^{-1}$ (short diameter / long diameter)

As for stem alignment, the angle of the axis of the stem and the femur within +/- 3° both in the anteroposterior and lateral views was regarded as the safe zone [5]. The alignment was measured with Image J 1.45 s (National Institute of Health, USA). JOA hip score was assessed in an unblinded fashion, mainly by the first author at the outpatient clinic before, three months after, and two years after surgery.

Statistical analysis

The first 50 cases were compared with the second 50 cases using Student's t-tests, Pearson χ^2 tests, and logistic regression analysis with multivariate and a forward stepwise selection (SPSS 16.0, Chicago, Illinois). A *p*-value <0.05 was considered significant.

Results

The implant survival rate was 99% in the 100 standard patients at the two-year follow-up; one revision surgery was required for a periprosthetic femoral fracture. The surgical complication rate possibly related to the traction table (categories 2 and 3) was 5%: three anterior dislocations, one periprosthetic femoral fracture, and one intraoperative perforation from femoral rasping. Mean surgical time (72.0 min versus 82.5 min, $p = 0.027$), rate of allogeneic blood transfusion (2% versus 24%, $p = 0.001$), and cup alignment in the safe zone (100% versus 88%, $p = 0.027$) were significantly improved in the second group compared to the first group (Table 2).

The surgical time was negatively correlated with the case number, with shorter surgical times as more cases were completed (Fig. 3). Both intraoperative and total estimated blood loss showed a positive correlation with the length of the surgery (Figs. 4 and 5). The cup inclination was 41.0° (range, 29° to 53°) and the anteversion was 16.8° (range, 5° to 30°) with 94% in the safe zone (Fig. 6). The preoperative JOA hip score significantly improved three months post-operatively, and continued to improve until two years both in the first group and the second group ($p = 0.001$, respectively, Table 2).

Category 1 surgical complications consisted of four sinking stems, two with excessive reaming of the acetabulum, two with cup migration, and one each with an insufficiency fracture of the ipsilateral calcaneus, the ipsilateral pubis, or the sacroiliac region. Category 2 consisted of one periprosthetic femoral fracture and one intraoperative perforation from femoral rasping. Category 3 consisted of three anterior dislocations. Seven patients died, but all deaths were unrelated to surgery: malignancy in four, cerebrovascular disease in two, and anaphylactic shock in one.

In the refractory group, longer surgical time and more blood loss was observed, and postoperative JOA hip score at three months was significantly lower than in the

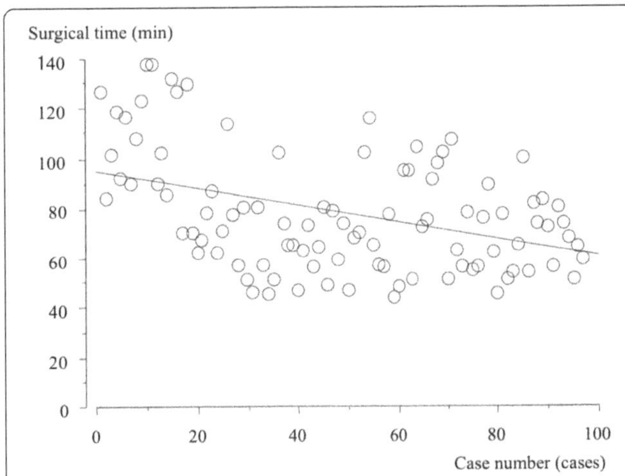

Fig. 3 Surgical time for the initial 100 cases in the standard group. A learning curve is indicated by decreasing time by case. (Surgical time [min]) = 94.1 - 0.34 × (cases), $R^2 = 0.176$, p = 0.001, simple regression analysis

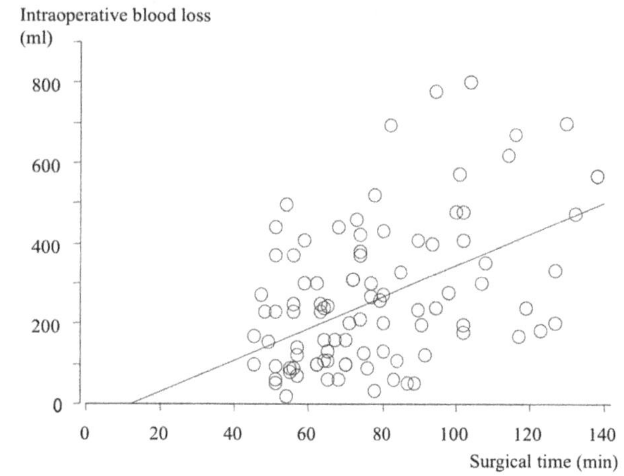

Fig. 4 Intraoperative blood loss and surgical time in the standard group. (Intraoperative blood loss [ml]) = 3.9 × (surgical time [min]) - 47.7, $R^2 = 0.251$, p = 0.001, simple regression analysis

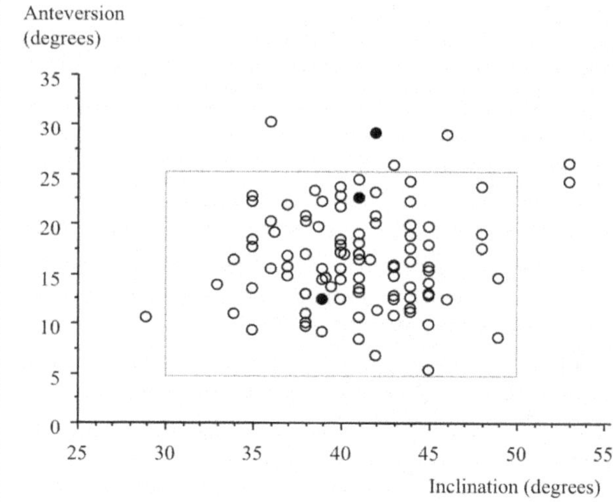

Fig. 6 Scatterplot of cup inclination and anteversion in the standard group. The square outlined by the dotted lines reflects Lewinnek's safe zone. The three black dots indicate dislocated hips

standard group (Table 1). However, the hip score was significantly improved at two years ($p = 0.001$).

Logistic regression analysis revealed that the rate of allogeneic blood transfusion decreased by 0.3 times for each 10 kg increase in patient weight and by 0.7 times with each decrease in surgical time by 10 min ($p = 0.017$), but increased 1.9 times for each 10 years of age ($p = 0.031$).

Discussion

This study showed a moderate success rate for the first experience with traction DAA with an implant survival rate of 99% at the two-year follow-up. Our surgical complication rate of 5% was within the range of those reported in the literature for DAA (range: 0 - 24%, Table 3) [1–3, 5, 6, 8–13, 15–18, 23, 24]. Sariali et al. reported that only 57 of 1764 hips (3.2%) had complications, which occurred in the first 250 cases, indicating an initial complication rate of 22.8% [9]. In a multicenter cohort study of 1277 hips, Bhandari et al. documented a complication rate of 14.5%, but the rate was two times higher for surgeons who had performed less than 100 cases [10]. The 99% implant survival rate was consistent with previous reports, which ranged from 84.8% to 100% [1, 2, 6, 8, 10–13, 15–18, 23, 24]. Spaan et al. [24] reported the worst revision rate of 15.2% (7 of 46 hips) in their early experience with DAA with manual leg control, and abandoned the technique. Jewett et al. [12] and Woolson et al. [23] also reported a relatively high revision rate of about 3%. de Steiger et al. clearly showed an improvement in the cumulative percent revision at two years with surgical experience: 3 to 4% in the first 50 operations, 2% in operations 51-100, and 1% for surgeons doing more than 100 operations [14]. Therefore, we believe that our initial outcome is acceptable.

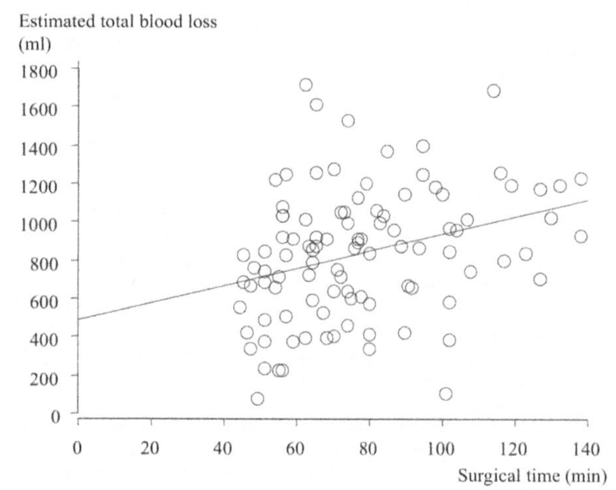

Fig. 5 Estimated total blood loss and surgical time in the standard group. (Estimated total blood loss [ml]) = 4.5 × (surgical time [min]) + 487.4, $R^2 = 0.098$, $p = 0.002$, simple regression analysis

It is true that safety and accuracy take priority over speed and efficiency, but surgical time is also important. DAA is technically demanding due to its minimal invasiveness and limited exposure from the intermuscular plane. However, surgical time decreases with the surgeon's experience. Previous reports showed that surgical time ranged from 55 min to 164 min [1, 3, 5, 6, 8–10, 13, 15–18, 23, 24]. In this study, surgical time declined from 83 min in the first 50 cases to 72 min in the second 50 cases. On the other hand, in refractory patients, 115 min were needed to complete the procedure. In the first author's experience, mean surgical time was 157 min using the direct lateral approach, 123 min for the anterolateral approach, and 132 min for the direct anterior approach with manual leg positioning. This

Table 3 Comparison of previous reports of THA via the DAA

Author name	Traction/ Manual	Number of patients	Implant survival rate	Surgical complication rate	Surgical time (min)	Follow-up period (months)
Sariali[9]	Traction	1764	NA	3.2%	72	NA
Bhandari[10]	Traction	1277	97.3%	14.5%	95	NA
Siguier[2]	Traction	926	99.6%	1.9%	NA	NA
Jewett[12]	Traction	800	96.8%	15.8%	NA	21
Hartford[11]	Traction	500	98.4%	5.0%	NA	3
Matta[5]	Traction	494	NA	4.0%	75	NA
Woolson[23]	Traction	247	97.2%	15.4%	164	8
Laude[8]	Traction	80	98.8%	3.8%	55	NA
Barret[13]	Traction	43	100%	0%	84	12
Kennon[1]	Manual	672	100%	10.4%	60	6
Seng[17]	Manual	182	97.8%	2.2%	73	NA
Homma[18]	Manual	120	100%	0.8%	117	20
Rachbauer[3]	Manual	100	NA	11.0%	105	3
Oinuma[15]	Manual	99	100%	4.0%	79	17
Nakata[6]	Manual	99	100%	5.1%	105	6
Restrepo[16]	Manual	50	100%	0%	56	24
Spaans[24]	Manual	46	84.8%	23.9%	84	12

The superscript number of the author name reflects the reference number. *NA* not applicable

study showed decreased surgical time in traction DAA with a positive learning curve.

Implant alignment is key to stability and long-term retention. The cup safe zone rate of 94% in this study was acceptable in comparison with previous reports, which ranged from 27% to 99% [5, 6, 13, 18, 23, 25]. The stem safe zone rate of 94% also was comparable to previous reports, which ranged from 22% to 98% [6, 13, 15, 18, 25]. Homma et al [18] reported the lowest safe zone rate of 27% for the cup and Kobayashi et al. [25] reported the lowest safe zone rate of 22% for the stem in DAA with manual leg control, even using fluoroscopy. Our excellent success rate might be due to three dimensional planning-assisted implant positioning, sufficient soft tissue release and exposure of the surgical site, and adjustment of pelvic tilt using fluoroscopic guidance. Care should be taken to obtain accurate imaging due to the limited field of view in fluoroscopy.

The dislocation rate after DAA has been reported to be 0 - 2.2% including both anterior and posterior dislocation [1, 2, 5, 6, 8–10, 12, 13, 15, 17, 18, 23–25]. Of three dislocations in this study, two were even in the safe zone (Fig. 6), but hyperextension of the hip led to anterior dislocation. We insist that patient education is still essential for THA with muscle sparing techniques.

The advantage of DAA is muscle sparing of the gluteus medius and minimus as well as the gluteus maximus and the tensor fascia lata, which serve as hip abductors and pelvic stabilizers [5]. Preservation of the posterosuperior capsule or the short external rotators is also expected in DAA. Anatomically, the piriformis inserts on the tip of the greater trochanter, and the obturator internus and externus insert on the medial aspect of the greater trochanter, running anteriorly to the piriformis [26, 27]. The surgeon should pay attention to the tension on the leg during hip extension for femoral procedure, as too much tension may cause fracture of the trochanter or femoral nerve palsy. Matta et al. [5] suggested that stems requiring straight reamers for canal preparation are more difficult because they require the most anterior mobilization of the femur to allow access down the canal. If further mobilization of the femur is necessary, it can be accomplished with further release of the capsule and conjoint tendon and piriformis sequentially for sufficient exposure [28].

The role of the traction table has been controversial in DAA. Siguier et al. [2] and Matta et al. [5] used a special traction table for DAA. Siguier et al. [2] reported a 2% surgical complication rate in 926 THAs by traction DAA from 1993 to 2000, excluding obese patients, muscular male patients, and patients who had previous hip surgery or severely dysplastic hips. Matta et al. [5] reported 93% of implants aligned in the safe zone, a 4% surgical complication rate, and 75 min of surgical time in 494 THAs by traction DAA from 1996 to 2005. They used a classic Smith-Petersen approach before 2002 and a mini-incision after 2002. Kennon et al. [1] and Oinuma et al. [15] utilized a bending function with a standard surgical table and manual leg control. The two surgical procedures are similar, but traction DAA has several advantages. First, a perineal post stabilizes the pelvis and this stability allows reliable positioning of the acetabular reamer and component [2]. Second, fluoroscopy is easily used with a traction table to provide immediate feedback about the reaming process, and to verify accurate implant alignment [5]. Third, sterilization and draping are much easier, and sterilized assistants to hold the leg are not necessary, saving time, medical resources and human resources.

There are several limitations to this study. First, because the first author was an inexperienced surgeon with DAA, and also with the new traction table, improved safety and efficacy was due to a combination of these two factors, and could not just be attributed to the traction table. In other words, there was a learning curve for DAA as well as for the use of the traction table. de Steiger et al. reported that 50 or more operations were required to reach a revision rate similar to that of a high volume surgeon with traction DAA, based on an Australian registry [14]. Second, this study showed only a short-term outcome with a two-year follow-up period. However, the follow-up periods found in the literature were within two years, and so the long-term outcome of DAA is unknown (Table 3). A longer-term follow-up is necessary because Eto et al. reported that the mean duration from primary to revision THA was 3.0 years [29].

Conclusions

The direct anterior approach with a novel mobile traction table showed a positive learning curve for surgical time, rate of allogeneic blood transfusion, and cup alignment in the safe zone.

Abbreviations

DAA: Direct anterior approach; Hb: Hemoglobin; JOA: Japanese Orthopedic Association; THA: Total hip arthroplasty; traction DAA: DAA with traction table

Acknowledgements

Not applicable.

Funding

This study was supported by collaboration between industry (Surgical Alliance, Tokyo, Japan) and academia (Chiba University, Japan), grants from Mitsubishi Tanabe Pharma Corporation (Osaka, Japan), and Chiba Prefectural Federation of Small Business Association.

Authors' contributions

JN conceived the study, participated in its design and wrote the manuscript as corresponding author. SH, SO and RA helped to conceive the study, participated in its design and coordination, and helped to draft the manuscript. TS, MS, and KT participated in the design of the study and help to create this study model. SO checked the final manuscript. All authors have read and approved this final submitted manuscript.

Competing interests

The first author (JN) has a financial relationship with Surgical Alliance (Tokyo, Japan) for collaboration between industry and academia, and has patents on the mobile traction table. The other authors do not have any conflict of interest.

Consent for publication

Not applicable.

Author details

[1]Department of Orthopaedic Surgery, Graduate School of Medicine, Chiba University, 1-8-1 Inohana, Chuo-ku, Chiba City, Chiba 260-8677, Japan. [2]Department of Bioenvironmental Medicine, Graduate School of Medicine, Chiba University, 1-8-1 Inohana, Chuo-ku, Chiba City, Chiba 260-8677, Japan. [3]Research Center for Frontier Medical Engineering, Chiba University, 1-33 Yayoi-cho, Inage-ku, Chiba City 263-8522, Japan.

References

1. Kennon RE, Keggi JM, Wetmore RS, Zatorski LE, Huo MH, Keggi KJ. Total hip arthroplasty through a minimally invasive anterior surgical approach. J Bone Joint Surg Am. 2003;85 Suppl 4:39–48.
2. Siguier T, Siguier M, Brumpt B. Mini-incision anterior approach does not increase dislocation rate: a study of 1037 total hip replacements. Clin Orthop Relat Res. 2004;426:164–73.
3. Rachbauer F, Nogler M, Krismer M. Minimally invasive single-incision anterior approach for total hip arthroplasty -early results. Minimally Invasive Total Joint Arthroplasty. Berlin, Heidelberg: Springer-Verlag Berlin Heidelberg; 2004. p. 54–59.
4. Smith-Petersen MN. Approach to and exposure of the hip joint for mold arthroplasty. J Bone Joint Surg Am. 1949;31:40–6.
5. Matta JM, Shahrdar C, Ferguson T. Single-incision anterior approach for total hip arthroplasty on an orthopaedic table. Clin Orthop Relat Res. 2005;441: 115–24.
6. Nakata K, Nishikawa M, Yamamoto K, Hirota S, Yoshikawa H. A clinical comparative study of the direct anterior with mini-posterior approach: two consecutive series. J Arthroplasty. 2009;24:698–704.
7. Judet J, Judet H. Anterior approach in total hip arthroplasty. Presse Med. 1985;14:1031–3.
8. Laude F. Total hip arthroplasty through an anterior Hueter minimally invasive approach. Interact Surg. 2006;1:5–11.
9. Sariali E, Leonard P, Mamoudy P. Dislocation after total hip arthroplasty using Hueter anterior approach. J Arthroplasty. 2008;23:266–72.
10. Anterior Total Hip Arthroplasty Collaborative Investigators, Bhandari M, Matta JM, Dodgin D, Clark C, Kregor P, Bradley G, Little L. Outcomes following the single-incision anterior approach to total hip arthroplasty: a multicenter observational study. Orthop Clin North Am. 2009;40:329–42.
11. Hartford JM, Knowles SB. Risk factors for perioperative femoral fractures: cementless femoral implants and the direct anterior approach using a fracture table. J Arthroplasty. 2016;31:2013–8.
12. Jewett BA, Collis DK. High complication rate with anterior total hip arthroplasties on a fracture table. Clin Orthop Relat Res. 2011;469:503–7.
13. Barrett WP, Turner SE, Leopold JP. Prospective randomized study of direct anterior vs postero-lateral approach for total hip arthroplasty. J Arthroplasty. 2013;28:1634–8.
14. de Steiger RN, Lorimer M, Solomon M. What is the learning curve for the anterior approach for total hip arthroplasty? Clin Orthop Relat Res. 2015;473:3860–6.
15. Oinuma K, Eingartner C, Saito Y, Shiratsuchi H. Total hip arthroplasty by a minimally invasive, direct anterior approach. Oper Orthop Traumatol. 2007; 19:310–26.
16. Restrepo C, Parvizi J, Pour AE, Hozack WJ. Prospective randomized study of two surgical approaches for total hip arthroplasty. J Arthroplasty. 2010;25: 671–9. e1.
17. Seng BE, Berend KR, Ajluni AF, Lombardi Jr AV. Anterior-supine minimally invasive total hip arthroplasty: defining the learning curve. Orthop Clin North Am. 2009;40:343–50.
18. Homma Y, Baba T, Kobayashi H, Desroches A, Ozaki Y, Ochi H, Matsumoto M, Yuasa T, Kaneko K. Safety in early experience with a direct anterior

approach using fluoroscopic guidance with manual leg control for primary total hip arthroplasty: a consecutive one hundred and twenty case series. Int Orthop. 2016 Mar;19 [Epub ahead of print].

19. ASA Physical Status Classification System. https://www.asahq.org/resources/clinical-information/asa-physical-status-classification-system. Accessed 29 Dec 2016.
20. Gross JB. Estimating allowable blood loss: corrected for dilution. Anesthesiology. 1983;58:277–80.
21. Lewinnek GE, Lewis JL, Tarr R, Compere CL, Zimmerman JR. Dislocations after total hip-replacement arthroplasties. J Bone Joint Surg Am. 1978;60: 217–20.
22. Kuribayashi M, Takahashi KA, Fujioka M, Ueshima K, Inoue S, Kubo T. Reliability and validity of the Japanese Orthopaedic Association hip score. J Orthop Sci. 2010;15:452–8.
23. Woolson ST, Pouliot MA, Huddleston JI. Primary total hip arthroplasty using an anterior approach and a fracture table: short-term results from a community hospital. J Arthroplasty. 2009;24:999–1005.
24. Spaans AJ, van den Hout JA, Bolder SB. High complication rate in the early experience of minimally invasive total hip arthroplasty by the direct anterior approach. Acta Orthop. 2012;83:342–6.
25. Kobayashi H, Homma Y, Baba T, Ochi H, Matsumoto M, Yuasa T, Kaneko K. Surgeons changing the approach for total hip arthroplasty from posterior to direct anterior with fluoroscopy should consider potential excessive cup anteversion and flexion implantation of the stem in their early experience. Int Orthop. 2016;40:1813–9.
26. Tamaki T, Nimura A, Oinuma K, Shiratsuchi H, Iida S, Akita K. An anatomic study of the impressions on the greater trochanter: bony geometry indicates the alignment of the short external rotator muscles. J Arthroplasty. 2014;29:2473–7.
27. Ito Y, Matsushita I, Watanabe H, Kimura T. Anatomic mapping of short external rotators shows the limit of their preservation during total hip arthroplasty. Clin Orthop Relat Res. 2012;470:1690–5.
28. Matsuura M, Ohashi H, Okamoto Y, Inori F, Okajima Y. Elevation of the femur in THA through a direct anterior approach: cadaver and clinical studies. Clin Orthop Relat Res. 2010;468:3201–6.
29. Eto S, Hwang K, Huddleston JI, Amanatullah DF, Maloney WJ, Goodman SB. The Direct Anterior Approach is Associated With Early Revision Total Hip Arthroplasty. J Arthroplasty. 2016. doi: 10.1016/j.arth.2016.09.012. [Epub ahead of print]

4

Bone preserving level of osteotomy in short-stem total hip arthroplasty does not influence stress shielding dimensions – a comparing finite elements analysis

Rene Burchard[1,2*], Sabrina Braas[2,3], Christian Soost[4], Jan Adriaan Graw[5] and Jan Schmitt[3,6]

Abstract

Background: The main objective of every new development in total hip arthroplasty (THA) is the longest possible survival of the implant. Periprosthetic stress shielding is a scientifically proven phenomenon which leads to inadvertent bone loss. So far, many studies have analysed whether implanting different hip stem prostheses result in significant preservation of bone stock. The aim of this preclinical study was to investigate design-depended differences of the stress shielding effect after implantation of a selection of short-stem THA-prostheses that are currently available.

Methods: Based on computerised tomography (CT), a finite elements (FE) model was generated and a virtual THA was performed with different stem designs of the implant. Stems were chosen by osteotomy level at the femoral neck (collum, partial collum, trochanter sparing, trochanter harming). Analyses were performed with previously validated FE models to identify changes in the strain energy density (SED).

Results: In the trochanteric region, only the collum-type stem demonstrated a biomechanical behaviour similar to the native femur. In contrast, no difference in biomechanical behaviour was found between partial collum, trochanter harming and trochanter sparing models. All of the short stem-prostheses showed lower stress-shielding than a standard stem.

Conclusion: Based on the results of this study, we cannot confirm that the design of current short stem THA-implants leads to a different stress shielding effect with regard to the level of osteotomy. Somehow unexpected, we found a bone stock protection in metadiaphyseal bone by simulating a more distal approach for osteotomy. Further clinical and biomechanical research including long-term results is needed to understand the influence of short-stem THA on bone remodelling and to find the optimal stem-design for a reduction of the stress shielding effect.

Keywords: Stress shielding, Short-stem, THA, Hip, Bone remodelling, Osteotomy level

* Correspondence: rene.burchard@uni-wh.de
[1]Department of Health, University of Witten/Herdecke, Witten, Germany
[2]Department of Trauma and Orthopaedic Surgery, Kreisklinikum Siegen, Siegen, Germany
Full list of author information is available at the end of the article

Background

During the last two decades, total hip arthroplasty (THA) has undergone significant technical changes. On the one hand, fixation of the implant has moved from cemented to cementless techniques and on the other hand (since the Mayo® stem) the development of short-stem prostheses has been established across the board [1, 2]. The main objective of every new development in THA is the longest possible survival of implant and bone-implant-interface. Apart from polyethylene abrasion, periprosthetic stress shielding is a scientifically proven phenomenon which leads to an inadvertent bone remodelling process [3–7]. While cementless procedures were developed to simplify stem revision, short stem designs were made to imitate a physiological stem behaviour and to reduce bone remodelling processes [8]. Therefore, almost every implant company offers at least one femoral short-stem-prosthesis in their THA product line.

Falez and colleagues have developed a classification of commercially available short hip stem prostheses referring to the level of osteotomy during THA (collum, partial collum, trochanter sparing, trochanter harming) (Fig. 1) [9]. They have extended the original classification from Feyen and Shimmin [10]. So far, many authors have analysed whether implanting the different hip stem prostheses result in significant preservation of bone stock. Preservation of bone stock is a relevant process for secure ingrowth of a standard stem in case revision surgery is needed after short stem implantation [6, 11–14].

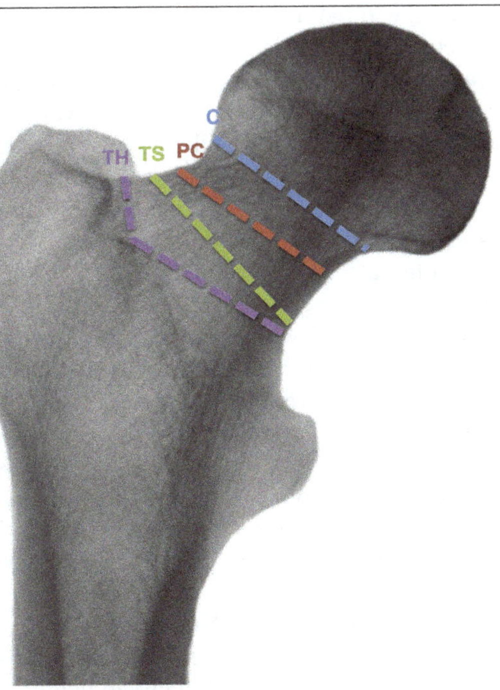

Fig. 1 Osteotomy levels of the different stem types (collum (C), partial collum (PC), trochanter sparing (TS), and trochanter harming (TH)

The aim of this preclinical study was to investigate if there are short-stem-design-depended differences of the stress shielding effects in each different type of short-stem THA implant according to the classification of Falez and colleagues. Using a previously validated data set, THA-stem dependent stress-shielding effects were analysed by virtual hip stem implantation within the framework of a finite element analysis (FEA) [15].

Methods

Based on computerised tomography (CT) by previous investigations a validated set of an in vivo scanned right femur of a female subject at the age of 75 was examined [15]. The scanner setting (Somatom® Plus-4, Siemens, Erlangen, Germany) was 140 kV, 206 mA, 17 s, spiral algorithm with recalculated slice thickness of 2 mm and a 512 × 512 pixel resolution.

The CT voxels were transferred to finite elements (FE) on a scale of 1:1 using the full information to generate the femoral model with an identical resolution of 0.66 m × 0.66 mm × 2 mm (FE and CT). The number of elements was approximately 250,000. Weinans et al. showed that differences of the stress shielding effect are independent to the density-modulus-relationship while using the same procedure for each investigation [16]. Therefore, the CT Hounsfield values (HU) were converted linearly into elastic moduli while bone was located between 170 and 1799 HU and transferred linearly to elastic moduli between 1500 and 15,000 MPa [17, 18].

Table 1 shows the different stem prostheses with their specifications including manufacturer, applied size, size-specific length, largest depth of the stem body and classification type by Falez and colleagues. The different stem designs were realised through a virtual implantation using the FE software Ansys® (Ansys 14.5.7, Ansys Inc., Canonsburg, USA). A geometrical matrix of each stem was generated and an automatic algorithm selected all elements of the bony model that belong to the matrix information [19]. The elements were assigned to an elastic modulus value of titanium alloy (110,000 MPa). FEA was performed on the cluster of the University of Siegen which provides 272 Intel-Xeon®-CPUs, 6.4 TB Working Space and 40 TB physical space. Therefore, the usable peak performance was above 17 TFLOPs.

For stress analysis, a weight-dependent head force was applied with a magnitude of 347% of the body-weight [20, 21]. The vertical axis (z) of the coordinate system was defined by the hip and knee joint centre and the frontal axis (x) by the dorsal aspect of the femoral condyles. So the head force was multiplied by -sin(15°) to obtain the x-component, by -sin(13°) to obtain the y- and by cos(15°) to obtain the z-component [22]. Because of their highly variable in vivo magnitude,

Table 1 Specifications of all investigated stems

Stem	Manufacturer	Stem-size	Type [1]	Length	max. Depth
Silent®	DePuy®, London, UK	24 × 45	collum	45 mm	24 mm
Metha®	B.Braun Aesculap®, Tuttlingen, Germany	2	partial collum	92 mm	19 mm
Nanos®	Smith&Nephew®, London, UK	2	partial collum	92 mm	17 mm
Aida®	implantcast®, Buxtehude, Germany	0	trochanter sparing	96 mm	16 mm
Fitmore®	Zimmer®, Warsaw, USA	A4	trochanter sparing	93 mm	14 mm
SMF®	Smith&Nephew®, London, UK	1	trochanter harming	90 mm	18 mm
Profemur Preserve®	MicroPort Orthopedics®, Arlington, USA	1	trochanter harming	91 mm	15 mm
Spotorno® *(standard)*	Zimmer®, Warsaw, USA	8	-	146 mm	17 mm

simulation of additional muscle forces was disregarded [16, 23].

The strain simulation process after applying the hip center force was performed with the gradient solver (default settings) of the FE software during the solution process. Similar to previously published work, slice by slice analysis was performed before linear analysis with full resolution [24, 25]. In addition, periprosthetic regions of interest (ROI) were defined according to Gruen et al. of each short-stem-type and according to the ROIs of a typical standard stem (CLS Spotorno®, Zimmer, Warsaw, USA) [26].

Statistical analysis was done by a Z-Test according to Paternoster [27] that compares regression parameters. The method estimates adequate fitting curves by different regression models. To find the best fitting curve we test for each type of prostheses a linear, quadratic, and cubic regression function and compare the resulting R^2 values. The highest R^2 value is equivalent for the best fit and shows the most adequate model for the underlying relationship. The estimated regression equations that fit the data best for all groups of prostheses are of the form

$$SED_{Change_{ik}} = \beta_{0k} + x_{ik}\beta_{1k} + x^2{}_{ik}\beta_{2k} + x^3{}_{ik}\beta_{3k} + e_{ik},$$

with i for the observations, k for the different groups, and x for the bone layers corresponding to the different ROI zones. e describes the error term and $\beta_0 - \beta_3$ are the estimated regression parameters that characterise the curves pattern. Correlations between the strain patterns and the length and depth of the implant were analysed by a correlation analysis. The results are calculated with statistical software package SPSS® Version 24 (IBM, Armonk, North Castle, New York, USA).

The Medical Ethics Committee of the University of Marburg approved this study (number of ethical approval: 84/96). Written informed consent was obtained from all study participants before participation.

Results

To evaluate the impact of the different short-stem THA-implants on periprosthetic bone structure, a classic strain analysis for every short-stem-type was performed. Figure 2 shows the results of the analysis (strain energy density (SED) change after virtual implantation) for each stem type including a standard reference stem and the native femur without prosthesis. While medial regions of the bone showed clear strain reductions by every stem, the SED in the lateral regions increased in most scenarios. Only in ROI 3 and 4 virtual implantation of the trochanter sparing type stems resulted in a stress-shielding phenomenon leading to lower strain values. In addition, geometrical ROIs of the standard stem (CLS Spotorno®) were taken for analysis in each short-stem scenario to demonstrate the influence of the different stems on a potential revision bone stock. Similar to the findings above, a clear shielding effect appeared only in medial bone regions. The trochanter-sparing effect in ROI 3 and 4 was seen after virtual implantation of the collum type stem. In summary the results demonstrate that implantation of a short-stem prosthesis reduced the stress shielding effect compared to implantation of standard stem.

To demonstrate strain patterns in full resolution, a graphical reprocessing of the data set used for the analysis shown in Fig. 3 was performed for the complete bone and for the methadiaphyseal area. Especially in the metadiaphyseal area short stems provide stability for an integration of a standard stem (Fig. 3b). In the trochanteric region, only the collum-type stem showed a biomechanical behaviour more similar to the native femur than any other stem type (Fig. 3a and b). In contrast, partial collum, trochanter harming and trochanter sparing models did not differ between each other for biomechanical behaviour. Furthermore, the three models provided less stress shielding with a lower SED than the standard stem. Additionally, individual data illustration of every stem is shown in Additional file 1 (Figure S3).

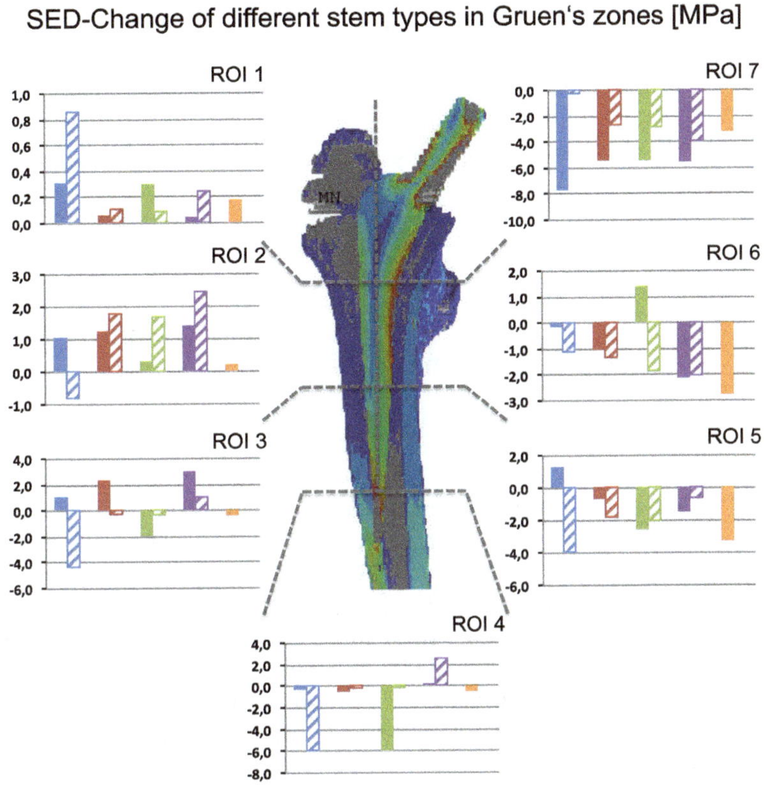

Fig. 2 SED-Changes [MPa] in every ROI according to Gruen and colleagues. The different stem types (collum (*blue*), partial collum (*red*), trochanter sparing (*green*), trochanter harming (*violet*), and standard (*orange*)) were taken for stress analysis. ROIs were defined by stem type (populated) and geometry of the standard stem (hatched)

To approve our findings shown in Fig. 3, we performed a statistical regression analysis of the stress patterns of every stem-type according to Falez and colleagues. The best fit with regard to the pattern-curves for every stem-type was analysed by a cubic regression line. Fitting curves are available in Additional file 1. To compare the different cubic patterns of the prostheses, a Z-test for pairwise comparisons was performed. Table 2 shows the calculated z-values for the differences of the regression parameters. The results show that the majority of the stem-types have different SED change patterns. Only the collum and standard type as well as the partial collum and the trochanter sparing type do not differ from each other. Thus, for this stem-types the progress of SED change is

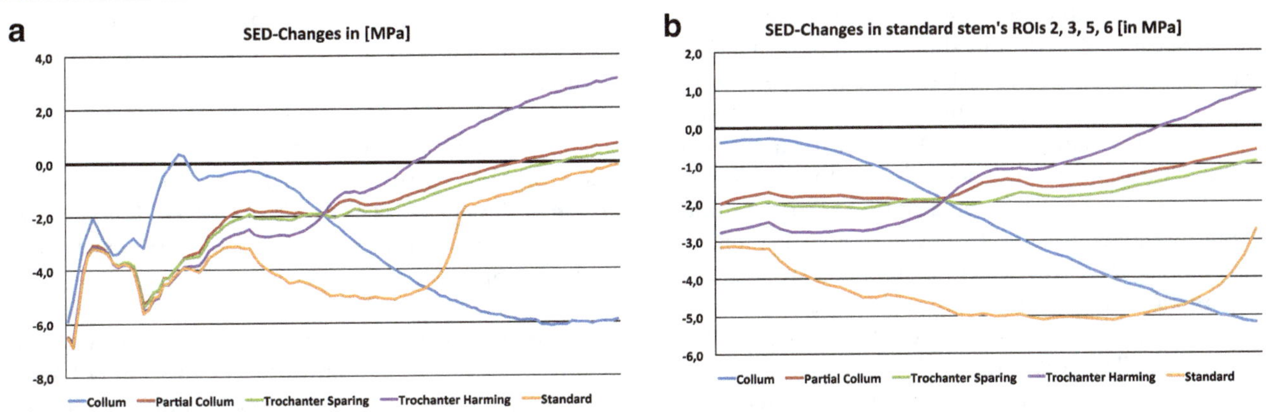

Fig. 3 SED-Changes [MPa] from the tip of the trochanter to the end of ROI 4 based on the CLS Spotorno® stem geometry (**a**) and from the tip of ROI 2&6 to the end of ROI 3&5 based on the CLS Spotorno® stem geometry (**b**). The different stem types (collum (*blue*), partial collum (*red*), trochanter sparing (*green*), trochanter harming (*violet*), and standard (*orange*)) were taken for stress analysis

Table 2 Statistical testing

	$\beta_{1k} - \beta_{1k}$	$\beta_{2k} - \beta_{2k}$	$\beta_{3k} - \beta_{3k}$
Collum vs. *trochanter sparing*	5.958***	−7.109***	5.961***
Collum vs. *trochanter harming*	9.651***	−10.456***	9.263***
Collum vs. *standard*	1.864	−0.656	−0.246
Partial collum vs. *trochanter sparing*	−0.217	0.247	−0.245
Partial collum vs. *trochanter harming*	4.997***	−5.063***	4.6434***
Partial collum vs. standard	−1.8472	3.517***	−4.575***
Trochanter sparing vs. *trochanter harming*	5.600***	−5.696***	5.238***
Trochanter sparing vs. *standard*	−1.840	3.643***	−4.803***
Standard vs. *trochanter harming*	6.109***	−7.613***	8.149***

*** $z \geq 3.29$ (two sided)

equal and can be estimated with the same regression parameters keeping in mind that they start from different initial levels.

Additionally, the correlation analysis shows no significant impact of the stem-length (p = 0.961) and the stem-depth (p = 0.243) (Table 1) on the overall change of SED. In summary the analysis demonstrated that the SED did not differ after implantation of partial collum, trochanter sparing, or trochanter harming stems.

Discussion

Currently, there are multiple designs of short-stem THA-prostheses available [2]. Different fixation-techniques defined by osteotomy level are supposed to provide a maximum of bone stock preservation until the first aseptic revision surgery [9, 28]. A surgeon's decision for a special stem design is often complicated by missing biomechanical data. The main objective of this study was to compare stems-designs of THA-prostheses for their impact on stress-shielding of the periprosthetic bone. Our findings show a stress-shielding prevention by common short-stems independent from the level of osteotomy.

In the current study, we used the previously validated FEA based on clinical data to show the impact of a short-stem THA-implant on stress shielding and bone remodelling [6, 7, 15]. Descriptive examinations can be performed by dual X-ray absorptiometry (DEXA), a technique that operates with lower radiation-doses than CT-based methods. However, DEXA could not be used for simulations in this study because it lacks several virtual implantation options. The transfer from bone density values to elastic modulus has been performed by different mathematical approaches [17, 29–32]. According to studies from Ciarelli and colleagues, it was possible to use a linear relationship because FE models provide consistent bony stress-shielding patterns and are independent of the used density-modulus-relationship [16, 17]. Because an identical specimen dataset was used for each simulation, common problems of a CT-based approach such as partial volume effects, fat errors, or metal artefacts had no impact on our conclusions. Because in the used model, the influence of muscle forces on the SED was not exactly clear, the applied hip forces were verified by telemetric in vivo measurements [33]. This led us to choose a simulation of an isolated resultant force on the centre of the hip joint.

Over decades most biomechanical THA studies used a classification of seven delineated sections (ROI) for quantification of zonal radiographic bone looseness described by Gruen and colleagues in 1979 [26]. Their study was based on a first essay of Salvati and colleagues from 1976 [34]. Gruen's classification is used for manual radiographic analyses and ensures a worldwide comparability of radiologic conclusions until today. Since in the digital era new powerful tools like computerized DEXA or CT-based data sets have arisen, it becomes easy to provide high-resolution results. Therefore, Joshi and colleagues used an approach with twelve ROIs [11]. In addition to this, we performed an analysis slice by slice taking into account the complete information without data compression. With this approach, we can provide full slice resolution with linear analysis.

In concordance with previous studies, results did not show a significant change of the periprostetic bone strain based on the length of the stem. In addition, a greater proximal dimension of the stem in the sagittal plane was not associated with any reduction in periprostetic bone strain [9, 35].

Falez and colleagues have provided a viable classification of different short-stem designs of THA-implants with regard to the level of osteotomy [9]. The intention of a force application as proximal as possible trough the femoral stem led to many developments on the prostheses market. Starting with a "hip resurfacing arthroplasty" (e.g. Burmingham Cap® model), multiple efforts were made to develop new hip stems with a reduced stress-shielding effect [14, 36, 37]. The "collum type" represents a stem type that can be implanted as proximal as possible behind a cap model. However, common complications like osteonecrosis or pitfalls during the surgical procedure led to an early fail of those implants. Therefore, most of the above mentioned stems are no longer available [35, 38]. Like others, our findings for the proximal section describe a strain energy loading close to a native bone. However, the middle and the distal section do not profit by this stem type [35]. Neither in our results nor in findings from other study groups, the advantage of a collum-type prosthesis in the proximal section could be reproduced by metaphyseal anchoring stems [6, 12].

Therefore, representative stems of the partial collum, the trochanter harming and the trochanter sparing types were studied clinically and biomechanically [8, 39–41]. Like in previous studies, we could demonstrate a reduced stress shielding effect of stort-stem implants in comparison to a standard stem implants [8, 39–42]. Similar to Götze and colleagues who detected a non-physiological strain loading by a partial collum type stem, our findings suggest that there is no advantage of force application located most proximally compared to an osteotomy approach located most distally [8]. Floerkemeier and colleagues could show as well that a lower resection even due to more similar strain patterns to a femur model without an implant which suggest that a maximum bone preservation at the femoral neck do not lead to a more physiological load [43]. However, in case of revision surgery, the metadiaphysal bone stock is relevant for optimal ingrowth of a secondary THA-implant using a standard stem design. For that case, an approach with a distal osteotomy is associated with a reduced stress-shielding effect. Similarly, Heller and colleagues could show that changes in stem positioning of short stem implants had no influence on stress shielding effects or the short-stem itself [44].

Using cubic patterns for mathematical description of the strain load into the femur bone, the results showed similar regression slopes for collum-type and standard prostheses indicating similar bone loss pattern for both stem types. However, it is important to note that the regression slopes only capture patterns of SED changes and not absolute differences. In addition, a difference between the partial collum and trochanter sparing type was not observed.

The current study is limited by the virtual approach of THA stem implantation. It is unclear how data obtained from implantation simulations with FE software translate into the clinical setting. Our findings should be validated in DEXA or cadaver studies as a next step to obtain further data on the biomechanical physiology of the different stem types. This information might be a prerequisite for design of a prospective clinical trail.

Conclusion

Based on the result of this study, we cannot confirm that the design of current short stem THA-implants leads to a different stress shielding effect with regard to the level of osteotomy. Somehow unexpected, we found a bone stock protection in metadiaphyseal bone by simulating a more distal approach for osteotomy. In the proximal bone only a collum THA-prosthesis could lead to this effect but so far there is no THA-implant on the marked that provides this kind of stem. Further clinical and biomechanical research including long-term results is needed to understand the influence of short-stem THA on bone remodelling and to find the optimal stem-design for reduction of the stress-shielding effect.

Acknowledgements
Not applicable.

Funding
No funding was received for this study.

Authors' contributions
RB, SB, and JS conceived and designed the experiments. RB and SB performed the experiments. RB, VO, JAG, and JS analysed the data. CS performed the statistical analysis. RB, JAG, and JS wrote the paper. All authors read and approved the final version of the manuscript.

Consent for publication
Not applicable.

Competing interests
The authors declare that they have no competing interests.

Author details
[1]Department of Health, University of Witten/Herdecke, Witten, Germany. [2]Department of Trauma and Orthopaedic Surgery, Kreisklinikum Siegen, Siegen, Germany. [3]Department of Orthopaedics and Rheumatology, University of Marburg, Marburg, Germany. [4]Department of Statistics an Econometrics, University of Siegen, Siegen, Germany. [5]Department of Anesthesiology and Operative Intensive Care Medicine (CCM, CVK), Charité – Universitätsmedizin Berlin, Freie Universität Berlin, Humboldt-Universität zu Berlin, and Berlin Institute of Health, Campus Virchow-Klinikum, Berlin, Germany. [6]Department of Orthopaedics and Trauma Surgery, Lahn-Dill-Kliniken Wetzlar, Wetzlar, Germany.

References

1. Morrey BF. Short-stemmed uncemented femoral component for primary hip arthroplasty. Clin Orthop. 1989;249(1):169–75.
2. Jerosch J. Differences between short stem prostheses. Orthopade. 2014;43:783. doi:10.1007/s00132-014-2308-0.
3. Oh I, Harris WH. Proximal strain distribution in the loaded femur. J Bone Joint Surg. 1978;60A:75–85.

4. Eng CA, Bobyn JD, Glassman AH. Porous-coated hip replacement. The factors governing bone ingrowth, stress shielding and clinical results. J Bone Joint Surg. 1987;69B:45–55.
5. Eng CA, Glassman AH, Suthers KE. The case for porous-coated hip implants. The femoral side. Clin Orthop. 1990;261:63–81.
6. Lerch M, Kurtz A, Stukenborg-Colsman C, Nolte I, Weigel N, Bouguecha A, Behrens BA. Bone remodelling after total hip arthroplasty with a short stemmed metaphyseal loading implant: finite elements analysis validated by a prospectice DEXA investigation. J Orthop Res. 2012;30(11):1822–9.
7. Lengsfeld M, Guenther D, Pressel T, Leppek R, Schmitt J, Griss P. Validation data for periprosthestic bone remodelling theories. J Biomech. 2002;35: 1553–64.
8. Götze C, Ehrenbrink J, Ehrenbrink H. Is there a bone-preserving bone remodelling in short-stem prosthesis? DEXA analysis with the Nanos total hip arthroplasty. Z Orthop Unfall. 2010 Aug;148(4):398–405. doi:10.1055/s-0030-1250151.
9. Falez F, Casella F, Papalia M. Current concepts, classification and results in short stem hip arthroplasty. Orthopedics 2015;38(3)SUPPL:S6-S13.
10. Feyen H, Shimmin AJ. Is the length of the femoral component important in primary total hip replacement? Bone Joint J. 2014;96-B(4):442–8.
11. Joshi MG, Advani SG, Miller F, Santare MH. Analysis of a femoral hip prosthesis designed to reduce stress shielding. J Biomech. 2000;33:1655–62.
12. Chen HH, Morrey BF, An KN, Luo ZP. Bone remodelling charateristics of a short-stemmed total hip replacement. J Arthroplast. 2009;24(6):945–50.
13. Zeh A, Pankow F, Röllinhoff M, Delank S, Wohlrab D. A prospective dual-energy X-ray absorptiometry study of bone remodelling after implantation of the Nanos short-stemmed prosthesis. Acta Orthop Belg. 2013;79(2):174–80.
14. Munting E, Verhelpen M. Fixation and effect on bone strain pattern of a stemless hip prosthesis. J Biomech. 1995;28:949–61.
15. Lengsfeld M, Burchard R, Guenther D, Pressel T, Schmitt J, Leppek R, Griss P. Femoral strain changes after total hip arthroplasty – patient-specific finite element analyses 12 years after operation. Med Phys Eng. 2005;27:649–54.
16. Weinans H, Sumner DR, Igloria R, Natarajan RN. Sensitivity of periprosthetic stress-shielding to load and the bone density-modulus relationship in subject-specific finite element models. J Biomech. 2000;33(7):809–17.
17. Ciarelli MJ, Goldstein SA, Kuhn JL, Cody DD, Brown MB. Evaluation of orthogonal mechanical properties and density of human trabecular bone from the major metaphyseal regions with materials testing and computed tomography. J Orthopaed Res. 1991;9(5):674–82.
18. Schmitt J, Lengsfeld M, Alter P, Leppek R. Use of voxel-oriented femur models for stress analysis. Generation, calculation and validation of CT-based FEM models. Biomed Tech. 1995;40:175–81.
19. Schmitt J, Lengsfeld M, Leppek R, Alter P. Fully automated generation of hip prosthesis voxel models of the femur for finite element analysis. Comparison of direct and subsequent prosthesis implantation. Biomed Tech. 1997;42(6):150–5.
20. Pauwels F. Femoral neck fracture. A mechanical problem. Z Orthop Chir. [Suppl] 1935;63:1–138.
21. Stolk J, Verdonschot N, Huiskes R. Hip-joint and abductor-muscle forces adequately represent in vivo loading of a cemented total hip reconstruction. J Biomech. 2001;34(7):917–26.
22. Lengsfeld M, Kaminsky J, Merz B, Franke RP. Sensitivity of femoral strain pattern analyses to resultant and muscle forces at the hip joint. Med Eng Phys. 1996;18(1):70–8.
23. Bergmann G, Bender A, Dymke J, Duda G, Damm P. Standardized loads acting in hip implants. PLoS One. 2016;11(5):e0155612. doi:10.1371/journal.pone.0155612.
24. Gross S, Abel EW. A finite element analysis of hollow stemmed hip prostheses as a means of reducing stress shielding of the femur. J Biomech. 2001;34(8): 995–1003.
25. Bobyn JD, Mortimer ES, Glassman AH, Engh CA, Miller JE, Brooks CE. Producing and avoiding stress shielding. Laboratory and clinical observations of noncemented total hip arthroplasty. Clin Orthop Relat Res. 1992;274:79–96.
26. Gruen TA, McNeice GM, Amstutz HC. "Modes of failure" of cemented stem-type femoral components: a radiographic analysis of loosening. Clin Orthop Relat Res. 1979;141:17–27.
27. Paternoster R, Brame R, Mazerolle P, Piquero A. Using the correct statistical test for the equality of regression coefficients. Criminology. 1998;4:859–66. doi:10.1111/j.1745-9125.1998.tb01268.x.
28. Ishaque BA, Gils J, Wienbeck S, Donle E, Basad E, Stürz H. Results after replacement of femoral neck prostheses - thrust plate prosthesis (TPP) versus ESKA cut prosthesis. Z Orthop Unfall. 2009;147(1):79–88. doi:10.1055/s-2008-1038992.
29. Carter DR, Hayes WC. The compressive behaviour of bone as a two-phase porous structure. J Bone Joint Surg Am. 1977;59(7):954–62.
30. Keller TS, Mao Z, Spengler DM. Young's modulus, bending strength, and tissue physical properties of human compact bone. J Orthop Res. 1990;8(4):592–603.
31. Snyder SM, Schneider E. Estimation of mechanical properties of cortical bone by computed tomography. J Orthop Res. 1991;9(3):422–31.
32. Rho JY, Hobatho MC, Ashman RB. Relations of mechanical properties to density and CT numbers in human bone. Med Eng Phys. 1995;17(5):347–55.
33. Bergmann G, Graichen F, Rohlmann A. Hip joint loading during walking and running, measured in two patients. J Biomech. 1993;26(8):969–90.
34. Salvati EA, Im VC, Aglietti P, Wilson PD Jr. Radiology of total hip replacements. Clin Orthop Relat Res. 1976;121:74–82.
35. Bishop NE, Burton A, Maheson M, Morlock MM. Biomechanics of short hip endoprostheses–the risk of bone failure increases with decreasing implant size. Clin Biomech. 2010;25(7):666–74. doi:10.1016/j.clinbiomech.2010.04.013.
36. Carrothers AD, Gilbert RE, Jaiswal A, Richardson JB. Birmingham hip resurfacing: the prevalence of failure. J Bone Joint Surg Br. 2010;92(10): 1344–50. doi:10.1302/0301-620X.92B10.23504.
37. Kaegi M, Buergi ML, Jacob HA, Bereiter HH. The thrust plate hip prosthesis: a follow-up of 15-20 years with 102 implants. J Arthroplast. 2016;31(5):1035–9. doi:10.1016/j.arth.2015.11.020.
38. Ender SA, Machner A, Pap G, Hubbe J, Grashoff H, Neumann HW. Cementless CUT femoral neck prosthesis: increased rate of aseptic loosening after 5 years. Acta Orthop. 2007;78(5):616–21.
39. Lerch M, von der Haar-Tran A, Windhagen H, Behrens BA, Wefstaedt P, Stukenborg-Colsman CM. Bone remodelling around the Metha short stem in total hip arthroplasty: a prospective dual-energy X-ray absorptiometry study. Int Orthop. 2012;36(3):533–8. doi:10.1007/s00264-011-1361-0.
40. Freitag T, Hein MA, Wernerus D, Reichel H, Bieger R. Bone remodelling after femoral short stem implantation in total hip arthroplasty: 1-year results from a randomized DEXA study. Arch Orthop Trauma Surg. 2016;136(1):125–30. doi:10.1007/s00402-015-2370-z.
41. McCalden RW, Korczak A, Somerville L, Yuan X, Naudie DD. A randomised trial comparing a short and a standard-length metaphyseal engaging cementless femoral stem using radiostereometric analysis. Bone Joint J. 2015;97-B(5):595–602. doi:10.1302/0301-620X.97B5.34994.
42. Gronewold J, Berner S, Olender G, Hurschler C, Windhagen H, von Lewinski G, Floerkemeier T. Changes in strain patterns after implantation of a short stem with metaphyseal anchorage compared to a standard stem: an experimental study in synthetic bone. Orthop Rev (Pavia). 2014;6(1):5211. doi:10.4081/or.2014.5211.
43. Floerkemeier T, Gronewold J, Berner S, Olender G, Hurschler C, Windhagen H, von Lewinski G. The influence of resection height on proximal femoral strain patterns after Metha short stem hip arthroplasty: an experimental study on composite femora. Int Orthop. 2013;37(3):369–77. doi:10.1007/s00264-012-1725-0.
44. Heller MO, Mehta M, Taylor WR, Kim DY, Speirs A, Duda GN, Perka C. Influence of prosthesis design and implantation technique on implant stresses after cementless revision THR. J Orthop Surg Res. 2011;6:20. doi:10.1186/1749-799X-6-20.

5

Combined application versus topical and intravenous application of tranexamic acid following primary total hip arthroplasty

Pei Zhang[1†], Yuan Liang[2†], Pengtao Chen[2], Yongchao Fang[2], Jinshan He[2,3*] and Jingcheng Wang[1,2,3*]

Abstract

Background: The use of intravenous (IV) or topical tranexamic acid (TXA) in total hip arthroplasty has been proven to be effective and safe in total hip arthroplasty. However, which of these two administration routes is better has not been determined. The combined administration of TXA has been used in total knee arthroplasty with satisfactory results. We hypothesized that combined application of TXA may be the most effective way without increased rate of thrombotic events such as deep vein thrombosis (DVT) and pulmonary embolisms (PE) in patients subjected to primary total hip replacement (THA). A meta-analysis was conducted to compare the efficacy and safety of the combined use of tranexamic acid (TXA) relative to topical or intravenous (IV) use alone for treatment of primary THA. The outcomes included total blood loss, postoperative hemoglobin decline, transfusion rates, and the incidence rates of deep vein thrombosis (DVT) and pulmonary embolisms (PE).

Methods: We searched electronic databases including PubMed, EMBASE, the Cochrane Library, Web of Science, the Chinese Biomedical Literature database, the CNKI database, and Wanfang Data until September 2016. The references of the included articles were also checked for additional potentially relevant studies. There were no language restrictions for the search. The data of the included studies were analyzed using RevMan 5.3 software.

Results: Seven studies met the inclusion criteria, encompassing a total of 1762 patients. Our meta-analysis demonstrated that total blood loss, postoperative hemoglobin decline, and transfusion rates were significantly lower for patients that received the combined treatment compared to patients that received either topical or intravenous administration of TXA. No statistical differences were found in the incidence of deep venous thrombosis (DVT) or pulmonary embolism (PE).

Conclusion: The group that received the combined treatment had lower total blood loss, postoperative hemoglobin decline, and transfusion rates without an increased rate of thrombotic events (DVT or PE). The topical or intravenous use of TXA in primary THA is generally considered to be safe and effective. This meta-analysis demonstrated that combined TXA application may be superior to topical or intravenous application of TXA alone. However, larger, high-quality randomized control trials are required for greater confidence in this finding.

* Correspondence: yzhjs163@163.com; wangjcyangzhou@163.com
[†]Equal contributors
[2]Department of Orthopedics, Clinical Medical College of Yangzhou University, Subei People's Hospital, Nantong West Road 98, Yangzhou 225001, China
[1]Dalian Medical University, Dalian, Liaoning 116044, China
Full list of author information is available at the end of the article

Background

Total hip arthroplasty (THA) is an effective surgical procedure for patients with end-stage hip diseases, but is always accompanied by substantial blood loss and high transfusion rates [1, 2]. Although allogenic blood transfusion may be beneficial to patients, it may induce considerable side effects, such as delay of hip functional recovery, adverse reaction to the transfusion, cardiovascular dysfunction, disease transmission, and joint infection [3–6]. Additionally, allogeneic blood transfusions are costly procedures [7]. Lately, the use of TXA has been expanded for use in THA procedures [8].

Tranexamic acid (TXA) is a synthetic amino acid analogue that acts as a competitive inhibitor of plasminogen and finally interferes with fibrinolysis [9]. TXA can decrease blood loss and reduce transfusion requirements, and has been successfully used in some surgical procedures including THA [8, 10–12]. Intravenous or topical TXA administration for total hip arthroplasty has been demonstrated to be effective and safe in total hip arthroplasty [8, 13–16]. However, which of these two administration routes may be more effective remains controversial due to different merits and drawbacks. The combined administration of TXA has been used in total knee arthroplasty with showed satisfactory results [17–19]. Therefore, we proposed a hypothesis that the combined application of TXA in THA may be the most effective administration strategy without increased rate of thrombotic events.

The efficacy and safety of combined application versus topical or intravenous application of tranexamic acid in THA remains controversial. To our knowledge, no meta-analysis had been previously reported. Therefore, we conducted this meta-analysis to compare these treatment strategies, evaluating outcomes of total blood loss, postoperative hemoglobin decline, transfusion rates, the incidence rate of deep vein thrombosis (DVT), and the incidence rate of pulmonary embolisms (PE).

Methods

Search strategy

We searched the electronic databases including PubMed, EMBASE, the Cochrane Library, Web of Science, the Chinese Biomedical Literature database, the CNKI database, and Wanfang Data until September 2016. The references of the included literatures were also checked for potentially relevant studies. There were no language restrictions. The data of the included studies were analyzed using RevMan 5.3 software. The key words used in search methods including "tranexamic acid", "total hip arthroplasty". We made a joint retrieval of free and subject words. The Boolean operators were used to combine them. The search results were showed in Fig. 1.

Selection criteria

Trials were eligible for inclusion if they met the following criteria: 1) Randomized controlled trials or retrospective control trials; 2) The study compared the efficacy and safety of combined application versus topical or intravenous application of tranexamic acid in primary THA; 3) The study evaluated at least one of the outcome measures of total blood loss, postoperative hemoglobin decline, transfusion rates, deep vein thrombosis (DVT) incidence, and pulmonary embolism (PE) incidence. Studies were excluded if: 1) Patients received other hemostasis treatment; 2) Patients had history of thrombotic events (PE or DVT).

Data extraction

The included studies were examined by two investigators and key data were extracted including first author's name, the published year, study type, sample size, mean age, anesthesia methods, TXA intervention, prosthesis type, prophylactic antithrombotic therapy, transfusion trigger, and surgical outcomes for the meta-analysis (including total blood loss, postoperative hemoglobin decline, transfusion rates, and postoperative complications: VT, PE). When disagreement existed, it was resolved by consulting another investigator.

Quality assessment

The quality of the randomized controlled trials was assessed according to the Cochrane risk assessment scale and included details of the methods of random sequence generation, allocation concealment, blinding, incomplete outcome data, selective outcome reporting, and other sources of bias. The Methodological Index for Non-Randomized Studies (MINORS) was used to assess non-RCTs. The assessments were performed by two investigators independently. Any disagreement was resolved by a third reviewer.

Statistical analysis

This meta-analysis was performed using RevMan 5.3. The heterogeneity level among included studies was assessed by using the value of P and I^2. If $I^2 < 50\%$, $P > 0.1$, this represented low heterogeneity between studies, and a fixed-effect model was used, otherwise, a random-effect model was used. For continuous outcomes, we calculated the mean difference (MD) with 95% confidence interval (CI). The risk difference (RD) with 95% CI was calculated for dichotomous data. If necessary, sensitivity analysis was conducted to identify the origins of the significant heterogeneity.

Results

Description of studies

The search of electronic database identified 498 potentially relevant references for preliminary review. After the scan of

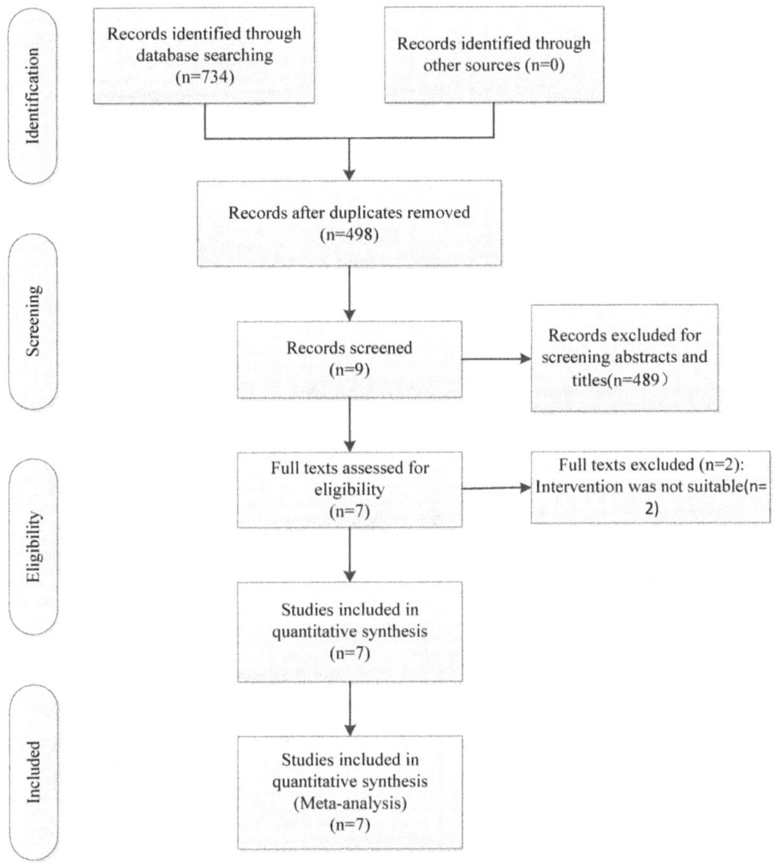

Fig. 1 The flow chart of studies selecting

titles and abstracts, 489 studies were excluded. After the full texts were assessed for eligibility, six RCTs and a retrospective study published between 2014 and 2016 were selected for inclusion [20–26]. The characteristics of the included studies are shown in Table 1.

The selected studies reported comparable baseline characteristics of treatment groups regarding age, gender, Body Mass Index (BMI), and preoperative laboratory parameters (red blood cell specific volume: Hct and hemoglobin: Hb). Six studies reported the transfusion trigger: less than 70 g/L for five studies and 80 g/L for the remaining study. For thromboprophylaxis, two studies used low molecular weight heparin (LMWH) combined with physical therapy, one used enoxaparin combined with physical therapy, one used enoxaparin and rivaroxaban, and one used rivaroxaban combined with physical therapy. Two studies did not report the use of thromboprophylaxis.

Risk of bias assessment

All included RCTs showed clear inclusion and exclusion criteria. In four [20, 22–24] of the included RCTs, the randomization algorithm was generated from a blinded biostatistician or a computer. In one RCT [26], the allocation concealment was performed using opaque sealed envelopes. One RCT [24] provided details of the double blinding for treatments and the blinding of outcome assessment. All RCTs reported complete outcome data. The results of the quality of the included RCTs are shown in Fig. 2. The MINORS scale was used to assess the retrospective study, as presented in Fig. 3.

Outcomes measures

Total blood loss (ml)

1) Comparisons between the combined group and the topical group.
   Six studies (1111patients) [20–23, 25, 26] investigated total blood loss. Heterogeneity was significant in the studies (P <0.00001; I^2 = 95%), so the random-effects model was used. The pooled result revealed that combined application of TXA significantly reduced total blood loss compared to topical application of TXA. (MD = −162, 95% CI: −265 to −60, P = 0.002. Figure 4a).
2) Comparisons between the combined group and the intravenous group.
   Seven studies (for a total of 1317 patients) [20–26] compared total blood loss. Heterogeneity was

Table 1 The characteristics of included studies

Study (year)	Number	Mean age	Anesthesia methods	TXA intervention	Prosthesis type	Thromboprophylaxis	Transfusion criteria
Xie 2016 [26]	70/70/70 (T/I/C)	62.2/59.5/60.5 (T/I/C)	General anesthesia	T:3 g; I: 1.5 g; C:1 g (IV) + 2 g (T)	Cementless	Enoxaparin + Physical therapy	Hb <7 g/dL
Yue 2015 [21]	136/238/357 (T/I/C)	60.3/62.6/61.9 (T/I/C)	–	T:3 g; I:15 mg/kg; TXA; C:15 mg/kg(IV) + 1.5 g (T)	Cementless	Low-molecular-weight heparin + Physical therapy	Hb <7 g/dL
Zhang 2015 [20]	34/34/34 (T/I/C)	65.2/63.4/64.7 (T/I/C)	–	T:0.1 g; I: I g; C:1 g(IV) + 0.1 g(T)	Cemented	Enoxaparin + rivaroxaban	Hb <7 g/dL
Zhao 2015 [25]	44/48/44 (T/I/C)	62.2/59.8/57.6 (T/I/C)	Continuous epidural anesthesia	T:1 g; I:1 g; C:1 g(IV) + 1 g(T)	Cementless	Rivaroxaban + Physical therapy	Hb < 8 g/dL
Lu 2016 [22]	141/141/141 (T/I/C)	66.8/66.0/65.0 (T/I/C)	General anesthesia	T: 2 g; I: 30 mg/kg TXA; C:30 mg/kg (IV) + 2 g (T)	Cementless	–	Hb <7 g/dL
Zhu 2016 [23]	20/20/20 (T/I/C)	58.0/60.4/62.0 (T/I/C)	–	T: 2 g; I: 15 mg/kg TXA; C:15 mg/kg (IV) + 2 g (T)	Cementless	–	–
Zeng 2016 [24]	50/50 (I/C)	54.0/53.6 (I/C)	–	I:15 mg/kg TXA; C:15 mg/kg (IV) + 1 g (T)	–	Low-molecular-weight heparin + Physical therapy	Hb <7 g/dL

C combined group, *T* topical group, *I* intravenous group, *IV* intravenous injection, *Hb* hemoglobin

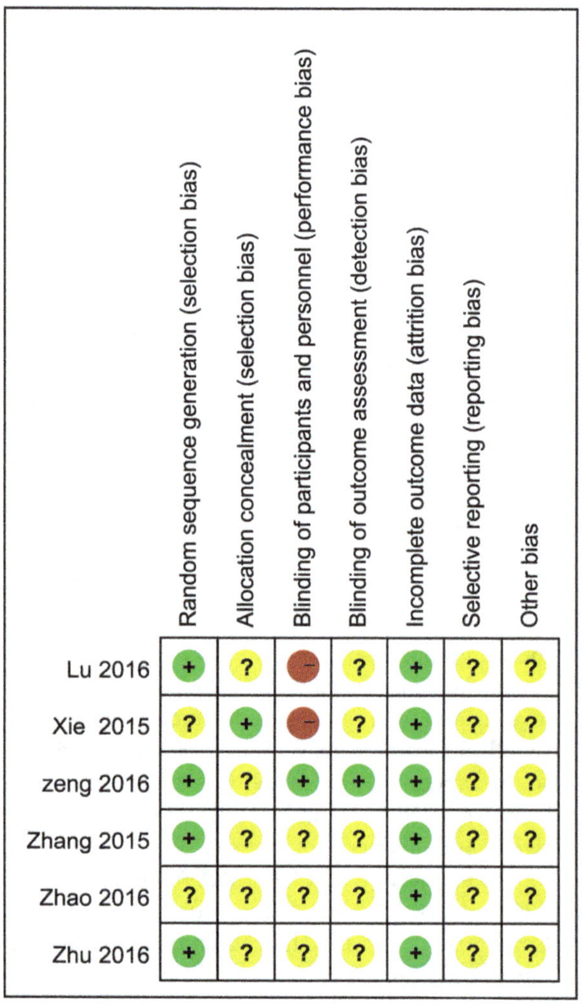

Fig. 2 The quality of the randomized controlled trials

significant in the studies (P =0.0001; I^2 = 78%), so the random-effects model was used. The pooled result revealed that the combined group exhibited lower total blood loss than the intravenous group (MD = −153, 95% CI: −201 to −105, P <0.00001. Figure 4b).

Postoperative hemoglobin decline (g/dl)

1) Comparison between the combined group and the topical group.
   Four reports (including 1003 patients) [21, 22, 25, 26] reported the outcome of postoperative hemoglobin decline. Significant heterogeneity was detected in the studies (P =0.007; I^2 = 75%), so the random-effects model was used. The pooled results showed that the combined application group showed postoperative hemoglobin decline (MD = −1.06, 95% CI: −1.30 to −0.82, P < 0.00001; Fig. 5a).
2) Comparison between the combined group and the intravenous group.
   Five studies (including 1209 patients) [21, 22, 24–26] reported the outcome of postoperative hemoglobin decline. Heterogeneity was significant in the studies (P =0.01; I^2 = 69%); so, the random-effects model was used. The pooled results showed that the combined application group exhibited lower postoperative hemoglobin decline (MD = −0.56, 95% CI: −0.78 to −0.34, P < 0.00001; Fig. 5b).

Transfusion rates

1) Comparison between the combined group and the topical group.

Quality assessment for non-randomized trials	Yue 2015
A clearly stated aim.	2
Inclusion of consecutive patients	2
Prospective data collection	2
Endpoints appropriate to the aim of the study	2
Unbiased assessment of the study endpoint	0
A follow-up period appropriate to the aims of study	2
Less than 5% loss to follow-up	2
Prospective calculation of the sample size	0
An adequate control group	2
Contemporary groups	2
Baseline equivalence of groups	2
Adequate statistical analyses	2
Total score	18

Fig. 3 Quality assessment for the non-randomized trial

Five studies (including 1071 patients) [20–22, 25, 26] compared transfusion rates. No significant heterogeneity was detected in the studies (P =0.97; I^2 = 0%). Therefore, the fixed-effects model was used for analysis. The results showed the combined application group had lower transfusion rates (RD = −0.05, 95% CI: −0.08 to −0.02, P = 0.0005; Fig. 6a).

2) Comparison between the combined group and the intravenous group.
Six studies (including 1277 patients) [20–22, 24–26] compared transfusion rates. No significant heterogeneity was detected in the studies (P =0.39; I^2 = 5%). Therefore, the fixed- effects model was used for analysis. The results showed that the combined application group had lower transfusion rates (RD = −0.04, 95% CI: −0.07 to −0.02, P = 0.0002; Fig. 6b).

Deep vein thrombosis (DVT)

1) Comparison between the combined group and the topical group.
Six articles (for a total of 1111 patients) [20–23, 25, 26] reported the incidence of DVT.

a

Study or Subgroup	Experimental Mean	SD	Total	Control Mean	SD	Total	Weight	Mean Difference IV, Random, 95% CI
Lu 2016	803.32	201.14	141	998.19	196.89	141	17.3%	-194.87 [-241.33, -148.41]
Xie 2015	776.75	188.95	70	905.07	237.7	70	16.5%	-128.32 [-199.45, -57.19]
Yue 2015	819.82	202.82	357	969.18	252.65	136	17.3%	-149.36 [-196.75, -101.97]
Zhang 2015	787	110	34	1,005	149	34	16.8%	-218.00 [-280.25, -155.75]
Zhao 2016	733.28	257.78	44	1,082.6	308.59	44	14.5%	-349.32 [-468.13, -230.51]
Zhu 2016	558	64.3	20	528.5	43.43	20	17.6%	29.50 [-4.51, 63.51]
Total (95% CI)			**666**			**445**	**100.0%**	**-162.74 [-265.17, -60.32]**

Heterogeneity: Tau² = 15216.95; Chi² = 107.12, df = 5 (P < 0.00001); I² = 95%
Test for overall effect: Z = 3.11 (P = 0.002)

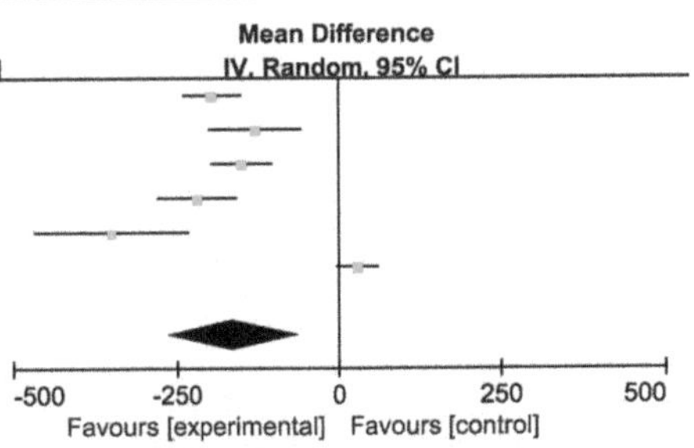

b

Study or Subgroup	Experimental Mean	SD	Total	Control Mean	SD	Total	Weight	Mean Difference IV, Random, 95% CI
Lu 2016	803.32	201.14	141	956.23	213.67	141	17.0%	-152.91 [-201.35, -104.47]
Xie 2015	776.75	188.95	70	878.03	210	70	14.8%	-101.28 [-167.46, -35.10]
Yue 2015	819.82	202.82	357	929.63	216.32	238	18.6%	-109.81 [-144.42, -75.20]
Zeng 2016	835.49	343.5	50	1,002.62	366.85	50	7.6%	-167.13 [-306.43, -27.83]
Zhang 2015	787	110	34	1,019	137	34	15.7%	-232.00 [-291.06, -172.94]
Zhao 2016	733.28	257.78	44	1,057.11	354.26	48	8.6%	-323.83 [-449.71, -197.95]
Zhu 2016	558	64.3	20	645.1	69.09	20	17.8%	-87.10 [-128.46, -45.74]
Total (95% CI)			**716**			**601**	**100.0%**	**-153.65 [-201.88, -105.42]**

Heterogeneity: Tau² = 2951.47; Chi² = 27.83, df = 6 (P = 0.0001); I² = 78%
Test for overall effect: Z = 6.24 (P < 0.00001)

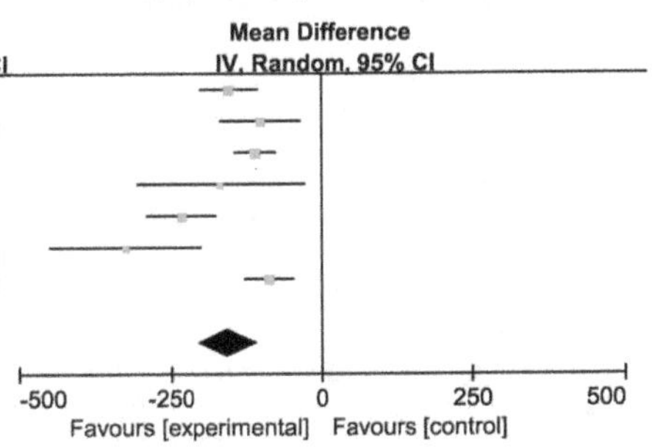

Fig. 4 **a**: The comparison between the combined group and the topical group in total blood loss. **b**: The comparison between the combined group and the intravenous group in total blood loss

a

Study or Subgroup	Experimental Mean	Experimental SD	Experimental Total	Control Mean	Control SD	Control Total	Weight	Mean Difference IV, Random, 95% CI
Lu 2016	2.821	1.106	141	4.189	0.8787	141	26.1%	-1.37 [-1.60, -1.13]
Xie 2015	2.98	0.78	70	3.89	0.72	70	25.3%	-0.91 [-1.16, -0.66]
Yue 2015	2.95	0.78	357	3.85	0.73	136	30.7%	-0.90 [-1.05, -0.75]
Zhao 2016	2.338	0.808	44	3.455	1.058	44	17.9%	-1.12 [-1.51, -0.72]
Total (95% CI)			**612**			**391**	**100.0%**	**-1.06 [-1.30, -0.82]**

Heterogeneity: Tau² = 0.04; Chi² = 12.10, df = 3 (P = 0.007); I² = 75%
Test for overall effect: Z = 8.73 (P < 0.00001)

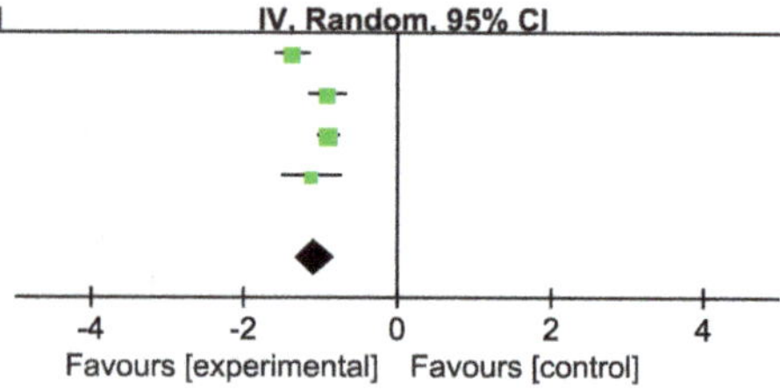

b

Study or Subgroup	Experimental Mean	Experimental SD	Experimental Total	Control Mean	Control SD	Control Total	Weight	Mean Difference IV, Random, 95% CI
Lu 2016	2.821	1.106	141	3.444	0.994	141	23.1%	-0.62 [-0.87, -0.38]
Xie 2015	2.98	0.78	70	3.36	0.78	70	22.4%	-0.38 [-0.64, -0.12]
Yue 2015	2.95	0.78	357	3.35	0.81	238	29.1%	-0.40 [-0.53, -0.27]
Zeng 2016	3.302	1.738	50	3.748	1.389	50	9.2%	-0.45 [-1.06, 0.17]
Zhao 2016	2.338	0.808	44	3.432	1.081	48	16.2%	-1.09 [-1.48, -0.71]
Total (95% CI)			**662**			**547**	**100.0%**	**-0.56 [-0.78, -0.34]**

Heterogeneity: Tau² = 0.04; Chi² = 12.95, df = 4 (P = 0.01); I² = 69%
Test for overall effect: Z = 5.00 (P < 0.00001)

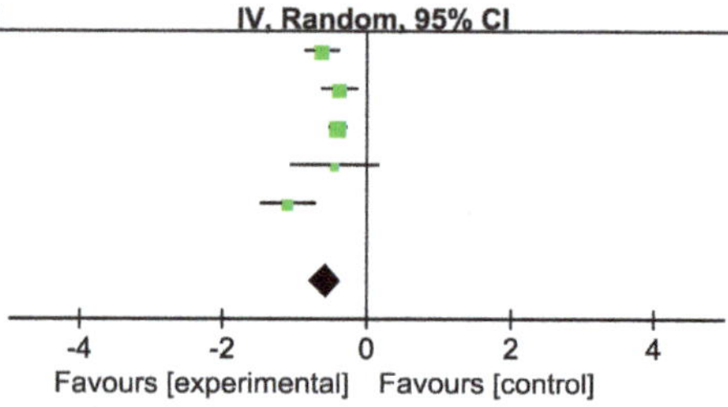

Fig. 5 a: The comparison between the combined group and the topical group in postoperative hemoglobin decline. **b**: The comparison between the combined group and the intravenous group in postoperative hemoglobin decline

a

Study or Subgroup	Experimental Events	Experimental Total	Control Events	Control Total	Weight	Risk Difference M-H, Fixed, 95% CI
Lu 2016	5	141	11	141	29.0%	-0.04 [-0.10, 0.01]
Xie 2015	0	70	4	70	14.4%	-0.06 [-0.12, 0.00]
Yue 2015	5	357	8	136	40.5%	-0.04 [-0.09, -0.00]
Zhang 2015	5	34	8	34	7.0%	-0.09 [-0.27, 0.10]
Zhao 2016	0	44	3	44	9.1%	-0.07 [-0.15, 0.02]
Total (95% CI)		**646**		**425**	**100.0%**	**-0.05 [-0.08, -0.02]**
Total events	15		34			

Heterogeneity: Chi² = 0.54, df = 4 (P = 0.97); I² = 0%
Test for overall effect: Z = 3.47 (P = 0.0005)

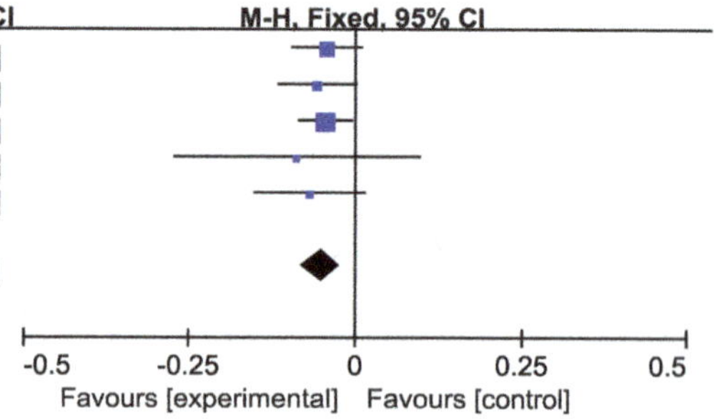

b

Study or Subgroup	Experimental Events	Experimental Total	Control Events	Control Total	Weight	Risk Difference M-H, Fixed, 95% CI
Lu 2016	5	141	9	141	22.5%	-0.03 [-0.08, 0.02]
Xie 2015	0	70	3	70	11.2%	-0.04 [-0.10, 0.01]
Yue 2015	5	357	10	238	45.6%	-0.03 [-0.06, 0.00]
Zeng 2016	1	50	8	50	8.0%	-0.14 [-0.25, -0.03]
Zhang 2015	5	34	9	34	5.4%	-0.12 [-0.31, 0.07]
Zhao 2016	0	44	2	48	7.3%	-0.04 [-0.11, 0.03]
Total (95% CI)		**696**		**581**	**100.0%**	**-0.04 [-0.07, -0.02]**
Total events	16		41			

Heterogeneity: Chi² = 5.25, df = 5 (P = 0.39); I² = 5%
Test for overall effect: Z = 3.75 (P = 0.0002)

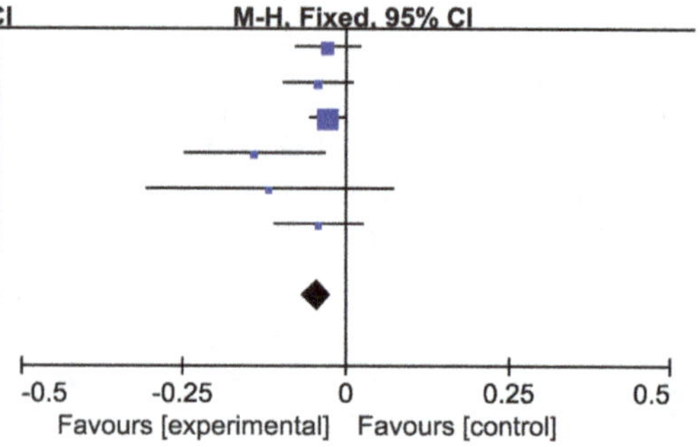

Fig. 6 a: The comparison between the combined group and the topical group in transfusion rates. **b**: The comparison between the combined group and the intravenous group in transfusion rates

No significant heterogeneity was found ($P = 0.87$; $I^2 = 0\%$), so the fixed-effects model was used. It showed no significant difference between the groups (RD = 0.00, 95% CI: −0.01 to 0.02, $P = 0.93$; Fig. 7a).

2) Comparison between the combined group and the intravenous group.
Seven articles (for a total of 1317 patients) [20–26] reported the incidence of DVT. No significant heterogeneity was found ($P = 1$; $I^2 = 0\%$), so the fixed-effects model was used. It showed no significant difference between the groups (RD = 0.00, 95% CI: −0.01 to 0.01, $P = 0.89$; Fig. 7b).

Pulmonary embolism (PE)

1) Comparison between the combined group and the topical group.
PE was reported in four included studies (1003 patients) [21, 22, 25, 26]. No significant heterogeneity was found ($P = 1$; $I^2 = 0\%$), therefore, the fixed-effects model was used. It manifested no significant difference between the treatments (RD = 0.00, 95% CI: −0.01 to 0.01, $P = 1$; Fig. 8a).
2) Comparison between the combined group and the intravenous group.
PE was reported in five included studies (1209 patients) [21, 22, 24–26]. No significant heterogeneity was found ($P = 1$; $I^2 = 0\%$), therefore, the fixed-effects model was used. It manifested no significant difference between the groups (RD = 0.00, 95% CI: −0.01 to 0.01, $P = 1$; Fig. 8b).

Discussion

To our knowledge, this is the first meta-analysis comparing the hemostatic efficacy and safety of the combined application of intravenous and topical application of tranexamic acid in primary THA. The most important finding of our meta-analysis was that the combined application of TXA was correlated with a significant lower total blood loss and transfusion requirements without increasing rate of thrombotic events (DVT or PE).

TXA has been shown to decrease blood loss and reduce transfusion requirements, and has been successfully used in surgical procedures including THA [8, 10–12]. Intravenous or topical TXA use alone has been demonstrated to be effective and safe in total hip arthroplasty [8, 13–16]. When TXA is given intravenously, it is widely distributed throughout the extracellular and intracellular compartment, and rapidly reaches a maximum plasma concentration (in 5 to 15 min) [26, 27]. Local fibrinolysis can be inhibited from the start of surgery [26]. Topical application of TXA may

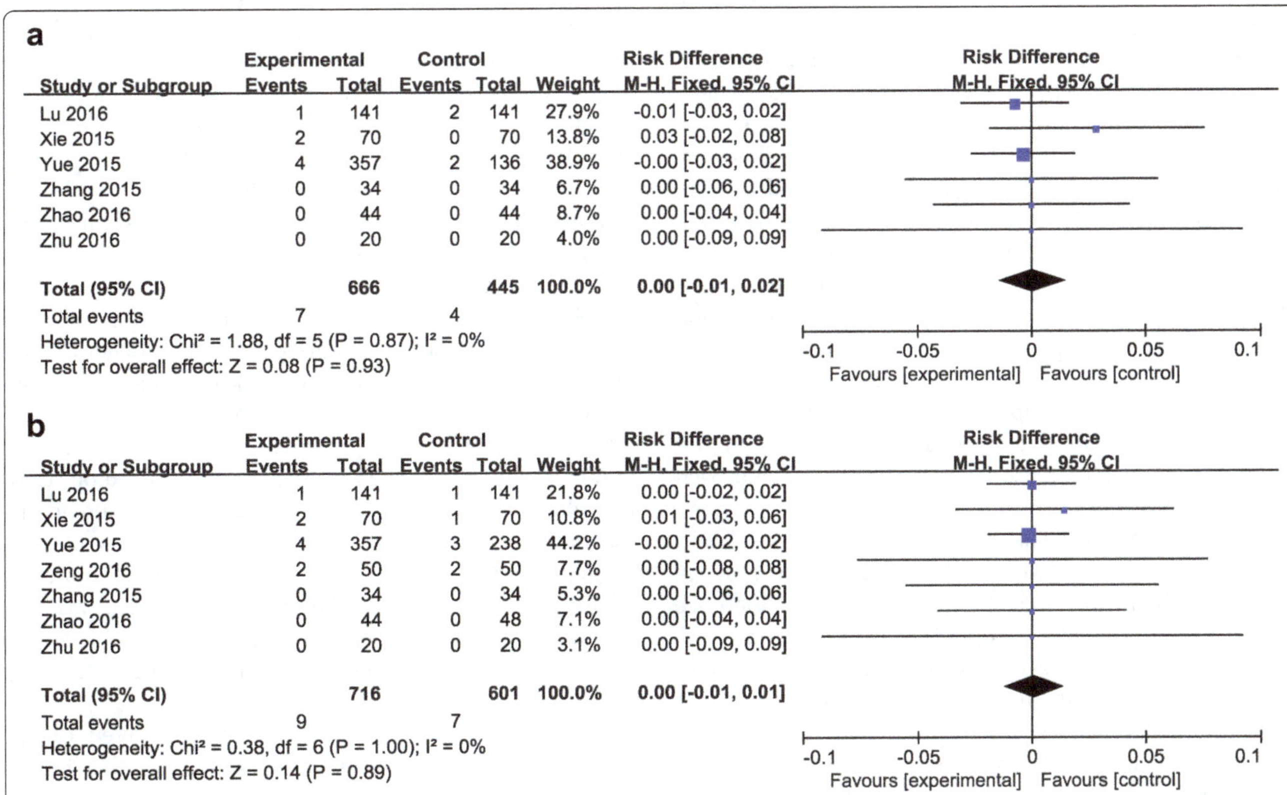

Fig. 7 **a**: The comparison between the combined group and the topical group in the incidence rate of DVT. **b**: The comparison between the combined group and the intravenous group in the incidence rate of DVT

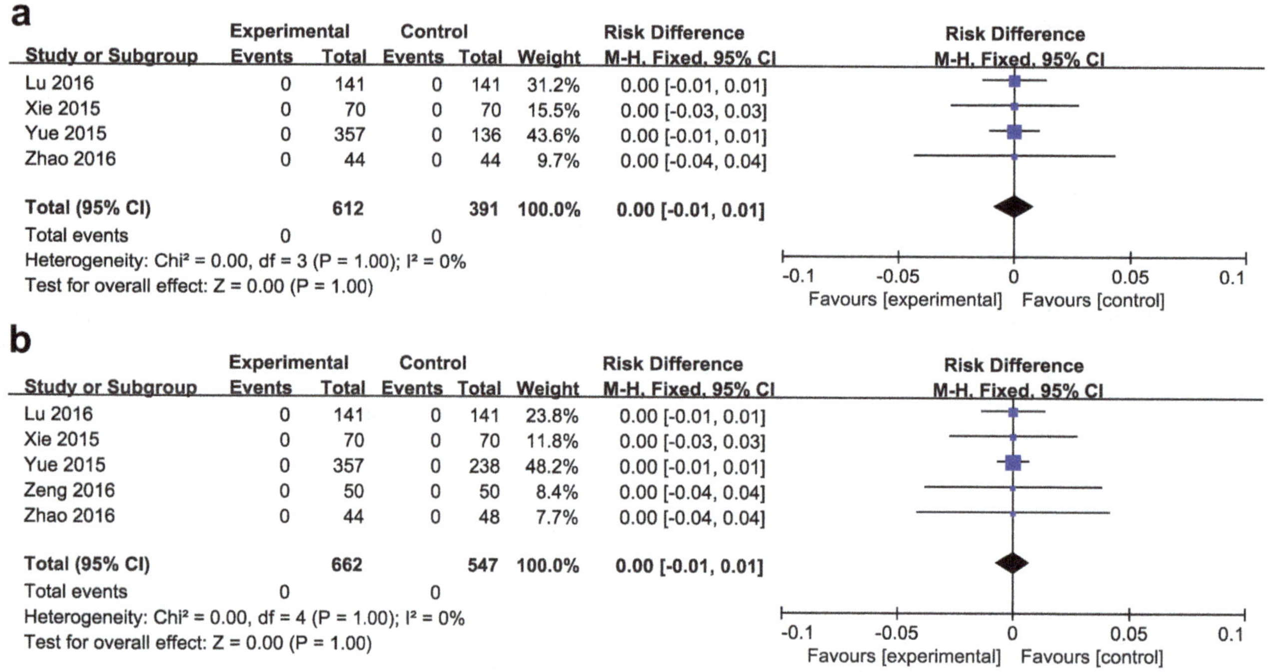

Fig. 8 a: The comparison between the combined group and the topical group in the incidence rate of PE. **b**: The comparison between the combined group and the intravenous group in the incidence rate of PE

maintain a maximum local level for hemostasis by maintaining fibrin clotting [26, 28]. The combined application of TXA has been used in total knee arthroplasty with satisfactory results [17–19]. To our knowledge, no meta-analysis has evaluated the efficacy and safety of combined application versus topical or intravenous administration of TXA in THA. The primary endpoints of our study included total blood loss, postoperative hemoglobin decline, and transfusion rates. Our results revealed that the combined group had lower total blood loss. Xie et al. [26] reported that compared to IV TXA or topical TXA, combined administration of TXA can additionally reduce total blood loss by 12 and 14%, respectively Zeng et al. [24] also reported that the combined group had significantly lower total blood loss than the intravenous group. The research results of Zhang et al. [20] and Zhao et al. [25] are consistent with our findings. Yue et al. [21] also favored a combined approach by retrospective study.

The result of our meta-analysis evaluating transfusion rates favored the combined group. Zhang et al. [20] reported that there was no statistically significant difference in transfusion rates for IV, topical, or combined administration of TXA. All the results of the remaining studies were consistent with the findings of our meta-analysis that the combined group had a lower transfusion rate.

Thrombotic complications could induce severe results and even death after THA, so it is urgent to determine whether combined application of TXA increases the rate of thrombotic events (DVT and PE). Many studies reported that topical or intravenous administration of TXA was not associated with an increased rate of thrombotic events [29–32]. In our meta-analysis, all the included studies reported no significant difference in the incidence rate of DVT or PE in the combined, topical, or intravenous treatment groups. This finding was in accordance with the results of our meta-analysis. Sensitivity analysis based on the study type also showed no statistical difference. Although the methods of thromboprophylaxis differed in the included studies, our study did not show any significant heterogeneity in DVT and PE among these studies. However, due to the small sample size and short follow-up in most of the included studies, larger studies with more patients and longer follow-up are required to confirm whether the combined treatment strategy is safe without increasing thrombotic events.

Significant heterogeneity was detected in some outcomes in our meta-analysis. The sensitivity analysis based on study type demonstrated no statistically significant difference in the outcomes. In four of the included RCTs, a blinded biostatistician or a computer generated the randomization algorithm. In one RCT,the allocation concealment was performed using opaque sealed envelopes. One RCT included details of the double blinding and the blinding of the outcome assessment.

There are several limits of this meta-analysis. We included a retrospective study in our analysis due to the limited amount of published RCTs. This inclusion decreased the evidence level of the meta-analysis to some extent. Although we searched electronic databases systematically, some relevant studies might have been missed due to publication bias. Additionally, the sample size was very small in most of the included studies.

In addition, there was clinical heterogeneity in the reports as follows: 1) Differences in surgical time, technique, approaches, and postoperative measures. 2) Different anesthesia methods, which can affect blood loss and transfusion requirements (general anesthesia was related with an increased rate of adverse events and blood transfusions compared with spinal anesthesia) [33, 34]. However, a larger sample size of patients and multicenter studies are required to confirm this conclusion. 3) Differences in the TXA dose, especially Zhang 2015 [20], there was insufficient data to perform subgroup analysis and the optimal dose still remains controversial. In order to clarify the contributions of all these identified issues, additional studies with larger sample sizes are needed.

The limitations of this study were as follows: 1) The relatively small sample size of each primary study, especially Zhu 2016 [23]; and there was significant heterogeneity in total blood loss and postoperative hemoglobin decline. However, we could not conduct subgroup analysis due to insufficient data.2)In some RCTs, the methods of random sequence generation, allocation concealment, blinding, and selective outcome reporting were unclear or not described, which may influence the stability of our outcomes to some extent. 3)A retrospective study was included due to the limitation of studies, which also lowered the robust analysis. 4) Differences in surgical time, technique, approaches, and postoperative measures may have influenced the results. 5) There is publication bias.

Conclusion

The group that received the combined treatment had lower total blood loss, postoperative hemoglobin decline, and transfusion rates without an increased rate of thrombotic events (DVT or PE). The topical or intravenous use of TXA in primary THA is generally considered to be safe and effective. This meta-analysis demonstrated that combined TXA application may be superior to topical or intravenous application of TXA alone. However, larger, high-quality randomized control trials are required for greater confidence in this finding.

Abbreviations

BMI: Body mass index; DVT: Deep vein thrombosis; Hb: Hemoglobin; Hct: Red blood cell specific volume; IV: Intravenous; PE: Pulmonary embolisms; THA: Total hip arthroplasty; TXA: Tranexamic acid

Acknowledgments

Not applicable.

Funding

Not applicable.

Authors' contributions

WJ and ZP conceived of the design of the study. LY and CP participated in the literature search, study selection, data extraction and quality assessment. FY and HJ participated in the design of the study and performed the statistical analysis. ZP finished the manuscript. All authors read and approved the final manuscript.

Competing interests

The authors declare that they have no competing interests.

Consent for publication

Not applicable.

Author details

[1]Dalian Medical University, Dalian, Liaoning 116044, China. [2]Department of Orthopedics, Clinical Medical College of Yangzhou University, Subei People's Hospital, Nantong West Road 98, Yangzhou 225001, China. [3]Department of Orthopedics, Clinical Medical College of Yangzhou University, Subei People's Hospital of Jiangsu Province, Yangzhou, China.

References

1. Bierbaum BE, Callaghan JJ, Galante JO, Rubash HE, Tooms RE, Welch RB. An analysis of blood management in patients having a total hip or knee arthroplasty. J Bone Joint Surg Am. 1999;81(1):2–10.
2. Saleh A, Small T, Chandran Pillai AL, Schiltz NK, Klika AK, Barsoum WK. Allogenic blood transfusion following total hip arthroplasty: results from the nationwide inpatient sample, 2000 to 2009. J Bone Joint Surg Am. 2014; 96(18):e155-e.
3. Carson JL, Duff A, Poses RM, Berlin JA, Spence RK, Trout R, et al. Effect of anaemia and cardiovascular disease on surgical mortality and morbidity: the lancet. Lancet. 1996;348(9034):1055–60.
4. Allain JP, Stramer SL, Carneiro-Proietti ABF, Martins ML, Silva SNLD, Ribeiro M, et al. Transfusion-transmitted infectious diseases. Biologicals. 2009;37(2):71–7.
5. Vamvakas EC, Blajchman MA. Transfusion-related mortality: the ongoing risks of allogeneic blood transfusion and the available strategies for their prevention. Blood. 2009;113(15):3406–17.
6. Newman ET, Watters TS, Lewis JS, Jennings JM, Wellman SS, Attarian DE, et al. Impact of perioperative allogeneic and autologous blood transfusion on acute wound infection following total knee and total hip arthroplasty. J Bone Joint Surg Am. 2014;96(4):279–84.
7. Shander A, Hofmann A, Ozawa S, Theusinger OM, Gombotz H, Spahn DR. Activity-based costs of blood transfusions in surgical patients at 4 hospitals. Transfusion. 2009;50(4):753–65.
8. Chen S, Wu K, Kong G, Feng W, Deng Z, et al. The efficacy of topical tranexamic acid in total hip arthroplasty: a meta-analysis. BMC Musculoskelet Disord. 2016;17:1–7.
9. Kazemi SM, Mosaffa F, Eajazi A, Kaffashi M, Daftari BL, Bigdeli MR, et al. The effect of tranexamic acid on reducing blood loss in cementless total hip arthroplasty under epidural anesthesia. Orthopedics. 2010;33(1):17.
10. Bonis MD, Cavaliere F, Alessandrini F, Lapenna E. Topical use of tranexamic acid in coronary artery bypass operations: a double-blind, prospective, randomized, placebo-controlled study. J Thorac Cardiovasc Surg. 2000; 119(3):575–80.
11. Strang CM, Hachenberg T. Current strategies to minimize of blood loss during radical prostatectomy. Anasthesiol Intensivmed Notfallmed Schmerzther. 2013;48(7-8):494–9. quiz 500–1.
12. Ngichabe S, Obura T, Stones W. Intravenous tranexamic acid as an adjunct haemostat to ornipressin during open myomectomy. A randomized double blind placebo controlled trial. Ann Surg Innov Res. 2015;9:10.
13. Mcconnell JS, Shewale S, Munro NA, Shah K, Deakin AH, Kinninmonth AW. Reduction of blood loss in primary hip arthroplasty with tranexamic acid or fibrin spray. Acta Orthop. 2011;82(6):660–3.
14. Martin JG, Cassatt KB, Kincaid-Cinnamon KA, Westendorf DS, Garton AS. Topical administration of tranexamic acid in primary total hip and total knee arthroplasty. J Arthroplasty. 2014;29(5):889–94.

15. North WT, Mehran N, Davis JJ, Silverton CD, Weir RM, Laker MW. Topical vs intravenous tranexamic acid in primary total hip arthroplasty: a double-blind, randomized controlled. Trial J Arthroplasty. 2015;31(4):1022–6.
16. Ueno M, Sonohata M, Fukumori N, Kawano S, Kitajima M, Mawatari M. Comparison between topical and intravenous administration of tranexamic acid in primary total hip arthroplasty. J Orthop Sci. 2015;21(1):44–7.
17. Wong J, Abrishami A, El BH, Mahomed NN, Roderick DJ, Gandhi R, et al. Topical application of tranexamic acid reduces postoperative blood loss in total knee arthroplasty: a randomized, controlled trial. J Bone Joint Surg Am. 2010;92(15):2503–13.
18. Karaaslan F, Karaoğlu S, Mermerkaya MU, Baktir A. Reducing blood loss in simultaneous bilateral total knee arthroplasty: combined intravenous–intra-articular tranexamic acid administration. A prospective randomized controlled trial. Knee. 2014;22(2):131–5.
19. Nielsen CS, Jans ØTØ, Foss NB, Troelsen A, Husted H. Combined intra-articular and intravenous tranexamic acid reduces blood loss in total knee arthroplasty: a randomized, double-blind, placebo-controlled trial. J Bone Joint Surg Am. 2016;98(10):835–41.
20. Zhang L, Wang DR, Zhao GP, Qin HX. T Efficacy of intravenous injection combined with topical tranexamic acid for hemostasis during primary total hip arthroplasty. J Pract Med. 2015;31(20):3358–60.
21. Yue C, Xie JW, Cai DF, Yang J, Zhou ZK, Pei FX. Efficacy and safety of intravenous injection combined with topical tranexamic acid for reducing perioperative bleeding during primary total hip arthroplasty: a retrospective study. CJBJS. 2015;8(1):44–8.
22. Lu C, Guo H, Hao YQ, Chen XS, Cai YZ, Xu P. A prospective randomized controlled study of tranexamic acid used in different ways to reduce blood loss in total hip arthroplasty. CJBJS. 2016;9(2):140–4.
23. Zhu C, Chu XB, Zhang JH. Different methods of tranexamic acid on reducing blood loss during total hip arthroplasty. J Jiangxi Univ TCM. 2016;28(1):47–9.
24. Zeng Y, Shen B, Yang J, Zhou ZK, Kang PD, Pei FX. Tranexamic acid administration in primary total hip arthroplasty: a randomized controlled trial of intravenous combined with topical versus single-dose intravenous administration. J Bone Joint Surg Am. 2016;98(12):983–91.
25. Zhao QB, Ren JD, Zhang XG, Wu HZ. Comparison of perioperative blood loss and transfusion rate in primary unilateral total hip arthroplasty by topical, intravenous application or combined application of tranexamic acid. CJTER. 2015;20(4):459–64.
26. Xie JW, Ma J, Yue C, Kang PD, Pei FX. Combined use of intravenous and topical tranexamic acid following cementless total hip arthroplasty: a randomized clinical trial. Hip Int. 2016;26(1):36–42.
27. Benoni G, Björkman DS, Fredin H. Application of pharmacokinetic data from healthy volunteers for the prediction of plasma concentrations of tranexamic acid in surgical patients. Clin Drug Investig. 1995;10(5):280–7.
28. Krohn CD, Sørensen R, Lange JE, Riise R, Bjørnsen S, Brosstad F. Tranexamic acid given into the wound reduces postoperative blood loss by half in major orthopaedic surgery. Eur J Surg Suppl. 2003;588:57–61.
29. Whiting DR, Gillette BP, Duncan C, Smith H, Pagnano MW, Sierra RJ. Preliminary results suggest tranexamic acid is safe and effective in arthroplasty patients with severe comorbidities. Clin Orthop Relat Res. 2014; 472(1):66–72.
30. Gillette BP, Desimone LJ, Trousdale RT, Pagnano MW, Sierra RJ. Low risk of thromboembolic complications with tranexamic acid after primary total Hip and knee arthroplasty. Clin Orthop Relat Res. 2012;471(1):150–4.
31. Hallstrom B, Singal B, Cowen ME, Roberts KC, Hughes RE. The Michigan experience with safety and effectiveness of tranexamic acid use in Hip and knee arthroplasty. J Bone Joint Surg Am. 2016;98(19):1646–55.
32. Sun X, Dong Q, Zhang YG. Intravenous versus topical tranexamic acid in primary total hip replacement: a systemic review and meta-analysis. Int J Surg. 2016;32:10–8.
33. Maurer SG, Chen AL, Hiebert R, Pereira GC, Di CP. Comparison of outcomes of using spinal versus general anesthesia in total hip arthroplasty. Am J Orthop (Belle Mead NJ). 2007;36(7):E101–6.
34. Basques BA, Toy JO, Bohl DD, Golinvaux NS, Grauer JN. General compared with spinal anesthesia for total hip arthroplasty. J Bone Joint Surg Am. 2015; 97(6):455–61.

6

Comparison of cortisol and inflammatory response between aged and middle-aged patients undergoing total hip arthroplasty

Jian Zhong, Hai-bo Si, Yi Zeng, Jing Yang, Zong-ke Zhou, Peng-de Kang, Fu-xing Pei and Bin Shen*

Abstract

Background: To investigate the differences in the perioperative serum cortisol, C-reactive protein (CRP) and interleukin-6 (IL-6) levels between aged and middle-aged patients undergoing total hip arthroplasty (THA).

Methods: Sixty patients (30 aged and 30 middle-aged) undergoing THA for osteoarthritis between August 2016 and January 2017 participated in this study. Blood samples were collected preoperatively and at 6 hours, 24 hours and 3 days after surgery to measure the cortisol, CRP and IL-6 concentrations. The clinical outcomes were assessed using the visual analogue scale (VAS) pain score and Harris hip score (HHS).

Results: No significant differences were found between the two groups before the operation in the cortisol, IL-6 and CRP levels; the VAS score; or the HHS. Cortisol was significantly lower at 6 hours after surgery in the aged group than in the middle-aged group ($P < 0.05$). IL-6 at 6 and 24 hours after surgery, CRP at 3 days after surgery and the VAS score at 6 and 24 hours after surgery in the aged group were significantly higher than those in the middle-aged group ($P < 0.05$). In the aged group, weak correlations were found between the cortisol concentration 6 hours after THA and the IL-6 level 24 hours after THA ($r = -0.37$, $P = 0.04$) and between the IL-6 level 6 hours after THA and the VAS score 24 hours after THA ($r = 0.42$, $P = 0.02$).

Conclusion: Aged patients showed lower cortisol levels at 6 hours after surgery and higher IL-6 levels at 6 and 24 hours after surgery than middle-aged patients undergoing THA.

Keywords: Arthroplasty, Hip, Cortisol, Aged, Middle aged

Background

Life expectancy has been prolonged considerably due to improved healthcare. The prevalence of osteoarthritis (OA) is almost 70% in women and 60% in men over the age of 65 years, and most people who suffer from OA display radiographic evidence and/or clinical symptoms [1, 2]. Total hip arthroplasty (THA) is an effective method to ease pain and improve the quality of life for people who suffer from serious pain and disability caused by OA [3–6].

However, surgeries can trigger stress responses, including a series of immunological, metabolic and hormonal changes [7–10]. As one crucial constituent of the stress response, cortisol secretion is inevitably increased after surgery [11, 12]. Human ageing causes homeostasis disturbances in all systems, with a progressive loss of structural and physiological integrity and function [13]. In particular, impairment of the suprachiasmatic nucleus, which affects the limbic region, hippocampus and hypothalamus, leads to adrenocortical secretion management disorders in aged people [14, 15].

Although several studies have compared cortisol levels between aged and middle-aged patients undergoing other operations, the conclusions have been inconsistent [16–19]. To the best of our knowledge, no study in the major English language medical databases has reported the cortisol levels of aged and middle-aged patients

* Correspondence: shenbin_1971@163.com
Department of orthopaedics, West China Hospital, Sichuan University, Chengdu 610041, People's Republic of China

undergoing THA. We performed this study to investigate differences in cortisol levels between aged and middle-aged patients undergoing THA and the relationship between endogenous cortisol and the inflammatory response after the operation. We hypothesized that aged patients undergoing THA would show a higher level of cortisol and lower interleukin-6 (IL-6) and C-reactive protein (CRP) levels postoperatively than middle-aged patients due to the anti-inflammatory effect of endogenous cortisol production.

Method

Patients

Patients aged over 40 years and scheduled for primary unilateral uncemented THA for OA between August 2016 and January 2017 were screened in this prospective, non-randomized, observational study. The exclusion criteria were as follows: senile dementia, steroid use within the past 6 months, chronic malnutrition, smoking, alcoholism, drug abuse, rheumatoid arthritis, hypertension, diabetes mellitus and other systemic diseases that would influence the neuroendocrine and inflammatory responses. The administration of non-steroidal anti-inflammatory drugs (NSAIDs) was suspended four weeks before the operation. Of the 68 eligible patients, 7 patients refused to participate, and 1 patient withdrew from this study. Finally, 60 patients were included in the study. The patients were divided into an aged group (over 65 years) and a middle-aged group (40–65 years). This study was conducted in accordance with the Declaration of Helsinki and approved by the local Ethics Committee. All patients gave informed consent prior to their inclusion in the study.

Surgical procedure

All surgeries were performed by one single experienced surgeon (B.S.). Generally, 1.5 g of cefuroxime was given within 30 min before the beginning of surgery, and general anaesthesia was used in all cases. The same operative technique was used. Through the posterolateral approach, the acetabular component was placed at 20° anteversion and 45° abduction, the femoral component was fixed at 15° anteversion, the capsular flap and the short external rotators were repaired in all cases, and wound drainage was indwelled in every patient.

Perioperative management

Preadmission counselling was given by qualified nurses, and the preliminary assessment was conducted by a doctor. Clear oral fluids were administered up to 3 h before the operation to minimize preoperative fasting. No sedative was used before surgery. One hundred milligrams of ropivacaine (100 mg: 10 ml) was diluted with 30 ml of saline and subcutaneously injected around the wound as a local infiltration analgesia.

Forty milligrams of parecoxib was given by intramuscular injection at 6 h after surgery. A second dose of 40 mg of parecoxib was given at 8:00 a.m. on postoperative day (POD) 1, followed by oral celecoxib (200 mg) every 12 h. Ten milligrams of rivaroxaban was given orally 8 h after the operation and then administered at 24-h intervals on the subsequent days provided that no bleeding events occurred.

At 8:00 a.m. on POD 1, wound drainage and the monitor were removed, and unrestricted food intake was permitted. Daily functional training, including walking and muscle power exercises, was guided and supervised by a physiotherapist.

Outcome assessments

Venous blood samples were collected in the morning of the day before surgery from each patient as baseline. The primary outcome was the serum cortisol level. Blood samples to measure the cortisol, CRP and IL-6 levels were obtained at 6 h, 24 h and 3 days postoperatively. After removing cells and debris by centrifugation, the samples were stored at −80 °C prior to the analysis. All measurements were performed at the clinical key laboratory of West China Hospital, which was certificated by the College of American Pathologists (CAP). CRP was measured using the rate nephelometric assay on the IMMAGE®800 Access immunoassay system (Beckman Coulter Inc., Brea, CA, USA) and reported in milligrams per litre (mg/L). IL-6 and cortisol were measured with electrochemiluminescence immunoassays (ECLIs) on the modular analytics E170 module (Roche Diagnostics, Mannheim, Germany) and were presented in picograms per millilitre (pg/mL) and nanomole per litre (nmol/L), respectively.

Visual analogue scale (VAS) pain scores (rest pain) were marked on the day of hospitalization and 6 h, 24 h, 2 days, and 3 days after surgery by a mediatinus (no pain = 0, worst pain = 10). The Harris hip scores (HHS) were obtained at the time of hospital admission and 3 months postoperatively to evaluate the early recovery effect. Adverse events were recorded at each follow-up.

Statistical analysis

Data were collected using Excel. Continuous variables are presented as the means and standard deviations (M ± SD). Dichotomous data are presented as numbers for each category. To compare data between two groups, the normality of all quantitative data was tested with the Shapiro-Wilk test. For normally distributed data, Levene's test for equality of variances was used to test the homogeneity of variances of matching data from two groups, and the two independent samples t-test was adopted if the variances were homogenous; otherwise, a *t*-test was performed. For non-normally distributed and ranked data, a nonparametric test (Mann-Whitney rank-sum test) was conducted. For enumeration data, the Chi-square test was employed. Because some of our variables (cortisol before and 24 h after surgery in the middle-aged group, IL-6 at 6, 24 h and 3 days after surgery in the middle-aged group, and CRP before and at 6 h after surgery in both groups) were not normally distributed, analysis of variance (ANOVA) of repeated measurement data was not used. Pearson's correlation coefficient and Spearman's rank correlation coefficient were calculated for variables with normal and non-normal distributions, respectively, within each group to analyse their possible correlations. The analyses were performed using the SPSS statistical software (Version 13.0, SPSS Inc., Chicago, IL, USA). For all comparisons, a P value <0.05 was considered significant.

Results

The patient screening and processing steps are illustrated in Fig. 1.

Patient demographics and operative information

The two groups were well matched for gender, height, weight, BMI, and operating time (Table 1).

Serial changes of cortisol

The mean preoperative cortisol levels did not significantly differ between the two groups. Six hours after surgery, serum cortisol increased from 314.84 ± 89.65 nmol/L and 291.93 ± 111 nmol/L at baseline to 701.85 ±

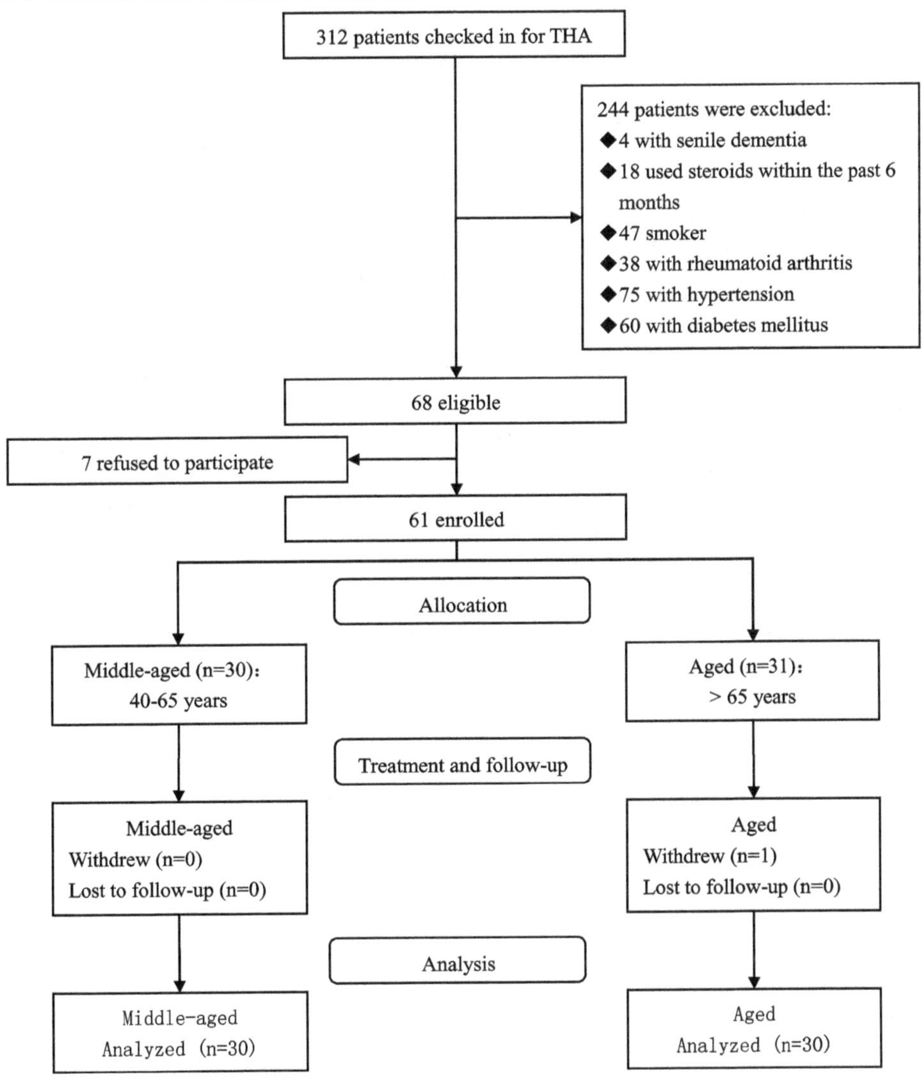

Fig. 1 The chart of patient flow in the study

Table 1 Demographic and operative information

Parameters	Middle-aged	Aged	$Z/\chi^2/t$	*P*
Age(yrs)	53.93 ± 7.40	71.80 ± 5.85	Z = −6.658	<0.001
Gender(M/F)	11/19	13/17	$\chi^2 = 2.411$	0.121
Height(cm)	167.77 ± 11.63	163.30 ± 9.10	*t* = 1.657	0.103
Weight(kg)	66.33 ± 11.88	65.67 ± 11.70	*t* = 0.219	0.827
BMI	23.44 ± 2.46	24.44 ± 2.62	*t* = −1.525	0.133
Operative time(min)	64.87 ± 10.10	63.77 ± 11.33	*t* = 0.397	0.693

156.32 nmol/L and 807.12 ± 161.34 nmol/L in the aged and middle-aged groups, respectively. Then, the cortisol concentrations dropped to 550.99 ± 210.73 nmol/L and 607.7 ± 214.31 nmol/L, respectively, at 24 h after the operation, which were still much higher than the baseline concentrations. The concentrations were almost the same at POD 3 (562.63 ± 142.7 nmol/L in the aged group and 609 ± 153.53 nmol/L in the middle-aged group) (Table 2). The preoperative serum cortisol concentrations and the cortisol levels at 24 and 72 h after surgery did not significantly differ between the two groups. However, serum cortisol was significantly lower six hours after the surgical procedure in the aged group than in the middle-aged group. Serum cortisol tended to be higher in the aged group preoperatively than in the middle-aged group; an opposite trend was seen postoperatively, although the differences were not significant except at 6 h after surgery (Fig. 2a).

Serum IL-6 levels

The IL-6 concentration was 3.54 ± 1.55 pg/ml for the aged group and 3.96 ± 1.59 pg/ml for the middle-aged group before surgery, both of which were within the normal range. These concentrations increased to 64.14 ± 16.43 pg/ml and 52.81 ± 29.16 pg/ml, respectively, 6 h after surgery and continued to rise until they peaked at 24 h after surgery (165.35 ± 50.50 pg/ml and 114.53 ± 56.78 pg/ml). At POD 3, these concentrations plummeted to lower but still above-normal levels (32.60 ± 13.42 pg/ml and 28.99 ± 15.01 pg/ml, respectively) (Table 2). In contrast to the changes in serum cortisol, serum IL-6 was lower before surgery and higher at 6, 24, and 3 days after surgery in the aged group than in the middle-aged group, but significant differences between the two groups were observed only at 6 and 24 h (Fig. 2b).

CRP concentration

The CRP levels were barely changed 6 h after THA compared with the preoperative measurements in both groups and fell within the normal range. The CRP concentration soared to 90.47 ± 22.44 mg/L (aged) and 81.56 ± 21.09 mg/L (middle-aged) 24 h after surgery and peaked at 119.40 ± 32.06 mg/L (aged) and 100.27 ± 25.34 mg/L (middle-aged) 3 days after the operation (Table 2). The aged group maintained higher blood CRP than the middle-aged group both before and after surgery, but the increments were subtle until 24 h after the operation in both groups. The difference became significant 3 days after surgery, at which time the blood CRP concentration was the highest within both groups. Additionally, the CRP concentration was virtually the same 6 h postoperatively and preoperatively (Fig. 2c).

VAS evaluation

The aged group scored 3.47 ± 1.46 in the preoperative VAS evaluation, whereas the middle-aged group scored 3.33 ± 1.32. Six hours after the operation, both groups experienced aggravated pain and scored 5.47 ± 1.11 and 4.87 ± 1.07, respectively. However, the scores in both groups decreased swiftly, with the aged group scoring

Table 2 Cortisol, IL-6 and CRP levels before and 6 h, 24 h and 3 days after THA

Parameters		Aged	Middle-aged	t/Z	*P*
Cortisol (nmol/L)	Preoperation	314.84 ± 89.65	291.93 ± 111.00	−1.38	0.17
	6 h	701.85 ± 156.32	807.12 ± 161.34	2.57	0.01
	24 h	550.99 ± 210.73	607.70 ± 214.31	−0.72	0.47
	POD3	562.63 ± 142.70	609.00 ± 153.53	1.21	0.23
IL-6 (pg/ml)	Preoperation	3.54 ± 1.55	3.96 ± 1.59	1.05	0.30
	6 h	64.14 ± 16.43	52.81 ± 29.16	−2.48	0.01
	24 h	165.35 ± 50.50	114.53 ± 56.78	−3.47	<0.01
	POD3	32.60 ± 13.42	28.99 ± 15.01	−1.21	0.23
CRP (mg/L)	Preoperation	3.35 ± 1.88	2.87 ± 1.27	−0.61	0.54
	6 h	3.70 ± 2.27	3.14 ± 1.88	−0.98	0.33
	24 h	90.47 ± 22.44	81.56 ± 21.09	−1.59	0.12
	POD3	119.40 ± 32.06	100.27 ± 25.34	−2.56	0.01

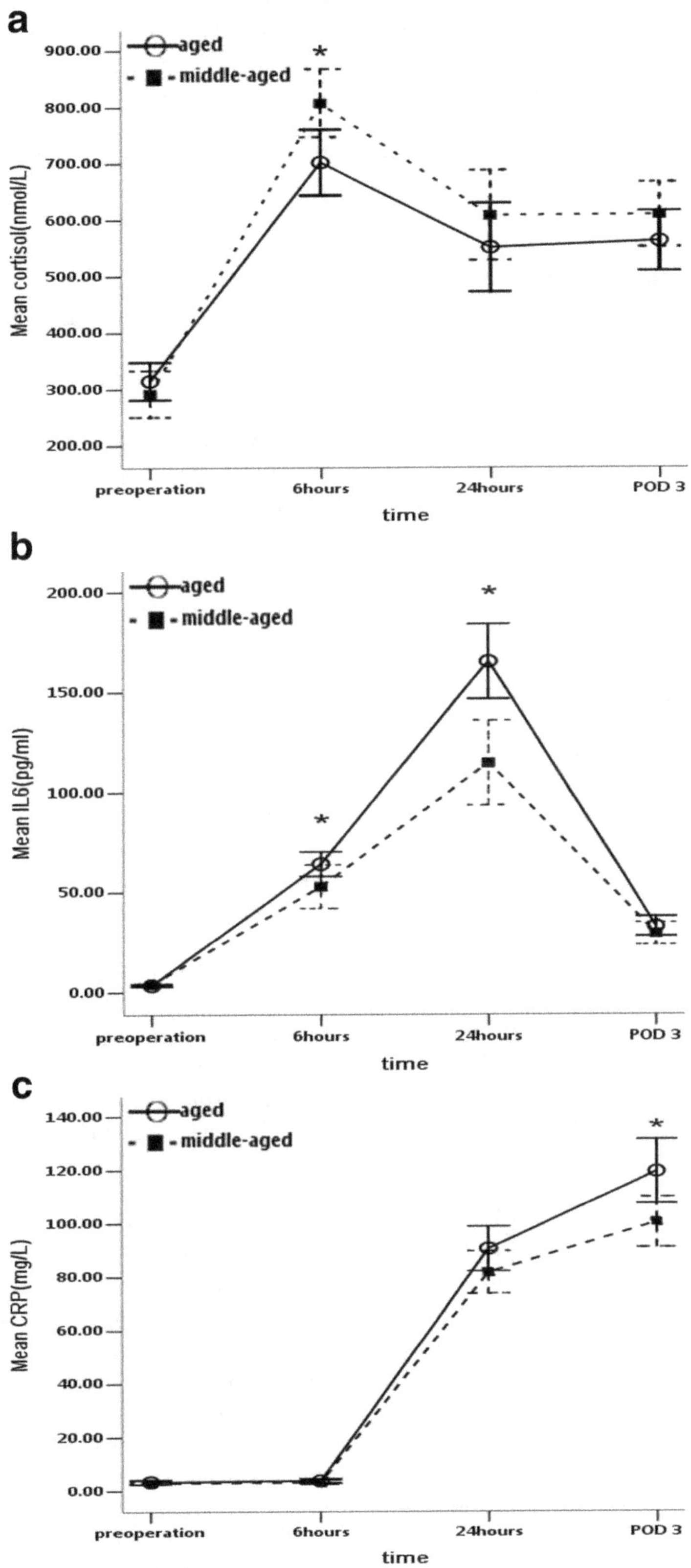

Fig. 2 The stress response (cortisol, **a**) and inflammatory response (IL-6 and CRP, **b** and **c**) of middle-aged and aged patients preoperatively and at 6 h, 24 h and 3 days after THA. Asterisk (*****) means the difference between the two groups reached statistical significance ($P < 0.05$)

slightly higher than their preoperative evaluation score (3.73 ± 0.98) and the middle-aged group scoring slightly lower than their preoperative rating (3.20 ± 1.19) 24 h after surgery. Then, the VAS scores in both groups fell to lower levels than their preoperative counterparts. The aged group felt more severe pain both before and after surgery than the middle-aged group, although significant differences were only shown at 6 and 24 h postoperatively, which was in accordance with the higher IL-6 levels in the aged group (Fig. 3a).

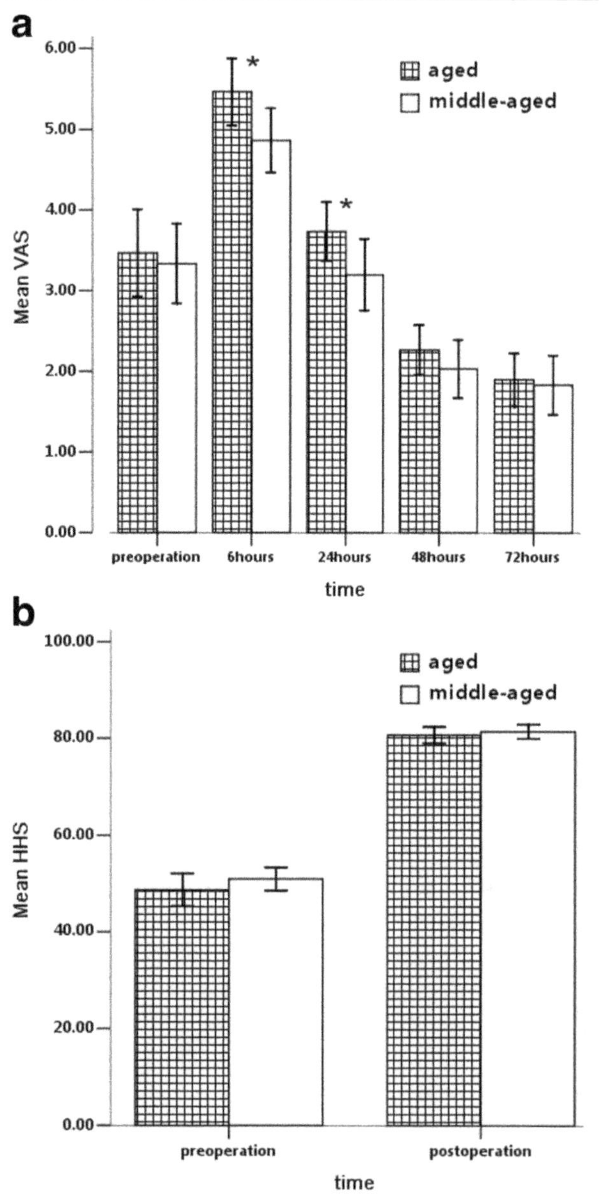

Fig. 3 a The pain assessment (VAS) of middle-aged and aged patients preoperatively and at 6, 24, 48 and 72 h after THA. **b** The function assessment (HHS) of middle-aged and aged patients preoperatively and at 3 months after THA. *: $P < 0.05$ comparing the two age groups

HHS evaluation

The middle-aged and aged groups scored 50.93 ± 6.40 and 48.67 ± 9.11, respectively, before THA and then 81.37 ± 3.94 and 80.67 ± 4.44, respectively, after THA. Both groups showed evident improvement in the hip function assessment after THA, but no significant differences between the two groups were shown before or after THA (Fig. 3b).

Possible correlations

The correlation analysis demonstrated only a possible weak correlation ($r = -0.37$, $P = 0.04$, Fig. 4a) between the cortisol concentration at 6 h and the IL-6 level at 24 h after THA in the aged group. A similar weak correlation ($r = 0.42$, $P = 0.02$, Fig. 4b) was detected between the IL-6 level at 6 h and the VAS score at 24 h after THA in the aged group. These correlations were not seen in the middle-aged group. Instead, the CRP concentration at 6 h after THA was weakly correlated with the VAS score at 24 h after THA in the middle-aged group ($r = 0.39$, $P = 0.04$, Fig. 4c). The rest of the data (including the cortisol, IL-6 and CRP levels; the VAS score at time points other than the aforementioned; and the HHS in both groups) were not correlated with each other.

Discussion

To the best of our knowledge, no study in the major English language medical databases has reported differences in cortisol secretion and inflammatory responses between aged and middle-aged patients receiving THA. In this prospective observational study, we aimed to investigate the differences in the serum cortisol, IL-6 and CRP levels between aged and middle-aged patients.

This present study found that aged patients undergoing THA showed lower serum cortisol and higher IL-6 and CRP levels and more serious pain after surgery than the middle-aged patients. However, the differences between the two groups did not influence the HHS score 3 months postoperatively. The reasons for these results may be as follows. First, ageing is an inevitable physiological process that is accompanied by hypofunction of multiple body systems [13] and is related to musculoskeletal and arthritic disorders [20]. As a result, aged people often suffer suprachiasmatic nucleus impairment, which affects the hippocampus and weakens its ability to modulate the adrenocortical circadian rhythmicity [21] and stress response [22], possibly resulting in decreased circadian fluctuation of cortisol secretion [23] and a smaller increment of the serum cortisol concentration in aged people after THA. Second, IL-6 and CRP have been broadly used as markers of the inflammatory response after operations [24]. Because CRP and IL-6 are both related to the seriousness of tissue trauma, they are also

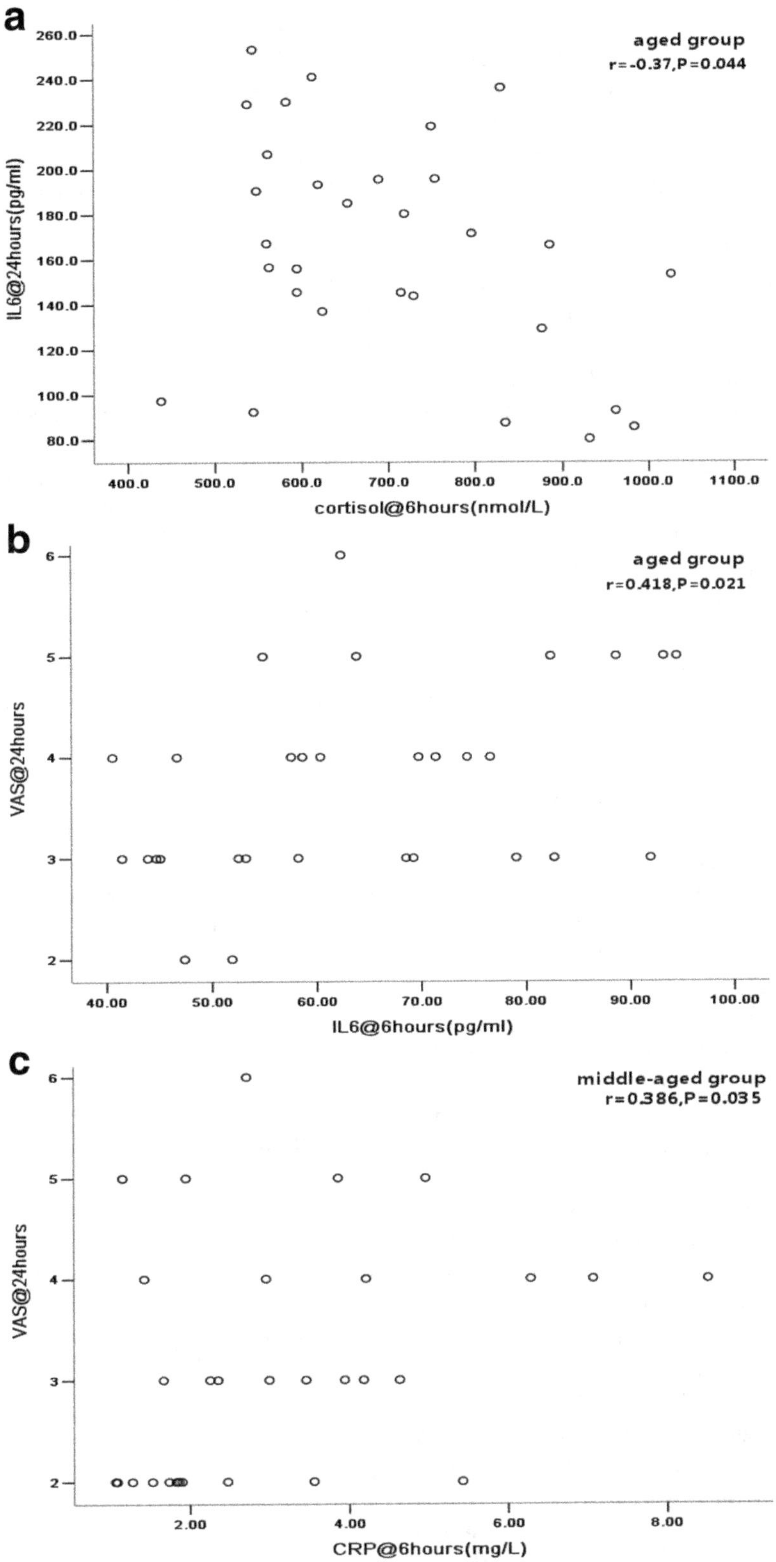

Fig. 4 **a** Correlation between cortisol at 6 h after THA and IL-6 at 24 h after THA in the aged group. **b** Correlation between IL-6 at 6 h after THA and VAS at 24 h after THA in the aged group. **c** Correlation between CRP at 6 h after THA and VAS at 24 h after THA in the middle-aged group

recognized as biomarkers of the extent of surgery [25]. As a major orthopaedic surgery, THA will trigger significant increases in the serum IL-6 and CRP concentrations, which is consistent with the results of our study. The aged group exhibited a stronger inflammatory response, suggesting that aged patients experienced a greater stress response. Hall GM et al. [26] reported that a lower IL-6 concentration more rapidly and exactly predicted the ability to walk 10 m and 25 m, whereas a lower CRP concentration was correlated with less pain at the time of discharge. Moreover, regardless of the nature of pain, all pain originates from inflammatory responses [27]. Thus, it is beneficial for the rehabilitation of aged patients to have a weaker inflammatory response. Third, the postoperative functional outcome of patients undergoing THA is affected by multiple factors and not only by endogenous or exogenous corticosteroids.

IL-6 and CRP are makers of inflammation, and inflammation triggers pain. Cortisol has anti-inflammatory effects; therefore, higher cortisol levels should suggest stronger anti-inflammatory efficacy and be directly correlated with lower IL-6 and CRP levels and indirectly correlated with the VAS score, at least in theory. However, in our study, only very weak correlations were found. These weak correlations could be coincidental correlations in our data. The small sample size may partially account for this unsatisfying result. There were several outliers in our data that could have weakened our results. Moreover, the use of NSAIDS for pain management could have inhibited the inflammatory response to a certain extent, thereby rendering the correlation weak or even non-significant.

Due to their potent effects on the inflammatory and immune responses, glucocorticoids have been broadly used to relieve the stress response caused by surgery [28]. In a prospective study comparing 40 patients undergoing elective total knee arthroplasty for OA, injection of a small dose of dexamethasone into the periarticular soft tissues significantly decreased the CRP concentration on the third postoperative day and IL-6 in the drainage fluid 24 h after the operation [29]. Peter et al. [30] found that the perioperative administration of corticosteroids significantly decreased serum IL-6 at 6 and 24 h after surgery. Additionally, glucocorticoids improved postoperative nausea and pain and shortened the length of hospitalization [29, 31]. In our study, the aged patients showed lower endogenous cortisol after surgery but suffered more severe pain at 6 h postoperatively, implying that endogenous cortisol could not relieve the stress response and that exogenous corticosteroid should be used to improve the postoperative outcome. Unfortunately, corticosteroid is also associated with adverse events, such as hyperglycaemia, poor wound healing, deep infection and delayed bone healing [32–36]. A meta-analysis by Toner AJ et al. confirmed that perioperative administration of glucocorticoids increased the blood glucose concentration [33]. In addition, even a single surge of perioperative blood glucose is directly related to infectious and non-infectious complications [34]. In animal models, glucocorticoids significantly impaired bone healing and reduced bone turnover [35, 36]. Although whether the perioperative use of corticosteroid produces adverse effects, such as impaired wound healing and deep infection, is controversial, some studies have suggested that low-dose and short-term administrations of corticosteroid should lessen these concerns [29–31, 37–40]. Glucocorticoid can relieve the stress response and alleviate postoperative pain but does not improve the functional outcome [38]. In the present study, there was no differences in the HHS between the two groups, implying that the postoperative functional outcome of patients undergoing THA was affected by multi-factors and not only by endogenous or exogenous corticosteroid.

Several limitations should be mentioned. The number of patients recruited in our study was small, and larger samples may be needed to reveal differences between some of the variables. Celecoxib and parecoxib were administered to the patients, which suppressed the inflammatory response and affected the serum IL-6 and CRP levels. The HHS may not have been sensitive enough to reflect minute differences in the surgical outcome and patient satisfaction between the two groups. Two other limitations of our study are the short observational time and the lack of standardized follow-up methodology. To confirm and validate the results of our study, studies with a large sample size and multi-centre randomized controlled trials are needed.

Conclusion

Aged patients undergoing THA exhibited a lower level of endogenous cortisol production at 6 h postoperatively and a more severe inflammatory response (IL-6 at 6 and 24 h and CRP at 3 days after surgery) and postoperative pain (VAS at 6 and 24 h after surgery). Further studies of perioperative glucocorticoid usage in aged patients should be conducted to demonstrate the benefits and possible side effects.

Abbreviations

CRP: C-reactive protein; HHS: Harris hip score; IL-6: interleukin-6.; NSAIDs: Non-steroidal anti-inflammatory drugs; OA: osteoarthritis; POD: Postoperative day; THA: Total hip arthroplasty; VAS: Visual analog scale

Acknowledgments

We thank all the patients for participation in our study, and we are grateful to the staff of our department for their support and contribution in this study.

Funding
No commercial, public, or nonprofit organizations financially supported this research.

Authors' contributions
JZ, BS designed this study. JZ and HS were responsible for gathering, analyzing and interpreting data, and writing the manuscript. JY and ZZ made contributions to revising the manuscript for crucial intellectual content. FP, YZ, and PK have contributed in the revision of the manuscript and interpretation of data. The final version of the text has been reviewed and approved by all authors.

Consent for publication
Not Applicable

Competing interests
The authors announce that they do not have any competing interests.

References

1. Goldring MB, Goldring SR. Osteoarthritis. J Cell Physiol. 2007;213:626–34.
2. Sarzi-Puttini P, Cimmino MA, Scarpa R, Caporali R, Parazzini F, Zaninelli A, Atzeni F, Canesi B. Osteoarthritis: an overview of the disease and its treatment strategies. Semin Arthritis Rheum. 2005;35:1–10.
3. Cremeans-Smith JK, Boarts JM, Greene K, Delahanty DL. Patients' reasons for electing to undergo total knee arthroplasty impact post-operative pain severity and range of motion. J Behav Med. 2009;32:223_33.
4. Fujita K, Makimoto K, Hotokebuchi T. Qualitative study of osteoarthritis patients' experience before and after total hip arthroplasty in Japan. Nurs Health Sci. 2006;8:81–7.
5. Hudak PL, Clark JP, Hawker GA, Coyte PC, Mahomed NN, Kreder HJ, Wright JG. "You're perfect for the procedure! Why don't you want it?" elderly arthritis patients' unwillingness to consider total joint arthroplasty surgery: a qualitative study. Med Decis Mak. 2002;22:272–8.
6. Toye FM, Barlow J, Wright C, Lamb SE. Personal meanings in the construction of need for total knee replacement surgery. SocSci Med. 2006;63:43–53.
7. Weissman C. The metabolic response to stress: an overview and update. Anesthesiology. 1990;73:308–27.
8. Cruickshank AM, Fraser WD, Burns HJ, Van Damme J, Shenkin A. Response of serum interleukin-6 in patients undergoing elective surgery of varying severity. ClinSci (Lond). 1990;79:161_5.
9. Wilmore DW, Long JM, Mason AD, Jr. Pruitt BA: Stress in surgical patients as a neurophysiologic reflex response. Surg Gynecol Obstet 1976, 142:257–269.
10. Chernow B, Alexander HR, Smallridge RC, Thompson WR, Cook D, Beardsley D, Fink MP, Lake CR, Fletcher JR. Hormonal responses to graded surgical stress. Arch Intern Med. 1987;147:1273–8.
11. Kellner M, Yassouridis A, Manz B, Steiger A, Holsboer F, Wiedemann K. Corticotropin-releasing hormone inhibits melatonin secretion in healthy volunteers–a potential link to low-melatonin syndrome in depression? Neuroendocrinology. 1997;65:284–90.
12. Desborough JP. The stress response to trauma and surgery. Br J Anaesth. 2000;85:109–17.
13. Lopez-Otin C, Blasco MA, Partridge L, Serrano M, Kroemer G. The hallmarks of aging. Cell. 2013;153:1194–217.
14. Ball MJ. Neuronal loss, neurofibrillary tangles and granulovacuolar degeneration in the hippocampus with ageing and dementia. A quantitative study. ActaNeuropathol. 1977;37:111–8.
15. Mani RB, Lohr JB, Jeste DV. Hippocampal pyramidal cells and aging in the human: a quantitative study of neuronal loss in sectors CA1 to CA4. Exp Neurol. 1986;94:29–40.
16. Langer P, Balazova E, Vician M, Martino E, Jezova D, Michalikova S, Moravec R. Acute development of low T3 syndrome and changes in pituitary-adrenocortical function after elective cholecystectomy in women: some differences between young and elderly patients. Scand J Clin Lab Invest. 1992;52:215–20.
17. Oyama T, Taniguchi K, Takazawa T, Matsuki A, Kudo M. Effect of anaesthesia and surgery on endocrine function in elderly patients. Canadian Anaesthetists' Society journal. 1980;27:556–9.
18. Arnetz BB. Endocrine reactions during standardized surgical stress: the effects of age and methods of anaesthesia. Age Ageing. 1985;14:96–101.
19. Blichert-Toft M, Christensen V, Engquist A, Fog-Moller F, Kehlet H, Madsen SN, Skovsted L, Thode J, Olgaard K. Influence of age on the endocrine-metabolic response to surgery. Ann Surg. 1979;190:761–70.
20. Mobasheri A, Matta C, Zakany R, Musumeci G. Chondrosenescence: definition, hallmarks and potential role in the pathogenesis of osteoarthritis. Maturitas. 2015;80:237–44.
21. Moberg GP, Scapagnini U, de Groot J, Ganong WF. Effect of sectioning the fornix on diurnal fluctuation in plasma corticosterone levels in the rats. Neuroendocrinology. 1971;7:11–5.
22. Conforti N, Feldman S. Effects of dorsal fornix section and hippocampectomy on adrenocortical responses to sensory stimulation in the rat. Neuroendocrinology. 1976;22:1–7.
23. Ferrari E, Cravello L, Muzzoni B, Casarotti D, Paltro M, Solerte SB, Fioravanti M, Cuzzoni G, Pontiggia B, Magri F. Age-related changes of the hypothalamic-pituitary-adrenal axis: pathophysiological correlates. Eur J Endocrinol. 2001;144: 319–29.
24. Ohzato H, Yoshizaki K, Nishimoto N, Ogata A, Tagoh H, Monden M, Gotoh M, Kishimoto T, Mori T. Interleukin-6 as a new indicator of inflammatory status: detection of serum levels of interleukin-6 and C-reactive protein after surgery. Surgery. 1992;111:201–9.
25. Demura S, Takahashi K, Kawahara N, Watanabe Y, Tomita K. Serum interleukin-6 response after spinal surgery: estimation of surgical magnitude. J Orthop Sci. 2006;11:241–7.
26. Hall GM, Peerbhoy D, Shenkin A, Parker CJ, Salmon P. Relationship of the functional recovery after hip arthroplasty to the neuroendocrine and inflammatory responses. Br J Anaesth. 2001;87:537–42.
27. Omoigui S. The biochemical origin of pain–proposing a new law of pain: the origin of all pain is inflammation and the inflammatory response. Part 1 of 3–a unifying law of pain. Med Hypotheses. 2007;69:70–82.
28. Holte K, Kehlet H. Perioperative single-dose glucocorticoid administration: pathophysiologic effects and clinical implications. J Am Coll Surg. 2002;195: 694–712.
29. Ikeuchi M, Kamimoto Y, Izumi M, Fukunaga K, Aso K, Sugimura N, Yokoyama M, Tani T. Effects of dexamethasone on local infiltration analgesia in total knee arthroplasty: a randomized controlled trial. Knee Surg Sports Traumatol Arthrosc. 2014;22:1638–43.
30. Sculco PK, McLawhorn AS, Desai N, EP S, Padgett DE, Jules-Elysee K. The effect of perioperative corticosteroids in Total hip arthroplasty: a prospective double-blind placebo controlled pilot study. J Arthroplast. 2016;31:1208–12.
31. Backes JR, Bentley JC, Politi JR, Chambers BT. Dexamethasone reduces length of hospitalization and improves postoperative pain and nausea after total joint arthroplasty: a prospective, randomized controlled trial. J Arthroplast. 2013;28:11–7.
32. Percival VG, Riddell J, Corcoran TB. Single dose dexamethasone for postoperative nausea and vomiting–a matched case-control study of postoperative infection risk. Anaesth Intensive Care. 2010;38:661–6.
33. Toner AJ, Ganeshanathan V, Chan MT, Ho KM, Corcoran TB. Safety of perioperative glucocorticoids in elective noncardiac surgery: a systematic review and meta-analysis. Anesthesiology. 2017;126:234–48.
34. Kiran RP, Turina M, Hammel J, Fazio V: The clinical significance of an elevated postoperative glucose value in nondiabetic patients after colorectal surgery: evidence for the need for tight glucose control? Ann Surg 2013, 258:599–604, 604-605.
35. Bissinger O, Kreutzer K, Gotz C, Hapfelmeier A, Pautke C, Vogt S, Wexel G, Wolff KD, Tischer T, Prodinger PM. A biomechanical, micro-computertomographic and histological analysis of the influence of diclofenac and prednisolone on fracture healing in vivo. BMC Musculoskelet Disord. 2016;17:383.
36. JH F, Bashutski JD, Al-Hezaimi K, Wang HL. Statins, glucocorticoids, and nonsteroidal anti-inflammatory drugs: their influence on implant healing. Implant Dent. 2012;21:362–7.
37. Salerno A, Hermann R. Efficacy and safety of steroid use for postoperative pain relief. Update and review of the medical literature. J Bone Joint Surg Am. 2006;88:1361–72.
38. Bergeron SG, Kardash KJ, Huk OL, Zukor DJ, Antoniou J. Perioperative dexamethasone does not affect functional outcome in total hip arthroplasty. ClinOrthopRelat Res. 2009;467:1463–7.

7

Relative survival following hemi- and total hip arthroplasty for hip fractures in Sweden

Szilard Nemes[1,2†], Dennis Lind[1,3*†], Peter Cnudde[1,2,4], Erik Bülow[1,2], Ola Rolfson[1,2] and Cecilia Rogmark[1,3]

Abstract

Background: Hip fractures are a common problem in the ageing population. Hip arthroplasty is the common treatment option for displaced intracapsular neck of femur fractures. Even though hip replacements are successful in restoring mobility, reducing pain and diminishing loss of health-related quality of life, the potential impact of a hip fracture on life expectancy as well as the postoperative mortality need consideration. The purpose of this study was to describe the mid-term relative survival rate for a cohort of Swedish patients whom underwent total- or hemiarthroplasty surgery following hip fracture. We also explored whether the survival rate is prosthesis-type specific and influenced by comorbidities, sex, socioeconomic and surgical factors.

Methods: Using prospectively collected information of the *Swedish Hip Arthroplasty Register*-linked database we identified 43,891 patients operated between 2005 and 2012. Patient- and surgery-specific data in combination with socio-economic data were available for this analysis. We studied relative survival rate and used multivariable modelling with Cox Proportional Hazards Model in Transformed Time.

Results: Compared to the Swedish general population the baseline excess hazard was very high in the first half year after the operation, thereafter the excess hazard decreased but remained non-negligible through the 8 years' follow-up period. The mortality rate of males was higher compared to women. Higher Elixhauser comorbidity index (ECI) was associated with worsening survival. However, patients who had ECI = 0 had higher mortality than patients with ECI =1 the first 420 days post fracture. Patients with a hemiarthroplasty had a worse survival than patients with a total hip arthroplasty. Of the hospital types considered university hospitals had lower survival rate. Younger patients had a greater loss of expected life span than patients who suffer hip fracture in their more advanced ages.

Conclusions: Swedish hip fracture patients who undergo arthroplasty surgery had a high excess hazard of dying in the first half year following surgery, and this excess hazard never subsided to negligible levels at least up to 8 years after surgery. Interestingly having no prior record of illnesses worsened the initial mortality. Men living alone had the highest long-term excess mortality.

Keywords: Hip fracture, Excess mortality, Relative survival, Hip arthroplasty

Background

From the onset of age 60 the residual life time risk for hip fracture for men and women is estimated to be around 5 and 10%, respectively [1]. The number of hip fractures are bound to increase as the population becomes older [2]. It is well-known that hip fracture patients have a high risk of dying, but the literature is not concordant on how large the excess mortality is, compared to the general population of the same age, on how long time the excess risk prevails or if there are differences between the sexes [3, 4]. In recent years, there has been an improvement in the immediate care of the hip fracture patient, with shorter time to surgery and mobilisation within the first postoperative day. There is however conflicting evidence as to whether this actually has led to reduced mortality. Pedersen et al. [5] found a significant decrease in 1-year mortality the last 35 years, whereas other studies on temporal trends did not [6, 7].

* Correspondence: dennis.lind@med.lu.se
†Szilard Nemes and Dennis Lind contributed equally to this work.
1Swedish Hip Arthroplasty Register, Centre of Registers Västra Götaland, Gothenburg, Sweden
3Department of Orthopedics, Lund University, Skane University Hospital, Malmö, Sweden
Full list of author information is available at the end of the article

The Swedish Hip Arthroplasty Registry (SHAR) provides a unique opportunity to study mortality on a large group of patients. Hip arthroplasty is considered the main treatment option for displaced femoral neck fractures for patients aged over 60 [8].

In this study, we aimed to identify the patients with the highest risk of dying after their fracture-related arthroplasty and to study the mortality, stratified by different patient, hospital and socioeconomic factors. Whilst previous studies have used the term absolute survival to study the increased risk, we intended to use techniques of relative survival analysis in an attempt to estimate and quantify the excess hazard introduced to our patients compared to the general population. We also studied if this excess hazard would either disappear in time, remain or continue to put the patient at higher risk of dying for several years after surgery.

Methods

Patients and methods

Since 2005 the SHAR registers hip fracture patients whom undergo both total and (or) hemiarthroplasty. We identified all patients operated between 2005 and 2012, and this patient group served as our study group. If a patient had sustained bilateral hip operations due to fractures, we only considered the first operation (Fig. 1). To adjust for confounding, accessible and relevant variables were collected from three registers. SHAR provided data about the patients' age at operation, sex, prosthesis type (hemiarthroplasty or total hip arthroplasty), and hospital type (rural, county, university or private). The SHAR is a Swedish quality register and has a high completeness (98%) and full coverage (100%) [8]. Date of death is continuously updated in SHAR. The risk of leakage out of the register was considered, however only a handful of patients are known to have asked for their data to be removed [9]. Emigration rate in this group of frail elderly Swedes can be considered very low, and similar to the general population of the same age. Those few patients who emigrated were censored as they were dead [9]. Using the Swedish unique 10 digit personal identity number we linked the data from SHAR to Statistics Sweden and the National Patient Register (NPR) (National Board of Health and Welfare) [10]. Statistics Sweden provided data about the patients' education and civil status, while the NPR delivered data about the patients' health status encoded as ICD-10 codes. Swedish hospitals are obliged by law to report all primary and secondary ICD-10-codes to the NPR for every contact with the hospital. Only individual with entries in all three registers were included. Individual ICD-10-codes were combined into Elixhauser comorbidity indices (ECI) for each patient [11, 12]. The ECI is an unweighted comorbidity index representing the number of present comorbidities out of 31 possible. The ICD-10-codes were identified from hospital based healthcare in the year before the index hospital admission. Patents without recorded visits were classified as patients without known comorbidity (i.e. Elixhauser = 0).

Statistical methods

We summarized continuous variables as means and standard deviations, categorical variables as counts and percentages. We used Student's t-test and $\chi 2$-test for group comparisons. In this paper we used relative survival analysis [13, 14] The measure of interest was cumulative relative survival function r(t). We estimated the cumulative relative survival function as $r(t) = \frac{S_O(t)}{S_P(t)}$.

Where $S_O(t)$ denotes the observed survival and $S_P(t)$ the population or expected survival at time t. We extracted the Swedish population or expected survival $S_P(t)$ from publicly available mortality tables tabulated for sex and age maintained by the Human Life-Table Database [15] and Human Mortality Data Base [16].

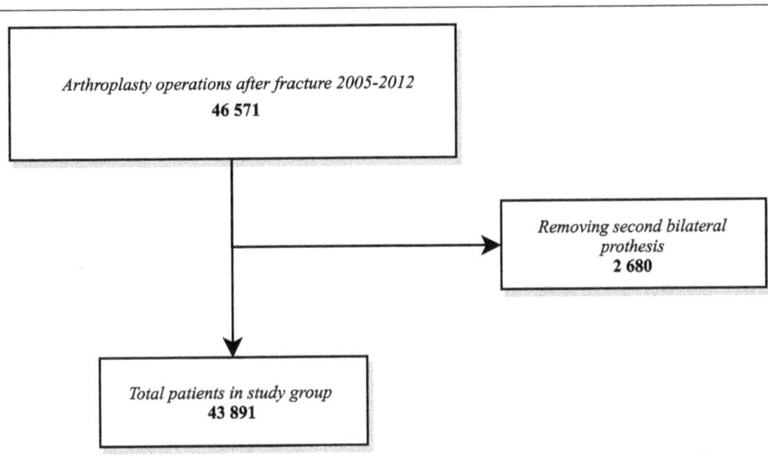

Fig. 1 Patient flowchart

The cumulative relative survival function r(t) can be any non-negative number. If r(t) = 1, then the observed survival of the studied group coincides with the expected or population survival. If r(t) > 1 then the observed survival of the studied group exceed the expected or population survival. If r(t) < 1 then the studied group experiences an excess mortality. We can partition the observed hazard for each individual $\lambda_O(t)$ into two additive components: $\lambda_O(t) = \lambda_P(t) + \lambda_E(t)$.

The age- and sex-specific baseline hazard is denoted by $\lambda_P(t)$. The difference between the baseline hazard and observed hazard, $\lambda_E(t)$ denotes the excess hazard of the study group.

Alongside with the cumulative relative survival, the excess hazard and the cumulative incidence curve served as the main methods of analysis. Additionally, we attempted to model the effect of clinical and patient related covariates with the help of multivariable Cox Proportional Hazards Model in Transformed Time [17]. We tested the assumption of proportionality with graphical examination and Brownian bridges [18]. We observed violation of the proportionality assumption for prosthesis type, age and ECI. We modelled these variables by the introduction of a step function that split the data in two epochs up to 14 months (420 days) and the subsequent period until end of study period. The multivariable regression analysis included interaction term between the aforementioned variables and the step function for time.

Results

In the SHAR a total of 43,891 patients with hip arthroplasty surgery due to hip fracture were identified between 2005 and 2012(Fig. 1.) There was a female predominance (70%) and the average age was 79 years for the survival group and 84 for the deceased group (Table 1).

As illustrated in Fig. 2 the baseline excess hazard of dying was elevated the first half year after the operation, thereafter the excess hazard decreased. However, it remained non-negligible trough the 8 years follow up period.

Table 1 Baseline demographic information for the study population stratified for survival status

	Alive	Dead	Total	*P*-value
Sample Size	22,575	21,316	43,891	
Sex: Female (%)	16,857 (74.7)	13,988 (65.6)	30,845	< 0.001
Age (mean & sd)	79.33 (9.17)	83.85 (7.77)		< 0.001
Hospital type (%)				< 0.001
University	5677 (25.1)	5916 (27.8)	11,593	
County	12,089 (53.6)	11,299 (53.0)	23,388	
Rural	3905 (17.3)	3351 (15.7)	7256	
Private	904 (4.0)	750 (3.5)	1654	
Prosthesis: Total hip arthoplasty (%)	7887 (34.9)	2690 (12.6)	10,577	< 0.001
Education (%)				< 0.001
Low	12,309 (54.5)	12,695 (59.6)	25,004	
Middle	6968 (30.9)	5740 (26.9)	12,708	
High	2793 (12.4)	1914 (9.0)	4707	
Missing	505 (2.2)	967 (4.5)	1472	
Civil status (%)				< 0.001
Couple	7971 (35.3)	6269 (29.4)	14,240	
Single	5489 (24.3)	4417 (20.7)	9906	
Widow	9071 (40.2)	10,620 (49.8)	19,691	
Missing	44 (0.2)	10 (0.0)	54	
Elixhauser index (mean & sd)	1.13 (1.35)	1.27 (1.53)		< 0.001
Elixhauser stratified (%)				< 0.001
0	9930 (44.0)	9534 (44.7)	19,464	
1	5448 (24.1)	4087 (19.2)	9535	
2	3754 (16.6)	3467 (16.3)	7221	
3+	3443 (15.3)	4228 (19.8)	7671	

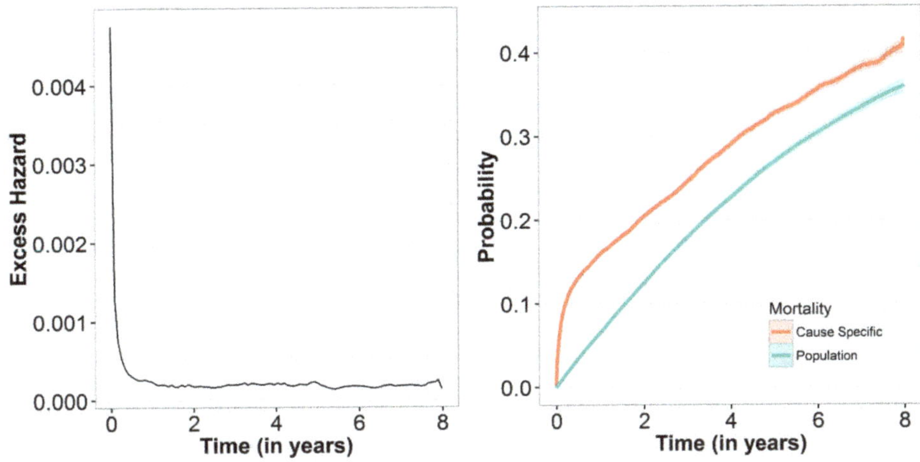

Fig. 2 Excess hazard and crude mortality curves for 43,891 Swedish hip fracture patients compared with the mortality rates of the Swedish general population

Age and sex

The mortality rate of males was higher, and both sexes had survival rates inferior than their peers from the general population (Fig. 3). Younger age, analysed as a continuous variable, led to an increased relative risk of dying, being more pronounced in the later period.

Elixhauser comorbidity index

In general, the higher the ECI the lower the survival was. But the group with a ECI of 1 had better survival during the first 420 days, compared with those with ECI of 0 (Fig. 3). Over time the negative effect of the increasing ECI on survival became more obvious.

Implant and hospital type

Patients with total hip arthroplasty had a better survival than patients with hemi-arthroplasty. Of the hospital types considered university hospitals had lower survival rate during the first 6 years, whilst patients operated at private, rural and county hospitals had similar survival rates. Over time, the impact of implant-type decreased (Fig. 3).

Socioeconomics

The separation of the survival rates for the different socioeconomic status was significant for education. Patients who completed higher levels of education had better survival that patients with low or middle education levels. (See Fig. 4) The later two categories had similar survival rates during the whole follow up period. Being married compared to being single and having higher achieved levels of education lowered the risk of death, however being a widow did not (Table 2). Multivariable relative survival regression corroborated most of the results of the univariate analysis.

Discussion

Main findings

Swedish hip fracture patients whom undergo hip arthroplasty had a high excess hazard of dying, up to 100 days after the operation compared with individuals in the general population of the same age and sex. This excess hazard diminished with time but never subsided to negligible levels. The mortality rate of hip fracture patients remained higher than the mortality rate of the general population during the whole 8 years' follow-up period.

Earlier papers have related the long-term mortality among hip fracture patients to the mortality rates in the general population [3, 4, 6, 19]. These studies highlighted an increased mortality among hip fracture patients compared with the general population using age and sex standardization. We used relative survival rate and multivariable modelling and could therefore relate every patient to the survival rate of members of the general population of the same age and sex.

The excess early mortality can possibly be explained by the comorbidities and frailty of hip fracture patients, aggravated by the injury and the surgery. The relationship between fracture and increased risk of death up to 8 years post-surgery, is more difficult to disentangle. Apart from the chronic disease status in this patient population, previous research has suggested that pain and fear of falling [20] is contributing to a decrease in activity and exercise and a decrease in walking distance [21], which in turn potentially contributes to a loss of independence and depression [22]. In order to improve outcomes following hip fracture surgery, it is imperative to identify modifiable factors that could possibly aid survival and function [23]. There have been promising results where an improved and close cooperation between orthopaedic surgeons and geriatricians have led to a reduction in mortality [24] aided by systematic and sustained quality improvement efforts [25, 26].

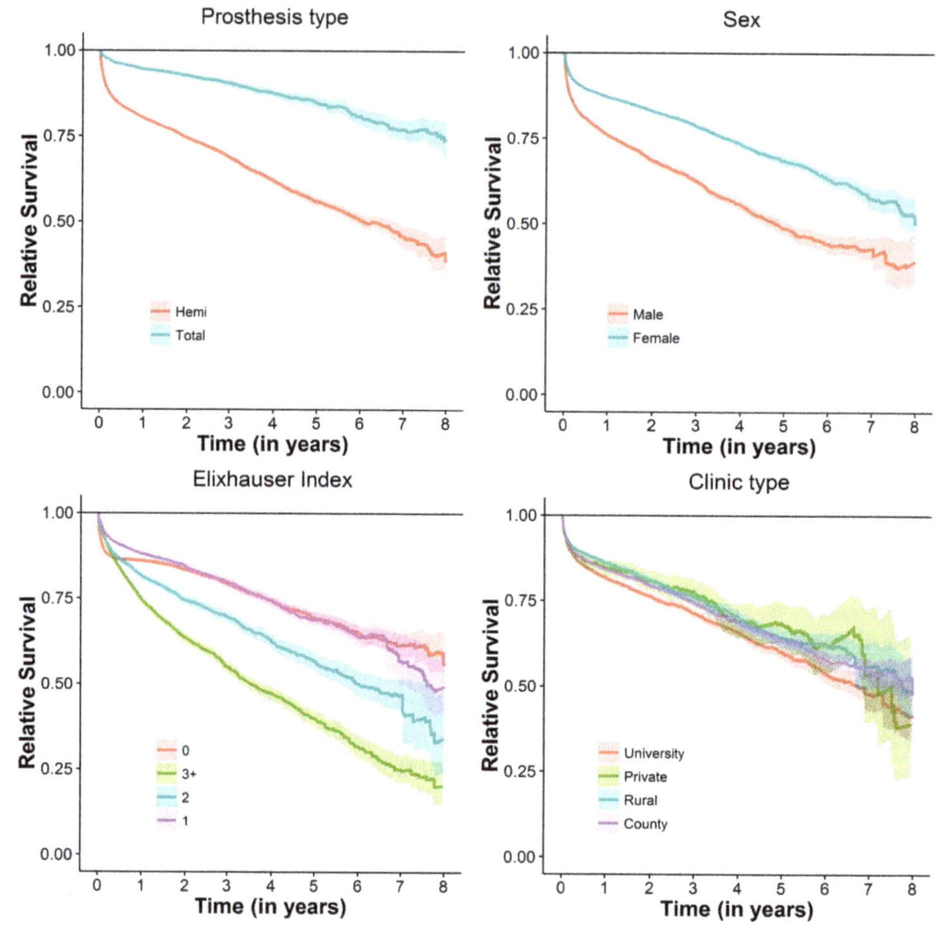

Fig. 3 Relative survival curves of 43,891 Swedish hip fracture patients stratified in patient and hospital related factors. If the survival curves deviates the horizontal reference line then the survival of the studied stratum differs significantly from the general population

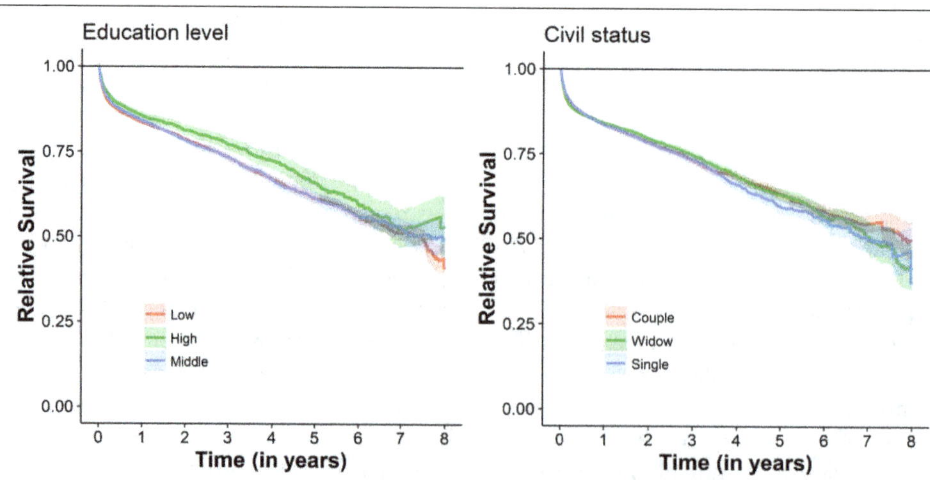

Fig. 4 Relative survival curves of 43,891 Swedish hip fracture patients stratified in Education level and Civil status. If the survival curves deviates the horizontal reference line then the survival of the studied stratum differs significantly form from the general population

Table 2 Multivariable relative survival regression analysis of survival of Swedish hip fracture patients

	HR	95% CI
Sex		
Female	*Ref*	
Male 0–420 days	2.48	2.37; 2.59
Male > 420 days	2.32	2.11; 2.55
Age		
0–420 days	0.94	0.94; 0.94
> 420 days	0.91	0.90; 0.92
Elixhauser 0–420 days		
0	*Ref*	
1	0.92	0.86; 0.97
2	1.23	1.16; 1.30
+3	1.47	1.39; 1.55
Elixhauser > 420 days		
0	*Ref*	
1	1.09	0.96; 1.24
2	1.30	1.15; 1.49
+3	1.75	1.55; 1.97
Year of operation		
0–420 days	1.00	0.99; 1.01
> 420 days	0.99	0.99; 1.01
Prosthesis		
Hemi	*Ref*	
Total 0–420 days	0.38	0.35; 0.41
Total > 420 days	0.54	0.46; 0.64
Hospital		
University	*Ref*	
County	0.95	0.92; 0.98
Rural	0.93	0.89; 0.97
Private	0.89	0.82; 0.95
Education		
Low	*Ref*	
Middle	0.99	0.96; 1.02
High	0.91	0.87; 0.95
Civil status		
Couple	*Ref*	
Single	1.08	1.03; 1.12
Widow	1.03	0.99; 1.06

Age

Advanced age is associated with an increase in mortality after hip fracture however, this may be due to the higher general mortality rates that comes with aging [27, 28], as we by relative survival analysis observed that age was positively associated with the relative survival. Patients who suffer a hip fracture in their younger years lost more of their expected life span than patients who had their fracture in more advanced age. This effect increased with the follow-up time. This finding suggests that especially in the younger hip fracture population, there could be a greater benefit of an improved collaboration between healthcare professionals within the hospital setting, general practitioners and the municipal social care.

Sex

The excess mortality of males was higher than for females. This was more evident in the beginning of the study period. Subsequently the excess sex-related differences in survival following hip fracture surgery follow a similar trends of the sex-related difference in survival of the general population. That men have a higher risk of dying after hip fracture is well known from the literature, and was shown also in an recent study [19]. It can be debated if this is induced by sex as an isolated variable, or if being male is a surrogate variable for comorbidity, unhealthy lifestyle or other confounders adding to their risk of both hip fracture and death.

Elixhauser comorbidity index

Generally patient comorbidity had a significant adverse effect on survival [28], even though moderate comorbidity may not be associated with an excess one-year-mortality [27–31]. The hazard rates increased with increased score of comorbidity, as measured by the ECI [32]. This effect became stronger with time. Interestingly, in the early period patients with ECI = 1 have higher survival rate than patients with ECI = 0, while after 420 days no such difference was seen. An attempted explanation could be that patients with known comorbidities are receiving increased medical attention prior to the surgery, improving their health status. The group of patients with an ECI = 0 may consist of two types of patients; really healthy individuals and those who are not, but never sought medical attention and as such have undiagnosed and/or untreated comorbidity. Assumingly, in the hip fracture population there are a number of patients neglecting their health. These patients may present with an unstable medical condition at the time of their hip fracture, and subsequently have a higher risk of dying. We believe our results could question the validity of comorbidity indices based on administrative patient registers. Besides sick individuals not being known to the healthcare, there is a possibility of misdiagnosis bias due to incorrect coding [33].

Hospital type

We found lower relative survival of patients treated at university hospitals. Similar results has been described in a Danish study [34], whilst a Canadian study found an improved survival in teaching hospitals compared to community hospitals [35]. Finally, a study from the USA concluded that hospital volume did not predict mortality, even though hospitals with high caseload had fewer complications [36]. Swedish university hospitals typically serve an urban population, so when comparing different hospitals, we also compare different populations. Based on the available evidence one could conclude that both hospital level and volume are blunt variables confounded by case-mix, level of competence of the staff and an unclear definition of what high volume is, making comparisons between different healthcare systems difficult.

Year of surgery

The year of surgery was not associated with any excess risk of mortality, indicating that during our study period the rate between hip fracture patients survival and the survival of the general population did not change. This finding is in agreement with the findings of Klop et al. [37]. In a systematic review on randomized clinical trials, Mundi et al. found similar mortality in hip fracture patients over time [6].

Implant type

Patients operated with total hip arthroplasty had lower mortality than those with hemi-arthroplasty. This is most probably a reflection of selection bias as choice of implant is based on patient frailty, age and activity level.

Socioeconomics

Solitary life style [38] and social deprivation [39] have been previously associated with increased mortality after hip fracture. In our study we found similar results, where being non-married brought on a slight increase in mortality. However, in our study being widowed had no adverse effect on mortality.

Strengths and limitations of the study

Other factors may influence mortality. Solbakken and collaborators [40] concluded that self-perceived health, smoking, and BMI predict mortality of hip fracture patients. Vosoughi and collaborators [41] reached similar conclusions regarding smoking and BMI and noted improved nutrition as modifiable factors. Hence, as our register data is limited in terms of such variables, our results could not be adjusted for those and might have to be interpreted with caution due to varying degree of validity [42].

The SHAR has an excellent completeness of over 98% [8], in combination with the large patient cohort are the main strengths of the present study. The additional access to socioeconomic and comorbidity data from governmental administrative registers further add to the strength [10]. Additionally, the use of relative survival analysis has an overarching advantage that, through a single measure, it indicates the degree to which a study sample corresponds to the general population with respect to health status and survival [43].

Perspective

Orthopaedic healthcare of today focuses on a timely and effective treatment of hip fracture patients. Post-operative care can also be of a fast-track nature, both reflecting new scientific knowledge and health economic challenges. Concerns have been raised whether a shorter length-of-stay is associated with an increase in mortality [44]. Our findings may assist the clinician to identify patients at risk of excess mortality. The patient without prior medical records or diagnoses can actually be more challenging than expected. A younger patient will suffer a risk of a greater expected life span loss than the more elderly patient and this should not be neglected. The same goes for singles and/or males. The hip fracture patient in general carries a highly increased risk of dying during several months after fracture, compared to the general population, and further closer follow-up care have to be provided after discharge from the hospital.

Conclusions

Hip fracture patients, in particular males, have a considerable excess hazard of dying compared with the general population. Younger patients have a greater loss of expected life span than patients who suffer hip fracture in their more advanced ages. Existing comorbidities, lower education and solitary life style all have an adverse effect on survival. The survival rates of hip fracture patients did not improve during a study period of 7 years.

Abbreviations

ECI: Elixhauser comorbidity index; SHAR: The Swedish Hip Arthroplasty Registry

Acknowledgements

The authors thank the coordinators in Gothenburg for their tireless efforts in the Swedish Hip Arthroplasty Register. We are also grateful to all the reporting clinics in Sweden.

Funding

The study has not received any specific funding.

Authors' contributions

Conceptual design: SN, DL, CR. Acquisition of data: SN, EB. Analysis of data: SN, EB, DL. Interpretation of data: DL, CR, PC, OR, SN, EB. Drafting of manuscript: DL, SN, CR, PC, EB, OR. Revising of manuscript: DL, CR, PC, EB, OR, SN. All authors read and approved the final manuscript.

Consent for publication
Not applicable

Competing interests
The authors declare that they have no competing interests.

Author details
[1]Swedish Hip Arthroplasty Register, Centre of Registers Västra Götaland, Gothenburg, Sweden. [2]Department of Orthopedics, Institute of Clinical Sciences, Sahlgrenska Academy, University of Gothenburg, Gothenburg, Sweden. [3]Department of Orthopedics, Lund University, Skane University Hospital, Malmö, Sweden. [4]Department of Orthopedics, Hywel Dda University Healthboard, Prince Philip Hospital, Bryngwyn Mawr, Llanelli, UK.

References

1. Nguyen ND, Ahlborg HG, Center JR, Eisman JA, Nguyen TV. Residual lifetime risk of fractures in women and men. J Bone Miner Res. 2007;22(6):781–8.
2. Rosengren BE, Karlsson MK. The annual number of hip fractures in Sweden will double from year 2002 to 2050: projections based on local and nationwide data. Acta Orthop. 2014;85(3):234–7.
3. Omsland TK, Emaus N, Tell GS, Magnus JH, Awad L, Holvik K, Forsmo S, Gjesdal CG, Schei B, Vestergaard P, et al. Mortality following the first hip fracture in Norwegian women and men (1999 – 2008). A NOREPOS study. Bone. 2014;63:81_6.
4. von Friesendorff M, McGuigan FE, Wizert A, Rogmark C, Holmberg AH, Woolf AD, Akesson K. Hip fracture, mortality risk, and cause of death over two decades. Osteoporos Int. 2016;27(10):2945–53.
5. Pedersen AB, Ehrenstein V, Szepligeti SK, Lunde A, Lagerros YT, Westerlund A, Tell GS, Sorensen HT. Thirty-five-year trends in first-time hospitalization for hip fracture, 1-year mortality, and the prognostic impact of comorbidity: a Danish nationwide cohort study, 1980–2014. Epidemiology. 2017;28(6): 898–905.
6. Mundi S, Pindiprolu B, Simunovic N, Bhandari M. Similar mortality rates in hip fracture patients over the past 31 years. Acta Orthop. 2014;85(1):54–9.
7. Jantzen C, Madsen CM, Lauritzen JB, Jorgensen HL. Temporal trends in hip fracture incidence, mortality, and morbidity in Denmark from 1999 to 2012. Acta Orthop. 2018;89(2):170–6.
8. Kärrholm JLH, Malchau H, Mohaddes M, Rogmark C, Rolfson O. Swedish hip arthroplasty register annual report 2015; 2016.
9. Cnudde P, Rolfson O, Timperley AJ, Garland A, Karrholm J, Garellick G, Nemes S. Do patients live longer after THA and is the relative survival diagnosis-specific? Clin Orthop Relat Res. 2018;476(6):1166–75.
10. Cnudde P, Rolfson O, Nemes S, Kärrholm J, Rehnberg C, Rogmark C, Timperley J, Garellick G. Linking Swedish health data registers to establish a research database and a shared decision-making tool in hip replacement. BMC Musculoskelet Disord. 2016;17(1):414.
11. Elixhauser A, Steiner C, Harris DR. Comorbidity measures for use with administrative data. Med Care. 1998;36(1):8–27.
12. Quan H, Sundararajan V, Halfon P, Fong A, Burnand B, Luthi J-C, Saunders LD, Beck CA, Feasby TE, Ghali WA. Coding algorithms for defining comorbidities in ICD-9-CM and ICD-10 administrative data. Med Care. 2005; 43:1130.
13. Pohar M, Stare J. Relative survival analysis in R. Comput Methods Prog Biomed. 2006;81(3):272–8.
14. Pohar M, Stare J. Making relative survival analysis relatively easy. Comput Biol Med. 2007;37(12):1741–9.
15. Human life table database. http://www.lifetable.de/. 10 Apr 2018.
16. Human mortality data base. http://www.mortality.org/. 10 Apr 2018.
17. Stare J, Henderson R, Pohar M. An individual measure of relative survival. J R Stat Soc: Ser C: Appl Stat. 2005;54(1):115–26.
18. Stare J, Pohar M, Henderson R. Goodness of fit of relative survival models. Stat Med. 2005;24(24):3911–25.
19. Jurisson M, Raag M, Kallikorm R, Lember M, Uuskula A. The impact of hip fracture on mortality in Estonia: a retrospective population-based cohort study. BMC Musculoskelet Disord. 2017;18(1):243.
20. Salkeld G, Cameron ID, Cumming RG, Easter S, Seymour J, Kurrle SE, Quine S. Quality of life related to fear of falling and hip fracture in older women: a time trade off study. BMJ. 2000;320(7231):341–6.
21. Magaziner J. Changes in functional status attributable to hip fracture: a comparison of hip fracture patients to community-dwelling aged. Am J Epidemiol. 2003;157(>11):1023–31.
22. Nightingale S, Holmes J, Mason J, House A. Psychiatric illness and mortality after hip fracture. Lancet. 2001;357(9264):1264–5.
23. Ariza-Vega P, Kristensen MT, Martín-Martín L, Jiménez-Moleón JJ. Predictors of long-term mortality in older people with hip fracture. Arch Phys Med Rehabil. 2015;96(7):1215–21.
24. Stenqvist C, Madsen CM, Riis T, Jorgensen HL, Duus BR, Lauritzen JB, van der Mark S. Orthogeriatric service reduces mortality in patients with hip fracture. Geriatr Orthop Surg Rehabil. 2016;7(2):67–73.
25. Lisk R, Yeong K. Reducing mortality from hip fractures: a systematic quality improvement programme. BMJ Qual Improv Rep. 2014;3(1):1–7.
26. Parker MJ. Reducing morbidity and mortality in the hip fracture patient group. Orthop Traumatol. 2016;30(2):153–8.
27. Gonzalez-Zabaleta J, Pita-Fernandez S, Seoane-Pillado T, Lopez-Calvino B, Gonzalez-Zabaleta JL. Comorbidity as a predictor of mortality and mobility after hip fracture. Geriatr Gerontol Int. 2016;16(5):561–9.
28. Smith T, Pelpola K, Ball M, Ong A, Myint PK. Pre-operative indicators for mortality following hip fracture surgery: a systematic review and meta-analysis. Age Ageing. 2014;43(4):464.
29. Hindmarsh D, Loh M, Finch CF, Hayen A, Close JC. Effect of comorbidity on relative survival following hospitalisation for fall-related hip fracture in older people. Australas J Ageing. 2014;33(3):E1–7.
30. Uriz-otano F, Pla-vidal J, Tiberio-lópez G, Malafarina V. Maturitas factors associated to institutionalization and mortality over three years , in elderly people with a hip fracture — an observational study. Maturitas. 2016;89:9–15.
31. Roche JJW, Wenn RT, Sahota O, Moran CG. Effect of comorbidities and postoperative complications on mortality after hip fracture in elderly people: prospective observational cohort study. BMJ. 2005;331(7529):1374.
32. Schnell S, Friedman SM, Mendelson DA, Bingham KW, Kates SL. The 1-year mortality of patients treated in a hip fracture program for elders. Geriatr Orthop Surg Rehabil. 2010;1(1):6–14.
33. Bülow E, Rogmark C, Cnudde P, Rolfson O, Garellick G, Nemes S. Comorbidity do not predict long-term mortality after total hip arthroplasty. Acta Orthop. 2017;14(Jun 14;1–6):1–6.
34. Kristensen PK, Thillemann TM, Johnsen SP. Is bigger always better? A nationwide study of hip fracture unit volume, 30-day mortality, quality of in-hospital care, and length of hospital stay. Med Care. 2014;52:1023.
35. Weller I, Wai EK, Jaglal S, Kreder HJ. The effect of hospital type and surgical delay on mortality after surgery for hip fracture. J Bone Joint Surg Br Vol. 2005;87(3):361–6.
36. Shah SN, Wainess RM, Karunakar MA. Hemiarthroplasty for femoral neck fracture in the elderly: surgeon and hospital volume-related outcomes. J Arthroplast. 2005;20:503.
37. Klop C, Welsing PMJ, Cooper C, Harvey NC, Elders PJM, Bijlsma JWJ, Leufkens HGM, De Vries F. Mortality in British hip fracture patients, 2000-2010: a population-based retrospective cohort study. Bone. 2014;66:171–7.
38. Kim S-M, Moon Y-W, Lim S-J, Yoon B-K, Min Y-K, Lee D-Y, Park Y-S. Prediction of survival, second fracture, and functional recovery following the first hip fracture surgery in elderly patients. Bone. 2012;50(6):1343–50.
39. Thorne K, Johansen A, Akbari A, Williams JG, Roberts SE. The impact of social deprivation on mortality following hip fracture in England and Wales: a record linkage study. Osteoporos Int. 2016;27(9):2727–37.
40. Solbakken SM, Meyer HE, Stigum H, Søgaard AJ, Holvik K. Excess mortality following hip fracture: impact of self-perceived health, smoking, and body mass index. A NOREPOS study. Osteoporos Int. 2017;28(3):881-87.
41. Emami ARVMJ, Mahdaviazad BPH. Factors increasing mortality of the elderly following hip fracture surgery: role of body mass index, age, and smoking. Musculoskelet Surg. 2017;101(1):25-29.
42. Lofthus CM, Cappelen I, Osnes EK, Falch JA, Kristiansen IS, Medhus AW, Nordsletten L, Meyer HE. Local and national electronic databases in Norway demonstrate a varying degree of validity. J Clin Epidemiol. 2005;58(3):280–5.
43. Hockey R, Tooth L, Dobson A. Relative survival: a useful tool to assess generalisability in longitudinal studies of health in older persons. Emerg Themes Epidemiol. 2011;8(1):3.

Endoscopic resection of acetabular screw tip to decompress sciatic nerve following total hip arthroplasty

Sun-jung Yoon[1*], Myung-sik Park[1], Dean K. Matsuda[2] and Yun Ho Choi[3]

Abstract

Background: Sciatic nerve injuries following total hip arthroplasty are disabling complications. Although degrees of injury are variable from neuropraxia to neurotmesis, mechanical irritation of sciatic nerve might be occurred by protruding hardware. This case shows endoscopic decompression for protruded acetabular screw irritating sciatic nerve, the techniques described herein may permit broader arthroscopic/endoscopic applications for management of complications after reconstructive hip surgery.

Case presentation: An 80-year-old man complained of severe pain and paresthesias following acetabular component revision surgery. Physical findings included right buttock pain with radiating pain to lower extremity. Radiographs and computed tomography imaging showed that the sharp end of protruded screw invaded greater sciatic foramen anterior to posterior and distal to proximal direction at sciatic notch level. A protruding tip of the acetabular screw at the sciatic notch was decompressed by use of techniques gained from experience performing endoscopic sciatic nerve decompression. The pre-operative pain and paresthesias resolved post-operatively after recovering from anesthesia.

Conclusions: This case report describes the first documented endoscopic resection of the tip of the acetabular screw irritating sciatic nerve after total hip arthroplasty. If endoscopic resection of an offending acetabular screw can be performed in a safe and minimally invasive manner, one can envision a future expansion of the role of hip arthroscopic surgery in several complications management after total hip arthroplasty.

Keywords: Endoscopic sciatic nerve decompression, Sciatic nerve neuropathy, Acetabular dome screw, Total hip arthroplasty

Background

Sciatic nerve irritation due to an acetabular screw following total hip arthroplasty (THA) is rare; the few reported were treated with revision procedure to remove an acetabular screw [1]. Recent reports of the orthopaedic literature document the use of endoscopic decompression of sciatic nerve entrapment syndrome/deep gluteal syndrome treatment [2]. Endoscopy allows for complete extrapelvic sciatic nerve visualization and safe nerve decompression in the deep gluteal space [3, 4]. This is the first documented case of completely endoscopic treatment of sciatic nerve irritation by a protruded acetabular dome screw following THA.

Case presentation

An 80-year-old man complained of severe pain and paresthesias following acetabular component revision surgery via the original posterolateral approach. The patient subsequently complained of right leg pain and paresthesias. The symptoms were exaggerated during initial hip flexion and internal rotation that limited ambulation. Physical findings included right buttock pain with radiating pain to the ipsilateral lower extremity. Radiographs and computed tomography imaging (Figs. 1, 2, 3, and 4) showed an acetabular screw tip protruding into the greater sciatic foramen in an anterior to posterior and

* Correspondence: sunjungyoonkos@gmail.com
[1]Department of Orthopedic Surgery, Research Institute of clinical medicine of Chonbuk National University, Biomedical Research Institute of Chonbuk National University Hospital, 54907 Gunji-Ro 20, Dukjin-Gu, Chonbuk, Jeonju, South Korea
Full list of author information is available at the end of the article

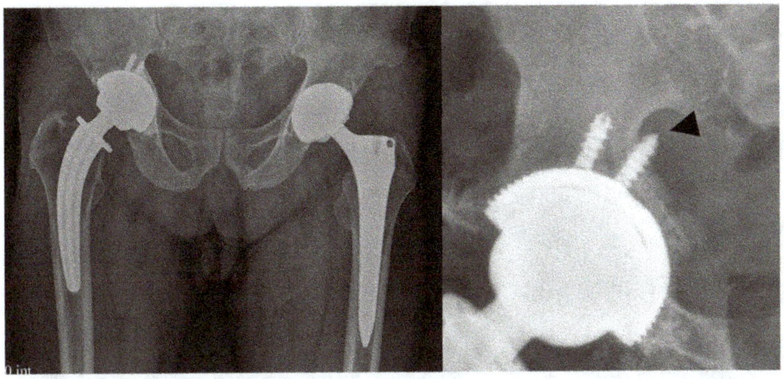

Fig. 1 Preoperative hip radiographs (anteroposterior view; Left, iliac oblique view; Right) with protruded dome screw (arrowhead) into sciatic notch

distal to proximal direction at the level of the sciatic notch. The screw was 30 mm in length and positioned at posterior-inferior acetabular quadrant. Magnetic resonance imaging demonstrated tenting of the right piriformis muscle tented by the end of screw. Mechanical irritation of the sciatic nerve screw was suspected.

Eight months after the aforementioned surgery, the patient underwent supine hip arthroscopy without distraction on a fracture table (Hana®, Mizuho OSI). The operating table was tilted right side upward to increase accessibility of ipsilateral buttock. An anterolateral viewing portal and poster lateral working portal were developed without incident. For deep gluteal space visualization, a 70-degree high definition long arthroscope with adjustable length cannulas were utilized. The cannula was opened to maintain the fluid flow when utilizing the radiofrequency probe. Fluid pressure was set to 60 mmHg with intermittent pressure increases up 80 mmHg. After endoscopic greater trochanteric bursectomy, the repaired piriformis from previous revision surgery was well visualized (Fig. 5). Endoscopic visualization of the sciatic nerve revealed a hypo vascular appearance, with entrapped by repaired the piriformis muscle and adjacent fibrous tissue. Endoscopic dynamic testing demonstrated sciatic nerve hypomobility with limited excursion during hip flexion and extension in internal and external rotation. The repaired piriformis tendon was tenotomized and more adjacent scar tissue was observed. Endoscopic resection of fibrovascular bands and adhesions between the piriformis muscle and posterior acetabular wall was performed without incident, allowing visualization of the protruding screw tip penetrated through the piriformis muscle (Fig. 6). Endoscopic piriformis muscle dissection and adhesiolysis was performed, improving visualization of the screw tip adjacent to the supero-lateral aspect of the sciatic nerve. No sciatic nerve intra-substance splitting or tearing was observed, supporting the diagnosis of sciatic nerve irritation without direct nerve injury. Via endoscopic and intermittent multiplanar fluoroscopic visualization, further dissection was performed proximally and distally to prevent inadvertent injuries to the sciatic nerve and the superior gluteal neurovascular bundle. Partial osteoplasty of the sciatic notch with a motorized burr performed under endoscopic guidance. Endoscopic resection of the offending screw tip was performed with a 5.5 mm motorized round burr (Fig. 7). The adjustable cannula protected the adjacent superior gluteal vessels from iatrogenic harm. The screw was scored from the superolateral direction to minimize the risk of unexpected injury by the burr after decorticating the sciatic notch. The protruded screw tip was completely resected and subsequently recontoured to a smooth surface. The screw tip was removed enbloc with an arthroscopic grasper (Fig. 8). Generated metallic debris

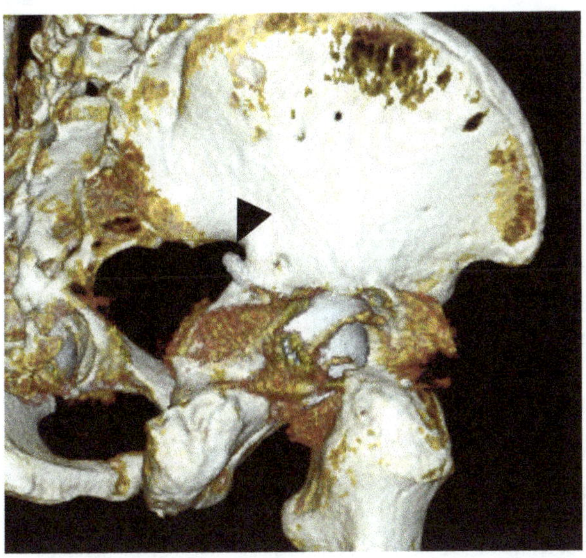

Fig. 2 Oblique 3-dimensional computed tomography reconstruction showing an acetabular screw protruded into sciatic notch (arrowhead)

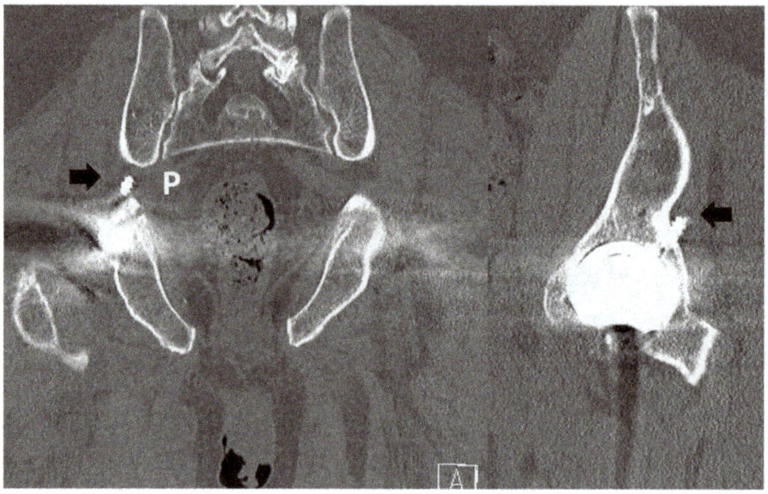

Fig. 3 Coronal and computed tomography views of right hip showing sciatic notch area occupied by an acetabular screw (arrow). The protruded screw was placed superiorly than piriformis muscle (P)

were removed via suction through the burr cannula. All visible metallic debris was removed. Dynamic arthroscopic and fluoroscopic examinations confirmed successful decompression of the acetabular screw with an immediate visible improvement in sciatic nerve vascularity and excursion. Key procedural steps of this arthroscopic procedure are shown as Additional file 1: Endoscopic technique.

After this endoscopic surgery, immediate hip range of motion was begun with a continuous passive motion machine. The pre-operative pain and paresthesias resolved post-operatively after recovering from anesthesia. The patient advanced to household ambulation without upper extremity aids at 1 postoperative week despite recommendations for 2 weeks of ambulation using crutches. By 3 months postoperatively, he had returned to full activities. At 6 months postoperatively, he had a negative active and passive piriformis test and he remained pleased with the outcome. Postoperative imaging included radiographs and computed tomography scans with 3-dimensional reconstruction demonstrating complete resection of the offending portion of the acetabular screw.

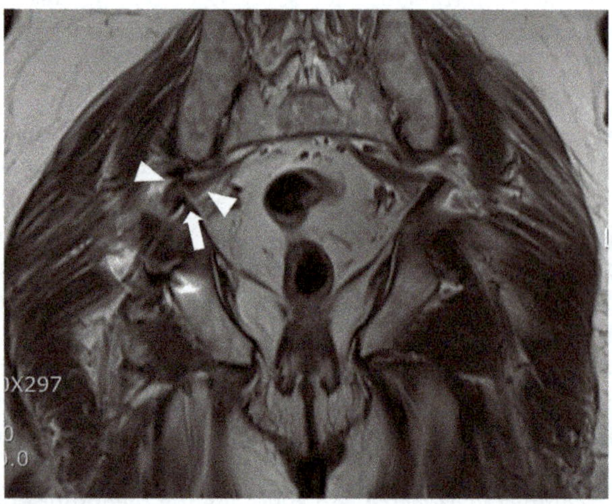

Fig. 4 T2 turbo spin echo magnetic resonance image displaying a screw protrusion (arrowhead) and irritated piriformis muscle (arrow)

Discussion

Nerve lesions following total hip arthroplasty (THA) are disabling complications occurring in 0.06 to 2.2% of arthroplasties [5, 6]. Hardware-induced sciatic nerve neuropathies are rarely reported [1, 6]. If placed in the

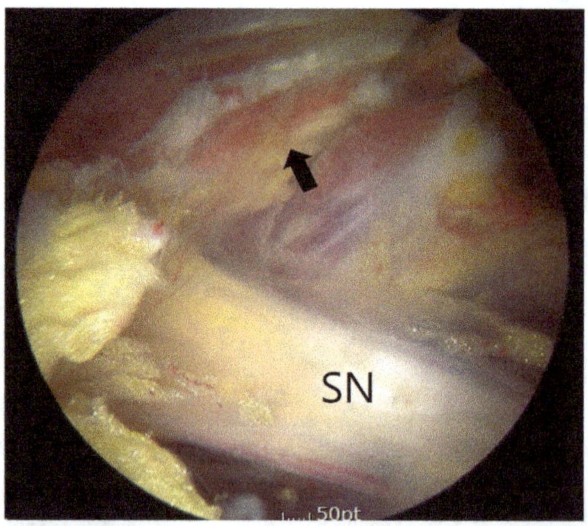

Fig. 5 Endoscopic view from anterolateral portal of right hip (supine, upward tilt ipsilateral hip) showing repaired piriformis in previous surgery (arrow). Sciatic nerve (SN) is pale and loss of perineural fat. It is better visualized in the accompanying video

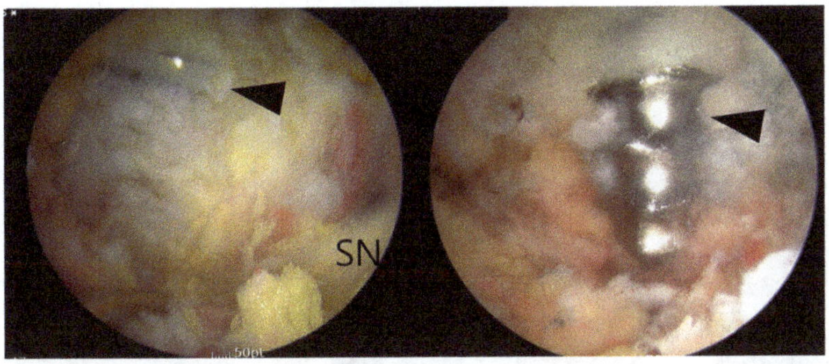

Fig. 6 Endoscopic view from anterolateral portal of right hip (supine, ipsilateral upward tilt) showing screw tip (arrow) protruding from posterior column into sciatic notch being irritated sciatic nerve (SN)

posterior superior quadrant, the screws may be directed toward the sciatic nerve [7]. Mechanical irritation should be suspected in cases of any sign of sciatic neuropathy after THA. The treatment of nerve injuries is tailored its causation. In most cases, the cause is unknown and treatment is directed toward managing symptoms rather than reversing the nerve injury [8]. Open sciatic nerve exploration with dissection of nerve bundle and burr-decompression of the screw has been reported [9]. A protruding acetabular screw can tether the sciatic nerve, restricting its excursion. Endoscopic resection of an offending acetabular screw has now been described. Indeed, had this protruded screw not been resectable by endoscopic means, open exploration and screw removal or resection may have been required. Some advantages of deep gluteal space endoscopy as a minimally invasive procedure are demonstrated in this case report. Decreasing morbidity with minimal blood loss while avoiding re-revision surgery with hip dislocation was facilitated. Moreover, early joint mobilization, relatively rapid postoperative rehabilitation, and outstanding cosmesis were realized. Surgical skills gained from experience with endoscopic technique for deep gluteal syndrome exploration and comfort with the 70 degree arthroscope aided the performance of this surgery. Careful management of endoscopic fluid pressure minimized risk of iatrogenic fluid extravasation into the intra-abdominal and/or retroperitoneal spaces.

An expandable cannula facilitated safe resection of the protruding screw tip while avoiding injury to the adjacent superior gluteal nerve and sciatic nerve. Circulating endoscopy fluid might decrease thermogenesis during metal-on-metal burring of the offending screw. In addition, generated metallic debris is removed immediately through suction system attached burr and cannula to minimize bodily retention with possible adverse consequences.

The decision to remove rather than try to preserve the piriformis muscle was influenced by the surgeon's experience with deep gluteal space exploration often performed for sciatic nerve decompression.

Relevant suggestions and pearls are summarized in Table 1.

For this patient, resection of offending screw tip using endoscopy was considered first, because the acetabular component implanted revision surgery had bony ingrowth without evidence of loosening. Although sciatic nerve irritation from a protruding acetabular screw is rare and its described treatment even rarer, the endoscopic techniques described herein may have broader

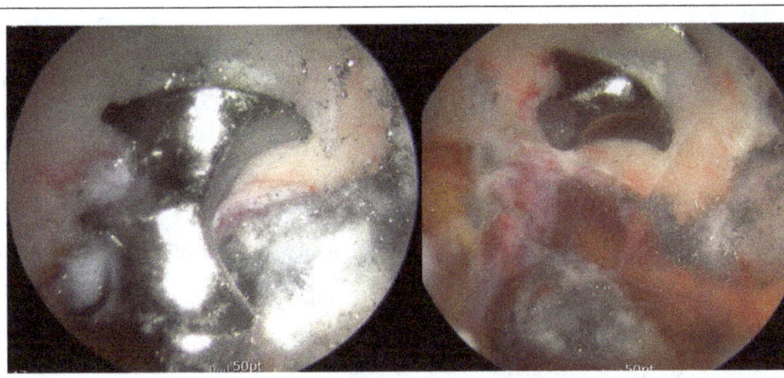

Fig. 7 Endoscopic view from anterolateral portal of right hip (supine) showing an acetabular screw being cut proximally by arthroscopic burr

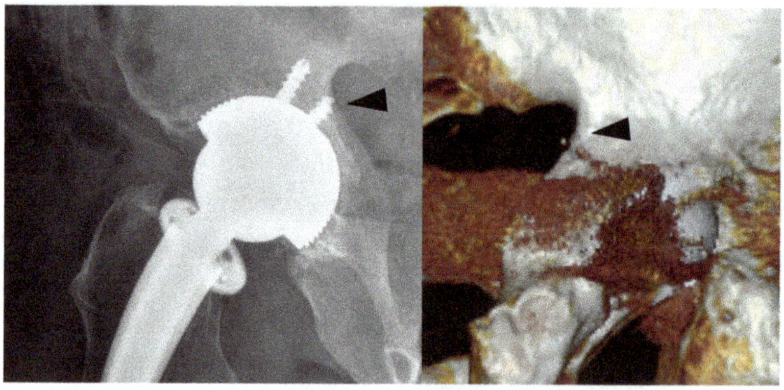

Fig. 8 Postoperative radiography and 3-dimensional computed tomography reconstruction showing the resected acetabular screw at sciatic notch level

applications. Recent interest in hip arthroscopy along with more advanced techniques gained from the endoscopic management of sciatic nerve entrapment syndrome/deep gluteal syndrome have allowed the application of minimally invasive hip surgery for conditions once thought treatable only by open sciatic nerve exploration, screw resection and/or revision hip arthroplasty. The endoscopic exploration and screw resection described herein enables less invasive surgery permitting early joint motion, accelerated rehabilitation, and potential outpatient management. Beyond iliopsoas tenotomy, endoscopic treatment may expand to other complication of THA including protruding screws causing adjacent neurovascular compromise.

Table 1 Pearls for endoscopic resection of protruded acetabular screw irritating sciatic nerve

Perform preoperative assessment of feasibility approaching the location of screw.
Perform accurate preoperative self-assessment of surgical experience and arthroscopic skills.
Consider patient position (supine or lateral) allowing for manual manipulation of the lower limb at the knee and hip joints for the full assessment of sciatic nerve excursion
Lateral position may facilitate ease of conversion to open surgery
Prepare for possible open resection of screw or revision total hip arthroplasty (rather than endoscopic resection) if endoscopic method fails.
Consider fluoroscopic guidance to identify and confirm resection of the protruding screw.
Mobilize and development of soft tissue around sciatic notch.
Consider sciatic notch osteoplasty to expose proper cutting level of the screw.
Pay careful attention to safe position of burr to prevent superior gluteal neurovascular bundle and sciatic nerve injury (may require several accessory portals).
Circulating fluid during burr resection of screw may minimize thermogenesis and metallic debris retention.
Confirm adequate resection and smooth recontour of the screw by arthroscopic dynamic testing while envisioning the sciatic nerve
Allow early mobilization of hip commensurate with symptomatic improvement.

Conclusion

A protruding acetabular screw at the sciatic notch was decompressed by use of techniques gained from experience performing endoscopic sciatic nerve decompression. Expandable cannula was used to protect superior gluteal neurovascular bundle proximally and sciatic nerve distally, followed by exposure of screw using an arthroscopic shaver.

Abbreviation

THA: Total hip arthroplasty

Funding

This paper was supported by Fund of Biomedical Research Institute, Chonbuk National University Hospital.

Authors' contributions

SY wrote the manuscript including the literature review. MP is an experienced hip surgeon with an interest in the sciatic nerve injury, and had made substantial contributions to conception and design. DM had been involved in revising the manuscript critically. YC guided the literature search and anatomic considerations. All authors have read and approved the final manuscript.

Consent for publication

Written informed consent was obtained from the patient for publication of this Case report and any accompanying images. A copy of the written consent is available for review by the Editor of this journal.

Competing interests

The authors declare that they have no competing interests.

Author details

[1]Department of Orthopedic Surgery, Research Institute of clinical medicine of Chonbuk National University, Biomedical Research Institute of Chonbuk

National University Hospital, 54907 Gunji-Ro 20, Dukjin-Gu, Chonbuk, Jeonju, South Korea. [2]DISC Sports and Spine Center, Marina del Rey, CA, USA. [3]Department of Anatomy, Medical School, Institute for Medical Sciences, Chonbuk National University, Jeonju 561-180, South Korea.

References

1. Park JH, Hozack B, Kim P, Norton R, Mandel S, Restrepo C, et al. Common peroneal nerve palsy following total hip arthroplasty: prognostic factors for recovery. J Bone Joint Surg Am. 2013;95:e55.
2. Martin HD, Shears SA, Johnson JC, Smathers AM, Palmer IJ. The endoscopic treatment of sciatic nerve entrapment/deep gluteal syndrome. Arthrosc J Arthrosc Relat Surg Off Publ Arthrosc Assoc N Am Int Arthrosc Assoc. 2011; 27:172–81.
3. Martin HD, Reddy M, Gómez-Hoyos J. Deep gluteal syndrome. J Hip Preserv Surg. 2015;2:99–107.
4. Park M, Yoon S-J, Jung S, Kim S-H. Clinical results of endoscopic sciatic nerve decompression for deep gluteal syndrome: mean 2-year follow-up. BMC Musculoskelet Disord. 2016;17:218.
5. Brown GD, Swanson EA, Nercessian OA. Neurologic injuries after total hip arthroplasty. Am J Orthop Belle Mead NJ. 2008;37:191–7.
6. Vastamäki M, Ylinen P, Puusa A, Paavilainen T. Late hardware-induced sciatic nerve lesions after acetabular revision. Clin Orthop. 2008;466:1193–7.
7. Wasielewski RC, Cooperstein LA, Kruger MP, Rubash HE. Acetabular anatomy and the transacetabular fixation of screws in total hip arthroplasty. J Bone Joint Surg Am. 1990;72:501–8.
8. Schmalzried TP, Noordin S, Amstutz HC. Update on nerve palsy associated with total hip replacement. Clin Orthop. 1997;344:188–206.
9. Xu LW, Veeravagu A, Azad TD, Harraher C, Ratliff JK. Delayed presentation of sciatic nerve injury after Total hip arthroplasty: neurosurgical considerations, diagnosis, and management. J Neurol Surg Rep. 2016;77(3):e134–8.

9

Impact of acetabular reaming depth on reconstruction of rotation center in primary total hip arthroplasty

Pu Shao[1], Zhizhou Li[1], Modi Yang[1], Yuzhuo Wang[3], Te Liu[2], Yuhui Yang[1], Lian Duan[1], Jinlan Jiang[2*] and Jianlin Zuo[1*]

Abstract

Purpose: To study the impact of acetabular reaming depth on reconstruction of rotation center (RC) in unilateral primary total hip arthroplasty (UPTHA) and guide individualized preoperative design.

Methods: 200 postoperative standard bilateral hip anteroposterior radiographs after UPTHA were included, which were collected from January, 2013 to June, 2017 in our hospital. Osteonecrosis of femoral head was the only diagnosis in this cohort. The parameters were measured on the anteropoterior radiographs by using RadiAnt DICOM viewer.

Results: The average of the thickness of the teardrop is about 6.13 ± 1.42 mm. The parameter a (the difference value of the distance of bilateral RC and midline) was positively correlated with the parameter e (the acetabular reaming depth), and the Pearson correlation coefficient was 0.49 when $P = 0.05$. Furthermore, the value of parameter (e) was 8.25 mm when a2 (the distance from the center of the prosthesis femoral head to the vertical line across the midpoint of pubic symphysis) equaled a1 (the distance from RC of the healthy femoral head to the vertical line across the midpoint of pubic symphysis).

Conclusions: The reaming depth of the acetabulum could influence the reconstruction of RC during UPTHA. When the medial margin of the cup was placed about 2 mm to the lateral border of the ipsilateral teardrop (the bottom of the ovum), the rotation center would be accurately restored.

Keywords: Total hip arthroplasty, Rotation center, Acetabulum, Reaming depth, Teardrop

Introduction

It is now acknowledged that total hip arthroplasty (THA) is one of the most successful procedures in the field of orthopeadics, which is widely applied to the treatment of many hip joint diseases resulted in dysfunction of hip joint [1]. Maximization of the prosthesis life is the most significant issue for orthopedic surgeons [2].

Among the influencing factors for successful restoration of joint, accurate biomechanical reconstruction of the femur and acetabulum is essential for satisfactory function achievement [3–5]. In order to reduce the occurrence of many postoperative complications it is necessary to Reproduce, as close as possible, normal or near-normal mechanics. One of the most important steps in achieving this is to transfer the hip joint RC into the true acetabulum [6–8]. The native acetabulum is subhemispherical in most cases, but the acetabular components used for THA are hemispherical, which inadvertently leads to displacement of RC when the acetabular component is fully implanted [9, 10]. Hence, it is very vital for hip replacement to reconstruct RC of femoral head prosthesis in the anatomical position of the acetabulum side. Moreover, the RC of hip is also pivotal for recovery of muscle function [4, 11–15], joint stability [16–19], and hip prostheses longevity [20–23]. If RC of femoral head prosthesis is not placed at the anatomical position, it may also lead to patients with

* Correspondence: jiangjl2003@hotmail.com; jlzuojianlin@163.com
[2]Scientific Research Centre of China-Japan Union Hospital of Jilin University, 126 xiantai street, Changchun 130033, People's Republic of China
[1]Department of Orthopedics, China-Japan Union Hospital of Jilin University, 126 xiantai street, Changchun 130033, People's Republic of China
Full list of author information is available at the end of the article

unequal limb length, unequal femoral eccentricity, etc. Over time it will cause the muscles to lose their original function, the joints are unstable, and eventually the loosening of the prosthesis.

So, the depth of acetabular prosthesis implantation becomes a main factor infecting the position of RC. Despite advances in surgery technique, the landmark of acetabular reaming depth for anatomic restoration of RC remains uncertain. In this paper, standard bilateral hip anteroposterior radiographs after unilateral primary THA (UPTHA) were used to clarify the accurate acetabular reaming depth for anatomically reconstructing RC of hip joint during THA.

Methods

General information

In this study, 200 standard bilateral hip anteroposterior radiographs after UPTHA were collected from January 2013 to June 2017 in our hospital. As shown in Table 1, there were 116 males and 84 females in all subjects. Among them, there were 97 patients on the left side and 103 patients on the right side. The average age was 58.1 years (from 24 to 80 years). The inclusion criterions applied was as follow: Patients with unilateral osteonecrosis of femoral head while the contralateral hip joint was normal. The exclusion criterions used were as follow: 1 Patients with unilateral or bilateral acetabular or femoral developmental dysplasia; 2. Patients with unilateral or bilateral hip joint fracture history.

X-ray and measurements

The standard bilateral hip anteroposterior radiographs were gathered after UPTHA. The criteria for taking the radiographs were as follow: The patients were supine on the photography table, with median sagittal plane coincided with the cassette midline, the lower limbs were fully extended, and were placed in internal rotation about 15°. The X-ray filter was used. The tube distance was 100 cm. The center of the beam was focused on the point 3 cm below the pubic symphysis midpoint, and the beam was vertically injected into the cassette. The position was controlled so as to make the bilateral obturator foramens isometrical and the tip of coccyx locating at the level and in the center of the pubic symphysis. The longitudinal axes of bilateral femurs were parallel to each other and to the longitudinal central axis of the pelvis.

Table 1 General information of the 200 patients

Item	Classification	Number	Percentage
Sexuality	Male	116	58%
	Female	84	42%
Age	<40	12	6%
	40–60	100	50%
	>60	88	44%
Operation Side	Left	97	48.5%
	Right	103	51.5%

As shown in Fig. 1, RadiAnt DICOM viewer (version 1.9.16, 32-bit, developed by Medixant Company in Poland in 2009) was applied to measure the following parameters on the above mentioned postoperative standard bilateral hip anteroposterior radiographs. First a transverse line passing through the lower edges of bilateral teardrops were drawn. Then the following measurements were made: a1. The distance from RC of the healthy femoral head to the vertical line across the midpoint of pubic symphysis; a2. The distance from the center of the prosthesis femoral head to the vertical line across the midpoint of pubic symphysis; b1. The diameter of the healthy femoral head; b2. The diameter of the femoral head prosthesis; c. The thickness of the teardrop on the contralateral side; d. The distance between the vertical lines tangent to the medial margins of the femoral head prosthesis and the acetabular prosthesis; e. The distance between the vertical lines tangent to the medial margins of the acetabular prosthesis and the medial border of the ipsilateral teardrop, which was defined as the horizontal reaming depth.

Correction and standardization of the measurements

After the measurement of the above parameters, the value correction was done. Parameter b2, the diameter of the femoral head prosthesis, was a known data, which could be retrieved from the patient chart. So, the ratio of the true value and the measured value of the femoral head prosthesis could be obtained in each case, which was named as correction coefficient. By multiplying each patient's data by the corresponding correction coefficient, the true value of each parameter could be obtained in each case. Standardization of the measured data was subsequently carried out in order to make the results comparable among the 200 patients with different heights and weights. After the measurements and corrections, the ratio of the diameter of the largest to the diameter of every other femoral head, called standardized coefficient, was obtained. Then, by multiplying the true value of each parameter with the standardized coefficient the standard value of each parameter was acquired.

Statistical analysis

SPSS 22.0 was applied for statistical analysis. Pearson correlation analysis was used to analyze the correlation between the parameter (a) ($a = a2 - a1$) and the parameter (e), and the pattern of relevant scatter plot was drawn. The illustration of relationship of parameter (e) and parameter (a) was further progressed by regression analysis.

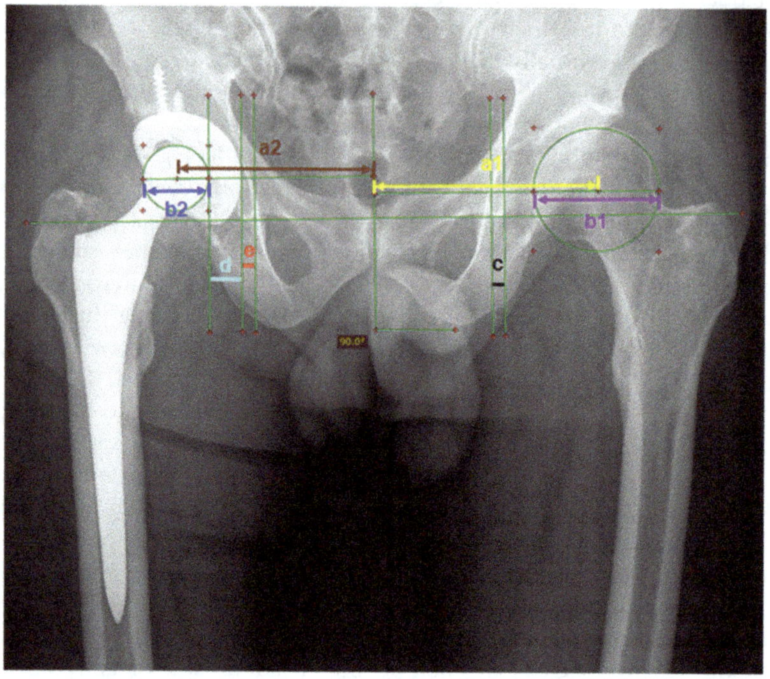

Fig. 1 Postoperative measurement: the distance between the center of rotation of the healthy femoral head to the vertical line across the midpoint of pubic symphysis (a1); the distance between the center of the prosthesis femoral head to the vertical line across the midpoint of pubic symphysis (a2); the diameter of the healthy femoral head (b1); the diameter of the prosthesis femoral head (b2); the thickness of the teardrop(c); the distance between the medial edge of prosthesis femoral head and the medial edge of the acetabular cup (d); the distance between the medial edge of the acetabular cup and the medial edge of teardrop (e)

Results

The diameter of the largest femoral head on the healthy side was 55.5mm. After the Pearson correlation analysis is performed for parameter a (the difference value of the distance of bilateral RC and midline) and parameter e(the distance between the vertical lines tangent to the medial margins of the acetabular prosthesis and the medial border of the ipsilateral teardrop), it can be concluded that the parameter (a) was positively correlated with the parameter (e), and the Pearson correlation coefficient was 0.49, when $P = 0.05$. That is to say the parameter (e) is increased with an increase in the parameter (a). As shown in Fig. 2, the pattern of the relevant scatter plot was suggested that the parameter (a) was positively correlated with the parameter (e). In addition, the regression analysis was further shown that the coefficients of the independent variables passed the statistical test at a confidence level of 0.05. The regression equation was finally established as follow:

$$e = 8.25 + 0.17 \times (a2\text{-}a1)$$

Hence, when the RC of the operated hip was restored anatomically in the horizontal direction, that is (a) = 0, the distance between the medial tangent line of the acetabular prosthesis and that of the lateral border of the ipsilateral teardrop, that is e, equaled 8.25 mm. This result was got at the condition that the diameter of the femoral head was 55.5 mm. Because of the medial margin of the teardrop cannot be seen during operation, we measured the thickness of teardrop, which is 6.13 mm ± 1.42 mm. Then we drew the conclusion that when the medial margin of the cup was about 2 mm (8.25 mm minus 6.13 mm equals about 2 mm) lateral to the lateral margin of the ipsilateral teardrop the rotation center of the operated hip would be anatomically restored.

Discussion

In all precedures of preoperative plan for THA, the anatomical reconstruction of acetabular RC is a very important target [24, 25]. The position of RC of the operated hip was the most important factor for the stress and function of the soft tissue around the hip joint. And in the anatomical reconstruction of the horizontal of the RC, the horizontal reaming depth of the acetabulum plays a very important role. The ideal position of acetabular prosthesis mainly depended on the femoral head size and the neck diameter. For the long-term service life of the prosthesis, the acetabulum should be placed in its anatomical position to normally inclusion of the acetabular prosthesis and restore the

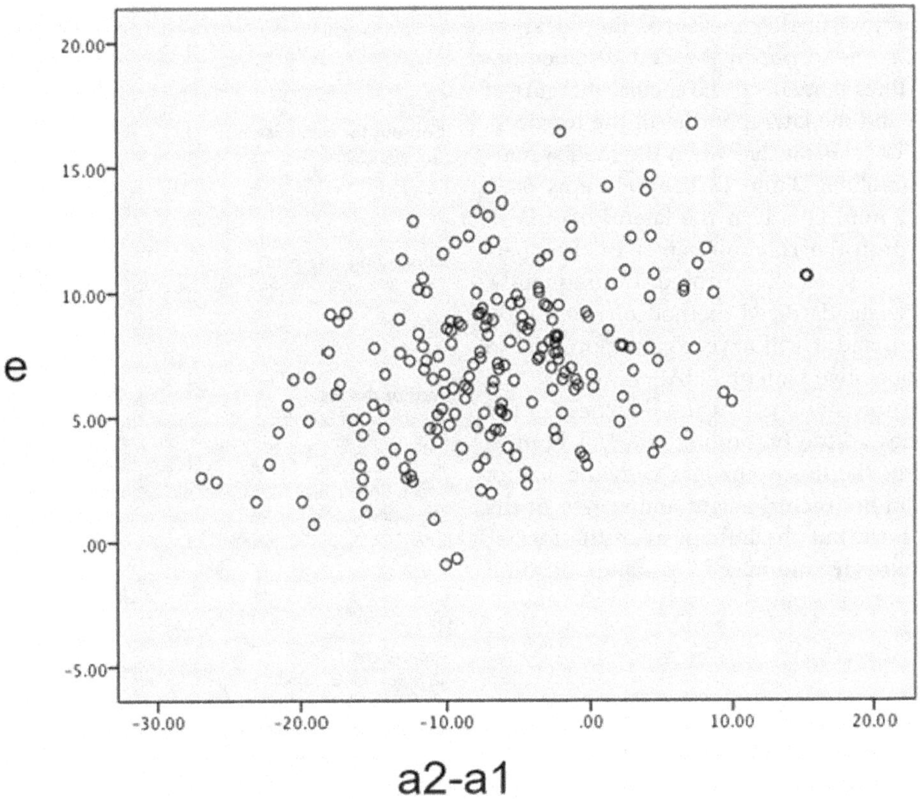

Fig. 2 The pattern of linear correlation scatter plot of the reaming depth (e) and the difference value of the distance of bilateral RC and midline (a2 - a1)

length of the limb [26]. In the existing literature reports, no one has studied the goal of the ideal depth of acetabular reaming. The acetabular reaming depth affects the position of the RC in horizon direction. If the reaming depth is too deep or too shallow, it may affect the survivorship of the prosthesis by changing the force torque of the reconstructed hip. There is no uniform standard for acetabular prosthesis depth in THA, so far. In this paper, standard bilateral hip anteroposterior radiographs after unilateral primary THA (UPTHA) were used to clarify the accurate acetabular reaming depth for anatomically reconstructing RC of hip joint during THA. And it will have a great potential in individualized preoperative plan of THA.

In this paper, the distance (a2) between the RC of operated and midline can be divided into three parts: the radius of femoral head component (half of b2), the thickness of acetabular cup (d) (including metal acetabular cup and high molecular polyethylene liner), and the reaming depth (e) (the distance between the medial tangent line of the acetabular component and that of the medial border of the ipsilateral teardrop) in the postoperative anteroposterior radiographs of THA. Because the radius of femoral head component and the thickness of acetabular component were two constant values, after the data correction and standardization, the reaming depth (e) became the only one variable affecting the reconstruction of RC. In this paper, we did correction to exclude influence of the magnification of the radiographs by calculating the ratio of the true value of the femoral head prosthesis (was a known data, which could be retrieved from the patient chart.) and the measured value of the femoral head prosthesis. Then we performed standardization to exclude influence of bone size on the measurements. We used diameter of the largest healthy femoral head (55.5 mm) in the 200 patients as the standard, the measurements of other patients were then multiplied by the ratio of the diameter of the corresponding femoral head to that of the largest femoral head (55.5 mm). By balancing different sizes of bone from this cohort of patients, we could analyze if there were linear correlations between the parameters. According to statistical analysis, it was suggested that the reaming depth (e) in horizon direction would be 8.25 mm under the condition that the diameter of healthy femoral head was 55.5 mm and RC was restored anatomically (a1 = a2).

It is well known that the medial margin of teardrops is visible in the radiographs imaging but invisible in the surgery procedure. But the lateral border of the teardrop is visible in the surgery procedure. It is the bottom of the ovum. Therefore, we further measured the thickness of the teardrop(c), so as to obtain the best distance between the vertical lines tangent to the medial margins of the acetabular cup and the lateral border of the teardrop. Then we drew the conclusion that when the medial margin of the cup was about 2 mm (8.25 mm minus 6.13 mm equals about 2 mm) lateral to the lateral margin of the ipsilateral teardrop the rotation center of the operated hip would be anatomically restored. Consequently, in this work, a new standardized method of restoration of RC was provided, and it will have a great potential in individualized preoperative plan of THA.

The limitation of this study is that the thickness of the cup prosthesis varies a little bit among different brands, and the thickness of the linear changes with the size of the cup. And we did not record height and weight of the patients in this cohort. But the influences of the former two factors were already minimized by standardization of the data.

Conclusion

We found that the reaming depth of the acetabulum influence the reconstruction of RC during THA. In the procedures of individualized preoperative plan, the distance between the medial tangent line of the acetabular prosthesis and that of the medial border of the ipsilateral teardrop, e = 8.25 mm, when the diameter of the healthy femoral head was 55.5 mm. Because of the average thickness of the normal teardrop(c) is 6.13 ± 1.42 mm, we can conclude that when the medial margin of the cup was placed about 2 mm to the lateral border of the ipsilateral teardrop (the bottom of the ovum), the rotation center would be accurately restored.

Abbreviations

RC: Rotation center; THA: Total hip arthroplasty; UPTHA: Unilateral primary total hip arthroplasty

Acknowledgements

None

Funding

"This work was supported and funded by the National Nature Science Foundation of China (No. 81701811)."

Authors' contributions

PS, ZL, MY and YW completed the data measurement. TL, YY and LD completed the statistical analysis. PS completed the article writing. At last JZ and JJ completed the article changes. After the review comments were sent back, JJ completed the revision of the manuscript according to the reviewer's request. All authors read and approved the final manuscript.

Consent for publication

Not applicable.

Competing interests

The authors declare that they have no competing interests.

Author details

[1]Department of Orthopedics, China-Japan Union Hospital of Jilin University, 126 xiantai street, Changchun 130033, People's Republic of China. [2]Scientific Research Centre of China-Japan Union Hospital of Jilin University, 126 xiantai street, Changchun 130033, People's Republic of China. [3]Department of Orthodontics, School and Hospital of Stomatology, Jilin University, Changchun 130021, People's Republic of China.

References

1. Bhaskar D, Rajpura A, Board T. Current concepts in Acetabular positioning in Total hip Arthroplasty. Indian J Orthop. 2017;51(4):386–96.
2. Bouffard V, Begon M, Champagne A, Farhadnia P, Vendittoli PA, Lavigne M, Prince F. Hip joint center localisation: a biomechanical application to hip arthroplasty population. World J Orthop. 2012;3(8):131–6.
3. Kiyama T, Naito M, Shinoda T, Maeyama A. Hip abductor strengths after total hip arthroplasty via the lateral and posterolateral approaches. J Arthroplast. 2010;25(1):76–80.
4. Asayama I, Chamnongkich S, Simpson KJ, Kinsey TL, Mahoney OM. Reconstructed hip joint position and abductor muscle strength after total hip arthroplasty. J Arthroplast. 2005;20(4):414–20.
5. Erceg M. The influence of femoral head shift on hip biomechanics: additional parameters accounted. Int Orthop. 2009;33(1):95–100.
6. Kilicoglu OI, Turker M, Akgul T, Yazicioglu O. Cementless total hip arthroplasty with modified oblique femoral shortening osteotomy in Crowe type IV congenital hip dislocation. J Arthroplast. 2013;28(1):117–25.
7. Erdemli B, Yilmaz C, Atalar H, Guzel B, Cetin I. Total hip arthroplasty in developmental high dislocation of the hip. J Arthroplast. 2005;20(8):1021–8.
8. Muratli KS, Karatosun V, Uzun B, Celik S. Subtrochanteric shortening in total hip arthroplasty: biomechanical comparison of four techniques. J Arthroplast. 2014;29(4):836–42.
9. Meermans G, Doorn JV, Kats JJ. Restoration of the Centre of rotation in primary total hip arthroplasty: the influence of acetabular floor depth and reaming technique. Bone Joint J. 2016;98-B(12):1597–603.
10. Kohnlein W, Ganz R, Impellizzeri FM, Leunig M. Acetabular morphology: implications for joint-preserving surgery. Clin Orthop Relat Res. 2009;467(3): 682–91.
11. Delp SL, Maloney W. Effects of hip center location on the moment-generating capacity of the muscles. J Biomech. 1993;26(4–5):485–99.
12. Doehring TC, Rubash HE, Dore DE. Micromotion measurements with hip center and modular neck length alterations. Clin Orthop Relat Res. 1999; (362):230–9.
13. Doehring TC, Rubash HE, Shelley FJ, Schwendeman LJ, Donaldson TK, Navalgund YA. Effect of superior and superolateral relocations of the hip center on hip joint forces An experimental and analytical analysis. J Arthroplasty. 1996;11(6):693–703.
14. Johnston RC, Brand RA, Crowninshield RD. Reconstruction of the hip. A mathematical approach to determine optimum geometric relationships. J Bone J Surg Am Vol. 1979;61(5):639–52.
15. McGrory BJ, Morrey BF, Cahalan TD, An KN, Cabanela ME. Effect of femoral offset on range of motion and abductor muscle strength after total hip arthroplasty. J Bone Joint Surg British Vol. 1995;77(6):865–9.

16. Kurtz WB, Ecker TM, Reichmann WM, Murphy SB. Factors affecting bony impingement in hip arthroplasty. J Arthroplast. 2010;25(4):624 634 e621–622.
17. Garcia-Rey E, Garcia-Cimbrelo E. Abductor biomechanics clinically impact the Total hip Arthroplasty dislocation rate: a prospective long-term study. J Arthroplast. 2016;31(2):484–90.
18. Sariali E, Klouche S, Mamoudy P. Investigation into three dimensional hip anatomy in anterior dislocation after THA. Influence of the position of the hip rotation Centre. Clin Biomech. 2012;27(6):562–7.
19. Timperley AJ, Biau D, Chew D, Whitehouse SL. Dislocation after total hip replacement - there is no such thing as a safe zone for socket placement with the posterior approach. Hip Int. 2016;26(2):121–7.
20. Callaghan JJ, Salvati EA, Pellicci PM, Wilson PD Jr, Ranawat CS. Results of revision for mechanical failure after cemented total hip replacement, 1979 to 1982. A two to five-year follow-up. J Bone Joint Surg Am Vol. 1985;67(7): 1074–85.
21. Karachalios T, Hartofilakidis G, Zacharakis N, Tsekoura M. A 12- to 18-year radiographic follow-up study of Charnley low-friction arthroplasty The role of the center of rotation. Clin Orthop Relat Res. 1993;296:140–7.
22. Lachiewicz PF, McCaskill B, Inglis A, Ranawat CS, Rosenstein BD. Total hip arthroplasty in juvenile rheumatoid arthritis. Two to eleven-year results. J Bone Joint Surg Am Vol. 1986;68(4):502–8.
23. Yoder SA, Brand RA, Pedersen DR, O'Gorman TW. Total hip acetabular component position affects component loosening rates. Clin Orthop Relat Res. 1988;(228):79–87.
24. Takamatsu T, Shishido T, Takahashi Y, Masaoka T, Tateiwa T, Kubo K, Endo K, Aoki M, Yamamoto K. Radiographic determination of hip rotation center and femoral offset in Japanese adults: a preliminary investigation toward the preoperative implications in Total hip Arthroplasty. Biomed Res Int. 2015;2015:610763.
25. Bjarnason JA, Reikeras O. Changes of center of rotation and femoral offset in total hip arthroplasty. Ann Trans Med. 2015;3(22):355.
26. Kluess D, Martin H, Mittelmeier W, Schmitz KP, Bader R. Influence of femoral head size on impingement, dislocation and stress distribution in total hip replacement. Med Eng Phys. 2007;29(4):465–71.

10

The effectiveness of inpatient rehabilitation after uncomplicated total hip arthroplasty

Justine M. Naylor[1,2,3*], Andrew Hart[1], Rajat Mittal[1], Ian A. Harris[1,2,3] and Wei Xuan[1,3]

Abstract

Background: Inpatient rehabilitation is an expensive option following total hip arthroplasty (THA). We aimed to determine if THA patients who receive inpatient rehabilitation report better hip and quality of life scores post-surgery compared to those discharged directly home.

Methods: Prospective, propensity score matched cohort involving 12 private hospitals across five Australian States. Patients undergoing THA secondary to osteoarthritis were included. Those receiving inpatient rehabilitation for reasons other than choice or who experienced significant health events within 90-days post-surgery were excluded. Comparisons were made between those who did and did not receive inpatient rehabilitation for patient-reported hip pain and function (Oxford Hip Score, OHS) and 'today' health rating (EuroQol 0–100 scale). Rehabilitation provider charges were also estimated and compared.

Results: Two hundred forty-six patients (123 pairs, mean age 67 (10) yr., 66% female) were matched on 19 covariates for their propensity to receive inpatient rehabilitation. No statistically nor clinically significant between-group differences were observed [OHS median difference (IQR): 0 (− 3, 3), $P = 0.60$; 0 (− 1 to 1), $P = 0.91$, at 90 and 365-days, respectively; EuroQol scale median difference 0 (− 10, 12), $P = 0.24$; 0 (− 10, 10), $P = 0.49$; 5 (− 10, 15), $P = 0.09$, at 35-, 90- and 365-days, respectively]. Median rehabilitation provider charges were 10-fold higher for those who received inpatient rehabilitation [median difference $7582 (5649, 10,249), $P < 0.001$]. Sensitivity analyses corroborated the results of the primary analyses.

Conclusion: Utilization of inpatient rehabilitation pathways following THA appears to be low value healthcare. Sustainability of inpatient rehabilitation models may be enhanced if inpatient rehabilitation is reserved for those most impaired or who have limited social supports.

Trial registration: ClinicalTrials.gov Identifier: NCT01899443.

Keywords: Arthroplasty, Arthroplasty, Hip, Rehabilitation, Physical therapy

Background

Total hip arthroplasty (THA) has been heralded as the 'operation of the Century' [1]. Large improvements in mobility and patient-reported outcomes are typically observed with changes far exceeding the small-to-moderate effects seen with non-surgical interventions for arthritis [2–4]. These changes are often experienced in the early subacute phase and improvements are evident regardless of underlying aetiology [3, 5, 6]. Such is the success of the operation, annual increases in the volume of surgery in Australia – as it has elsewhere - have been recorded by the Australian Orthopaedic Association National Joint Replacement Registry (AOANJRR) since 2003 [7]. Presently, over 36,000 THA procedures are undertaken annually in Australia with the majority (~ 60%) performed in the private sector [7]. In 2016, 87,733 primary THA procedures were performed in the United Kingdom (UK) [8]. In the United States (US), it is estimated that up to 562,000 THA cases may be undertaken annually by 2030 [9].

* Correspondence: Justine.Naylor@health.nsw.gov.au
[1]South Western Sydney Clinical School, University of New South Wales, Liverpool Hospital, Elizabeth Drive, Liverpool, NSW 2170, Australia
[2]South West Sydney Local Health District, Locked Bag 7103, Liverpool, NSW 2170, Australia
Full list of author information is available at the end of the article

Following surgery, physiotherapy-led exercise-based rehabilitation is often prescribed [10]. Evidence in support of such prescription is apparent when physiotherapy-led programs are compared to no or minimal intervention following THA. A recent systematic review of randomized trials concluded that physiotherapy-led exercise programs yielded better gait-related outcomes post-THA when compared to no intervention [10]. Interestingly, consistent with the evidence concerning the more intensive clinic-based rehabilitation programs following total knee arthroplasty (TKA) [11–15], clinic-based one-to-one or group-based programs have not been shown to be superior over monitored or unmonitored home-based programs for the recovery of mobility, function and health-related quality of life after THA [10, 16, 17]. Further, the evidence-base lacks randomized trials comparing inpatient-based rehabilitation with less intensive programs. This gap is important to address as utilization of inpatient rehabilitation is common and it is a comparatively costly pathway [18–20]. Recent Australian data from the private sector indicate the median referral rate per surgeon to inpatient rehabilitation is 29% (range 0–100%) [21]. Inpatient utilization rates vary internationally [22, 23], with reported rates as high as 81% (Japan) and 53% (US) and as low as 0% (Spain, Turkey) and 3% (UK) [24].

Only one randomized controlled trial (RCT) has been published aimed at determining the efficacy of inpatient therapy over a non-inpatient alternative following THA [25]. Eighteen days of inpatient rehabilitation was not more effective nor cost-effective compared to eigth domiciliary (physiotherapy) visits following THA or TKA (combined cohort).

Randomized trials are difficult to undertake in general, but they are particularly difficult to perform in the private healthcare sector where consumer and provider preferences are strong drivers of care delivery [26, 27]. This may partly explain why much of the evidence in this space - showing no superiority of the inpatient pathway - is predominantly provided by retrospective and prospective observational studies and administrative datasets [19, 28–30].

In light of the difficulty in performing an RCT, this study, using a propensity score (PS) matched cohort, aimed to determine whether privately insured THA patients who received inpatient rehabilitation, compared to those who did not, had better patient-reported joint and health scores across the first 12 months post-surgery. Informed by the high- and low-level evidence in this area, we hypothesized that the inpatient pathway would not procure superior patient-reported recovery to a level that was clinically meaningful over the alternative.

Methods

This study was nested within a national, prospective observational study involving 19 hospitals across five States [31] (ClinicalTrials.gov Identifier: NCT01899443). We have previously reported the results of a related PS matched cohort aimed at determining the effectiveness of a rehabilitation pathway involving inpatient rehabilitation compared to one not involving inpatient rehabilitation following TKA [32]. The PS is the probability of treatment assignment conditional on observed baseline characteristics [33–38]. Here, matching people on their probability of being allocated to inpatient therapy addresses treatment selection bias based on known patient characteristics.

Ethical approval and funding source

Ethical approval was provided by multiple ethics committees (see *Declarations*). Informed participant consent was obtained. The HCF Research Foundation funded the study, but had no role in study design or data analysis.

Sampling and hospital recruitment

Hospitals contributing to the AOANJRR [7] performing over 275 TKA or THA procedures in 2012, were eligible to participate in the larger study. Related publications describe the sampling procedure which procured 10 public and nine private hospitals [31, 32, 39].

Patient enrolment and eligibility

Patient enrolment and eligibility were identical to that described in an aforementioned study [32]. People awaiting arthroplasty secondary to osteoarthritis between August 2013–December 2014 were screened by site coordinators during their pre-admission review. Eligibility criteria for the larger study included primary surgery, no further arthroplasty planned within 3-months, and the ability to understand the protocol and be followed-up by telephone for 1 year. For this nested study, being privately insured was an additional inclusion criterion. Publicly insured patients were explicitly excluded because the few referred to inpatient rehabilitation (20/317, 6.3%) were primarily referred based on a clinical or social need (14/20). To reduce treatment selection bias and improve generalizability to uncomplicated THA, we also subsequently excluded the privately insured patients referred to inpatient rehabilitation due to slow progress, inadequate social supports (e.g living alone or without the help of an able carer), and those with conditions that would alter their rehabilitation pathway (e.g bilateral surgery or significant complication (defined below) up to 90-days post-surgery).

Data collection

Patient-level variables collected prior to surgery (baseline) included weight, height, insurance status, comorbid conditions including requirement for daily medication, education level, presence of other lower limb or back conditions impairing mobility and patient-reported outcomes measures (PROM). Additional patient-specific data via clinician-completed forms were collected by site coordinators - American Society of Anesthesiologists (ASA) scores, complications, length of stay (LOS), discharge destination, and reason for referral to inpatient rehabilitation if relevant. Patient-reported outcomes, including surveys, ongoing rehabilitation details, complication, and time-off-work (patient, carer) were obtained by researchers by telephone at 35, 90 and 365-days post-surgery. For quality control, clinician-collected data were re-abstracted from the medical record by researchers; significant patient-reported complications were verified by treating hospitals, surgeons or general practitioners.

Complications

Acute complications were stratified according to the Clavien-Dindo Classification whereby the code applied (1–5) is based on the type of care deviation necessitated by the complication [40]. People experiencing the more severe complications (coded ≥3) (e.g pulmonary emboli or dislocation), were excluded. Those experiencing a less severe complication, but one potentially affecting longer-term recovery (e.g neuropraxia) were also excluded. Patients experiencing any surgery-related complication requiring re-admission or any unrelated health event requiring hospital admission up to 90 days post-surgery, were also excluded.

Outcomes

The Oxford Hip Score (OHS) [41] and the Euroqol Visual Analogue Scale for health 'today' (EQVAS) [42, 43], were the primary outcomes. The EQVAS was obtained using a VAS at baseline and verbally at the time of follow-up as the methods have been shown to be equivalent in people awaiting arthroplasty [42].

Rehabilitation charges were determined from the perspective of the provider and the methodology is described elsewhere [32]. Table 1 summarizes the unit costs (AUD) applied for each rehabilitation 'type' encountered. Total provider charges for each participant were calculated based on the length of stay in a rehabilitation facility (where applicable), and the type and frequency of community-based therapy received up to 10-weeks post-surgery, including clinic, domiciliary, supervised hydrotherapy, and day hospital visits. Individuals in the 'No inpatient rehabilitation' group who also had no community-based rehabilitation were assigned $0 rehabilitation provider charges.

Analysis

The projected sample size for the larger study was ~ 2000. Assuming our recruitment pattern was consistent with patterns observed in the AOANJRR [7], we anticipated the definitive sample would comprise 40% THA recipients ($n = 800$), and most of those (60%) ($n = 480$) would be private insured. We conservatively predicted, therefore, our sample for this nested study would exceed 128 people (64 in each treatment group) which is what would be required (80% power, 0.05 significance level) to detect a minimal important between-group difference of 5 points (0.55 of the baseline SD) [41] in the OHS. A sample of 17 would be sufficient to detect a minimally clinically important improvement of 23 (1.36 SD [42, 43] baseline mean) for the EQVAS.

We assessed normality of the data prior to analysis. Mean, median and percentages were used to characterize the cohorts. Covariates of the unmatched cohorts were assessed using independent t-tests and χ^2, whilst covariates and outcomes in the matched (paired) cohorts were assessed using paired t-tests, Wilcoxon signed-rank tests and McNemar tests [33, 34].

Propensity score determination and subsequent matching were determined as follows:

i) PSs for the prediction of referral to inpatient rehabilitation were estimated for all eligible patients using unconditional logistic regression [33–35]. Here, the outcome was treatment group and model covariates included variables thought to influence treatment assignment prior to surgery or the primary outcomes [33–35]. Covariates included baseline Oxford and EQVAS scores, age, body mass index (weight [kg]/height [m]^2), gender, ASA scores,

Table 1 Unit charges assigned to each rehabilitation 'type' encountered

Rehabilitation 'type'	Unit charge	Comments
Inpatient rehabilitation, per night	$700	Based on 2015 private health insurance reimbursement figures. Note: The Australian Public Hospital Cost Report 2013 [46] cites $967.29 per night government. The figure used in this study was considered conservative.
Day Hospital, per visit	$255.15	Based on The Australian Public Hospital Cost Report 2013 [46] (clinic code 40.12, pg 112).
Private physiotherapy clinic visit	$74.90	Based on COMCARE 2015 [47] rates for a standard consultation or return visit. Same charge was applied regardless of group-based on one-to-one based care.
Domiciliary (hospital in the home) visit	$87.10	COMCARE 2015 [47] rate for a standard visit was used.
Physiotherapy supervised hydrotherapy visit	$74.90	Based on COMCARE 2015 [47] rates. Same charge was applied regardless of group-based or one-to-one based care.

Key: All charges in Australian dollars

comorbidity (any condition of the cardiovascular, renal, respiratory, endocrine, liver, central and peripheral nervous systems, and excluding musculoskeletal conditions), other lower limb or back problems limiting mobility, surgical approach ('anterior' or 'other'), and education level (Yr 8 or below, Yrs 9–10, Yrs 11–12, Degree qualified). We also included any measured variable that was found to be significantly different between the treatment groups prior to matching. For this reason, employment status was also used for matching.

ii) We assessed the distribution of the PSs across the two treatment groups using visual inspection and descriptive statistics to ensure there was sufficient overlap (area of common support [33–35]) in probabilities to receive inpatient rehabilitation.

iii) Using caliper matching without replacement [32, 33] we then used the PSs to match each patient who received inpatient rehabilitation in a 1:1 ratio with one who did not. A caliper distance of an absolute difference in PS of 0.05 was employed, equating to 0.28 of the pooled SD of the PSs for the unmatched cohorts. Successful matching was indicated by achieving a standardized mean difference (SMD) [34] between the groups < 0.20 for any given variable (differences < 0.1 are considered negligible [36]; differences up to 0.25 are considered tolerable [35]), and an absence of statistical significant difference ($p < 0.05$).

Variables not included in the matching were 'hospital' and 'surgeon'. The inclusion of these caused non-convergence of the estimate in the PS calculation owing to high correlation between surgeon or hospital and treatment group. To assess the influence of 'hospital' or 'surgeon' on primary outcomes, we performed multivariable linear regression analyses incorporating these variables.

As treatment allocation was not random, we considered the experience of a second arthroplasty (different joint) or later joint-related complication after 90 days as a potential between-group confounder of the primary outcomes. Thus, we conducted sensitivity analyses on the 365-day outcomes excluding persons who experienced such events.

We also performed sensitivity analysis using Rosenbaum bounds [37, 38] on the matched groups to determine the possible effect of unmeasured confounders on the conclusiveness of our results. A sensitivity parameter 'Gamma' was defined in the Rosenbaum bounds analysis. The Gamma indirectly informs how large the effect of the unmeasured confounder would need to be to change the conclusiveness of the matched results. The larger the gamma the more robust the result to an unobserved confounder. A Gamma of 1.2, for example, indicates that an unmeasured confounder would need to increase the likelihood of a patient being assigned to the inpatient group by a factor of 1.2 before the conclusiveness of the results are threatened [36, 44].

All analyses were conducted using SAS V9.4 (SAS Institute Inc. Cary, NC, USA) and the psens function in the rbounds package of R. No imputation was undertaken for missing data.

Results

Figure 1 summarizes cohort ascertainment. From an eligible sample of 431 privately insured primary, unilateral THA patients from 12 hospitals, 123 pairs were matched.

Unmatched cohort

In the unmatched cohort, a PS was estimable for 403 patients. The mean (SD) propensity score for the sample was 0.34 (0.18). Assessment of the overlap of the PSs across the unmatched groups revealed sufficient common support between the two treatment groups [Inpatient Group, $n = 136$ - mean 0.44 (0.18), min 0.06, max 0.85; Non-inpatient Group, $n = 267$ – mean 0.29 (0.16), min 0.02, max 0.85].

Unmatched versus matched cohorts

In the unmatched cohort, the inpatient rehabilitation group was older, had more males, had higher levels of comorbidity, and worse baseline OHSs (Table 2). Unadjusted comparisons between the two groups revealed significantly worse health scores at every time point and worse OHS at 90 days for the Inpatient Group (Additional file 1). Matching lowered the SMD for all but one covariate (it went from 0.10 to 0.11); the largest SMD was 0.14 (Table 3). Acute-care LOS was significantly longer in the Inpatient Group in both the unmatched (6.2 (2.2) vs 4.6 (1.7) days) and matched (5.9 (2.1) vs 5.0 (2.0) days) conditions.

Outcomes – Matched cohort only

35- and 90-days: Table 4 summarizes the comparisons between the matched groups. The Inpatient Group did not have superior outcomes at 35- or 90-days. Time-off-work outcomes were not significantly different. Median rehabilitation provider charges were significantly higher in the Inpatient Group regardless of whether inpatient provider charges were included in the calculation. The Inpatient Group received a greater number of physiotherapy sessions in the community (day hospital as well as clinic) [median difference 5 (IQR 9,0); Inpatient Group - 6 (IQR 2,10), Non-Inpatient Group 0 (IQR 0,3)] (Table 5). A greater proportion of the Inpatient Group were receiving community-based rehabilitation beyond week 10 (23.9% [95%CI 17.1–32.4] vs 12.2% [7.2–20.2]).

365-days: The Inpatient Group did not have superior outcomes at 365 days; the median OHS in both groups was the maximum score possible (48). Sensitivity analyses for the 365-day outcomes involving 114 pairs,

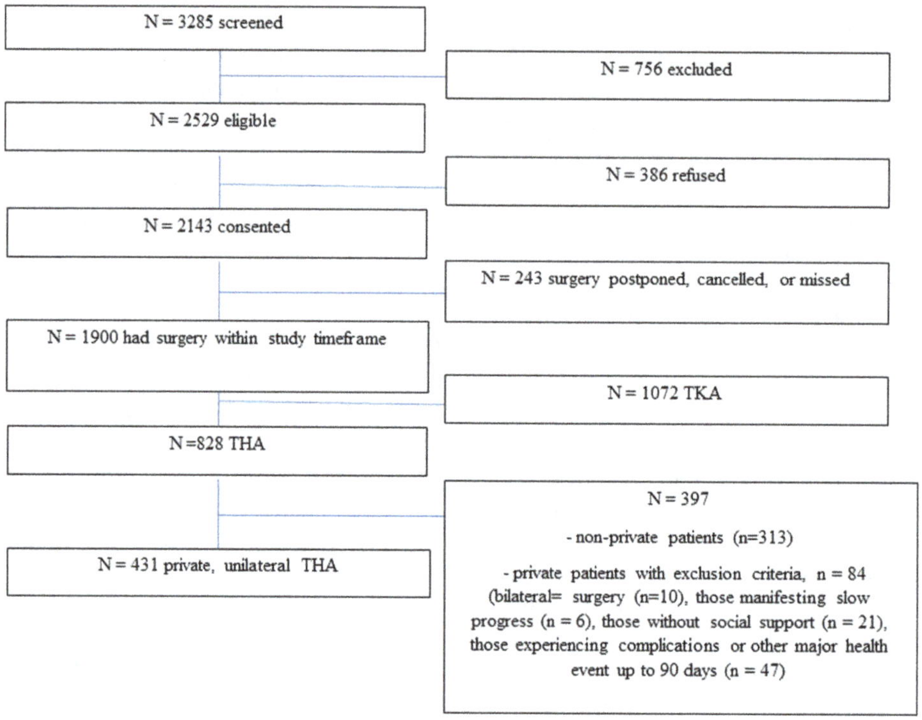

Fig. 1 Cohort ascertainment

yielded the same results (Additional file 2). In the analyses incorporating hospital and surgeon, neither significantly influenced the primary outcomes at any point (Additional file 3). Sensitivity analysis exploring the Rosenbaum bounds for the possible effect of unmeasured confounders yielded gamma values from 1.1 to 6.0 (Additional file 4).

Discussion

Results from a related PS matched cohort involving uncomplicated TKA recipients indicated that the inpatient rehabilitation pathway, compared to the non-inpatient pathway, did not provide superior patient-reported outcomes up to 1-year post-surgery [32]. The current study suggests the same is true for THA recipients. Importantly, the median between-group differences for the OHS and EQVAS were much smaller than the differences estimated to be clinically important. Further, the inpatient rehabilitation pathway was associated with far higher rehabilitation provider charges, and similar time-off -work outcomes for patients and carers. Overall, our findings align with the one aforementioned RCT conducted in this area involving hip arthroplasty [25], and highlight the impressive levels of patient-reported recovery typically seen after this surgery regardless of the rehabilitation pathway taken.

Our study has several strengths. The use of propensity-based scoring has allowed us to report the comparison between two rehabilitation pathways in simple, absolute terms of the outcomes whilst keeping measured covariates balanced between the groups. Most importantly, acceptable matching across all our measured covariates was achieved indicating that any differences in the outcomes observed are not attributable to confounding resulting from differences in these variables. Further, we removed other sources of 'noise' through our strict eligibility criteria, thus, between-group differences in the rate of complications or other major health events are not a source of bias. Finally, our cohort was derived nationally, thus, the characteristics of the unmatched and matched samples should reasonably reflect private patients who undergo THA in Australia.

Despite its advantages, a limitation of the PS method is that bias from unmeasured covariates that may be influencing treatment allocation or outcomes is not eliminated [33–37]. Here, surgeons and hospitals could be viewed as possible confounders. Our supplementary regression analyses, however, allowed us to adjust for the effect of these with neither having a significant effect on outcomes. We did not match on prosthesis type (as there were too many), though we did adjust for what may be considered more important (surgical approach). There is still a possibility that we have not accounted for all unknown confounders, but we think it unlikely we missed important ones. Our sensitivity analyses on the possible effect of unmeasured confounders indicate that an unknown confounder would need to change the

Table 2 Characteristics of total hip arthroplasty recipients: Pre-matching

	Inpatient Rehabilitation Group, *n* = 141	No Inpatient Rehabilitation Group, *n* = 290	Standardized Mean Difference	*P*-value
Age, mean (SD), y	68.7 (9.9)	63.7 (10.4)	0.50	< 0.001
Male, % (n)	68.1 (96)	47.6 (138)	0.42	< 0.001
BMI, mean (SD)	27.7 (4.9)	28.2 (4.9)	0.11	0.27
Education, % (n)				
1	1.4 (2)	1.4 (4)	0.0	0.97
2	21.3 (30)	18.3 (53)	0.08	0.46
3	56.7 (80)	51.4 (149)	0.11	0.30
4	20.6 (29)	29.0 (84)	0.20	0.06
ASA, % (n)				
1	9.2 (13)	19.1 (55)	0.29	0.009
2	54.6 (77)	62.2 (180)	0.15	0.14
3	33.3 (47)	17.4 (50)	0.37	< 0.001
4	2.8 (4)	1.4 (4)	0.10	0.30
Comorbidity, % (n)				
Nil	8.5 (12)	21.7 (63)	0.38	< 0.001
Yes, but no daily medication	5.0 (7)	11.4 (33)	0.24	0.03
Yes, with daily medication	86.5 (122)	66.9 (194)	0.48	< 0.001
Oxford Hip Score, mean (SD)	22.3 (9.2)	24.4 (8.6)	0.24	0.02
EuroQol VAS, mean (SD)	71.4 (19.0)	73.5 (16.3)	0.12	0.24
Other lower limb or back problems limiting mobility, % (n)	51.1 (72)	42.1 (122)	0.18	0.08
Anterior surgical approach	33.8 (48)	31.0 (90)	0.06	0.56
Paid employment, % (n)	31.2 (44)	44.1 (128)	0.27	0.01

Abbreviations: BMI body mass index, *ASA* American Society of Anesthesiology, Education 1 = nil formal; 2 = Year 10 or less; 3 = Year 11 or 12; 4 = Degree or greater; Comorbidity included any conditions of the cardiovascular, renal, respiratory, endocrine, liver, central and peripheral nervous systems, and excluding other musculoskeletal conditions. Note: Standardized mean difference was calculated using the following equation - Standardized Mean Difference[34] = $(\text{Mean1} - \text{Mean 2})/\sqrt{((\text{SD1})^2 + (\text{SD2})^2)/2}$

probability of being allocated to inpatient rehabilitation by at least a factor of 1.3 for five of our outcomes in order to change the statistical significance of the results. Further, if an unmeasured confounder changed a result from non-significant to significant, the effect could still favor discharge directly home. Given we have included many of the known potential confounders in our PS analysis and supplemented this with multiple regressions including 'surgeon' and 'hospital', we contend the important variables are covered. Further, we are not aware of any other unmeasured confounder that the literature points to that would lead us to change our conclusions. That our results concord with the one RCT conducted in this area [25] and several observational studies [28–30], it would appear we have not overlooked major confounding influences.

A potential limitation of our study is the lack of physical performance measures [45]. It remains to be seen if inpatient rehabilitation improves gait or strength more so than rehabilitation provided in other settings. We note gait outcomes have not been shown to be superior in supervised community-based settings compared to home programs when conducted within 8-weeks of surgery [10, 17]. It is possible the same is true for inpatient rehabilitation.

An important caveat is that our results apply to those who have had an uncomplicated recovery and to those for whom discharge destination was a choice. We contend then that the inpatient rehabilitation pathway remains an important option for those with complications, limited social supports, and poor progress acutely. Based on the criteria used here, we estimate that a small minority (approximately 14%) of privately insured patients may require inpatient rehabilitation based on these three conditions (9.1, 4.1 and 1.2% respectively) (Fig. 1). We note, however, recent data from the US suggest discharge to inpatient rehabilitation facilities following THA is associated with increased morbidity [23]. A reasonable approach, therefore, would be to avoid referral to inpatient facilities unless alternatives are exhausted.

A final important caveat is that our cost data pertain only to the first 90 days after surgery and only include rehabilitation provider charges. It is likely that there were continued cost differences beyond this time given a

Table 3 Characteristics of total hip arthroplasty recipients: Post-matching

	Inpatient Rehabilitation Group, *n* = 123	No Inpatient Rehabilitation Group, *n* = 123	Standardized Mean Difference	*P*-value
Age, mean (SD), y	67.8 (10.0)	66.9 (10.6)	0.09	0.48
Male, % (n)	64.2	68.3	0.09	0.50
BMI, mean (SD)	27.8 (4.8)	28.0 (5.1)	0.04	0.76
Education, % (n)				
1	1.6 (2)	1.6 (2)	0	1.0
2	20.3 (25)	22.80 (28)	0.06	0.64
3	55.3 (68)	51.2 (63)	0.08	0.52
4	22.8 (28)	24.4 (30)	0.04	0.76
ASA, % (n)				
1	10.6 (13)	7.3 (9)	0.11	0.37
2	59.4 (73)	61.0 (75)	0.03	0.79
3	28.5 (35)	28.5 (35)	0.0	1.0
4	1.6 (2)	3.3 (4)	0.11	0.70
Comorbidity, % (n)				
Nil	8.9 (11)	8.9 (11)	0	1.0
Yes, but no daily medication	4.9 (6)	3.3 (4)	0.08	0.52
Yes, with daily medication	86.2 (106)	87.8 (108)	0.05	0.71
Oxford Hip Score, mean (SD)	23.1 (8.9)	21.9 (8.2)	0.14	0.27
EuroQol VAS, mean (SD)	71.7 (19.4)	70.8 (16.8)	0.05	0.69
Other lower limb or back problems limiting mobility, % (n)	47.2 (58)	48.8 (60)	0.03	0.80
Anterior surgical approach	33.8 (42)	31.0 (38)	0.06	0.56
Paid employment, No. (%)	34.2 (42)	31.7 (39)	0.05	0.68

Abbreviations: BMI body mass index, *ASA* American Society of Anesthesiology; Education 1 = nil formal; 2 = Year 10 or less; 3 = Year 11 or 12; 4 = Degree or greater; Comorbidity included any conditions of the cardiovascular, renal, respiratory, endocrine, liver, central and peripheral nervous systems, and excluding other musculoskeletal conditions Note: Standardized mean difference was calculated using the following equation - Standardized Mean Difference[34] = (Mean1 – Mean 2)/$\sqrt{((SD1)^2 + (SD2)^2)/2}$

Table 4 Outcomes at 35, 90 and 365 days in the matched cohorts

	35 days				90 days				365 days			
	Inpatient	No Inpatient	*P*-value	Median difference	Inpatient	No Inpatient	*P*-value	Median difference	Inpatient	No Inpatient	*P*-value	Median difference
OHS median (IQR)					46 (41, 48	46 (41, 48)	0.60	0 (−3, 3)	48 (46, 48)	48 (46, 48)	0.91	0 (−1, 1)
EQVAS today, median (IQR)	80 (75, 90)	85 (80, 90)	0.24	0 (−10, 12)	85 (80, 95)	90 (80, 95)	0.49	0 (−10, 10)	85 (75, 95)	90 (80, 95)	0.09	5 (−10, 15)
Rehabilitation costs, $, median (IQR)					7620 (5796, 10,399)	0 (0, 225)	< 0.001	-$7582 (−10,249, −5649)				
Rehabilitation costs, $, excluding inpatient costs					$824 (87, 2041)	0 (0,225)	< 0.001	-$749 (− 1786, 0)				
Time off paid employment > 6 weeks, % (95% CI)					24 (17, 32)	21 (15, 30)	0.66	-2 (−13, 8)				
Carer time off paid employment, Yes/No, % (95%CI)	13 (8, 21)	13 (8, 21)	1.0	0 (−8, 8)								

Legend: *OHS* Oxford Hip Score, *EQVAS* EuroQol Visual analogue scale

Table 5 Profile of community-based supervised rehabilitation received amongst those who received it

	Inpatient Group			No Inpatient Group		
	%	No. of visits, mean (sd)	Median	%	No. of visits, mean (sd)	Median
Receiving community rehabilitation	79	8.7 (4.5)	8	35	5 .4 (3.7)	5
Type of community-based rehabilitation						
1-to-1 clinic	36	5.6 (4.4)	5	37	3.7 (2.4)	3
1-to-1 hydrotherapy	11	6.2 (3.2)	7	11	3.3 (1.3)	3
Group-based clinic	13	6.3 (2.9)	5	11	5.0 (3.6)	6
Group-based hydrotherapy	6	5.3 (3.8)	4	9	4.5 (2.6)	4
Domiciliary	1	1	1	40	6.2 (3.6)	7
Day Hospital program	62	8.7 (3.8)	8	6	7.0 (1.4)	7

Note: The data summarise attendance of those who had ongoing supervised rehabilitation after the acute hospital. Those who did not have ongoing supervised rehabilitation after discharge from hospital are excluded from these calculations. Interpretation example – 62% of those who had ongoing supervised rehabilitation after discharge from inpatient rehabilitation participated in a Day Hospital program compared to 6% of those who did not participate in inpatient rehabilitation. The percentages under 'type' are not additive as each type is not mutually exclusive

greater proportion of the Inpatient Group were still receiving community-based therapy beyond 10 weeks.

Conclusions

In conclusion, in the absence of sufficient high-level evidence to date, our study provides robust and useful signals concerning the comparative effectiveness and provider charges of a pathway that includes inpatient rehabilitation after uncomplicated THA. Consistent with the one published RCT in this space [25], our data indicate a rehabilitation pathway incorporating inpatient rehabilitation is not likely to be cost-effective for uncomplicated THA recipients. Our data and data elsewhere support the use of community-based and home-based programs to secure impressive levels of patient-reported recovery.

Additional files

Additional file 1: Unadjusted analyses. Unadjusted analysis between treatment group and outcome.

Additional file 2: Sensitivity analysis 1. Sensitivity analysis for 365 day outcomes.

Additional file 3: Sensitivity analysis 2. Sensitivity analysis to determine effect of 'hospital' and 'surgeon'.

Additional file 4: Sensitivity analysis 3. Sensitivity analysis to determine effect of the unmeasured confounders.

Abbreviations

95%CI: 95% confidence interval; AOANJRR: Australian Orthopaedic Association National Joint Replacement Registry; ASA: American Society of Anesthesiologists; AUD: Australian dollars; EQVAS: EuroQol Visual Analogue Scale; LOS: Length of stay; OHS: Oxford Hip Score; PS: Propensity score; RCT: Randomized controlled trial; SD: Standard deviation; SMD: Standardized mean difference; THA: Total hip arthroplasty; TKA: Total knee arthroplasty; UK: United Kingdom; US: United States; yr.: Year

Acknowledgements

Project manager – Helen Badge. Data entry - Shirley Cross, Carolyn Gray-Robens, Kristen Kovacic. Patients and hospitals participating in the study.

Funding

The study was funded by the HCF Research Foundation The funder did not have any influence on the study aims, design, analysis or write-up.

Authors' contributions

JMN – study conception, design, data collection, data collation, analysis, manuscript draft, final manuscript, obtainment of funding, supervision of contributors. RM – supervision of contributors, data collection, manuscript draft, approval of final manuscript. AH - data collection, data collation, analysis, manuscript draft, approval of final manuscript. IAH - manuscript draft, final manuscript, obtainment of funding, supervision of contributors. WX - analysis, manuscript draft, final manuscript, obtainment of funding. All authors read and approved the final manuscript.

Authors' information

JMN - PhD, BAppSc (Phty).
AH - MBBS.
RM - PhD, MBBS, MMed (Clin Epi).
IAH - PhD, MMed (Clin Epi), MBBS, FRACS (Orth).
WX - PhD

Consent for publication

Not applicable.

Competing interests

The authors declare that they have no competing interests.

Author details

[1]South Western Sydney Clinical School, University of New South Wales, Liverpool Hospital, Elizabeth Drive, Liverpool, NSW 2170, Australia. [2]South West Sydney Local Health District, Locked Bag 7103, Liverpool, NSW 2170, Australia. [3]Ingham Institute of Applied Medical Research, Westfields Liverpool, PO Box 3151, Liverpool, NSW 2170, Australia.

References

1. Learmonth ID, Young C, Rorabeck C. The operation of the century: total hip replacement. Lancet. 2007;370(9597):1508–19.
2. Vissers MM, Bussmann JB, de Groot IB, Verhaar JAN, Reijman M. Physical functioning four years after total hip or knee arthroplasty. Gait Posture. 2013;38:310–5.
3. Naylor JM, Harmer AR, Heard RC, Harris IA. Patterns of recovery following knee and hip replacement in an Australian cohort. Aust Health Rev. 2009;33: 124–35.

4. Ng CY, Ballantyne JA, Brenkel IJ. Quality of life and functional outcome after primary total hip replacement. A five-year follow-up. J Bone Joint Surg Br. 2007;89:868–73.
5. Yuasa T, Maezawa K, Nozawa M, Kaneko K. Cementless total hip arthroplasty for patients with rheumatoid arthritis: a more than 10-year follow-up. Eur J Orthop Surg Traumatol. 2016;26:599–603.
6. Colo E, Rijnen WH, Gardeniers JW, van Kampen A, Schreurs BW. Satisfying results of primary hip arthroplasty in patients with hip dysplasia at a mean follow-up of 20 years. Clin Orthop Relat Res. 2016;474:2462–8.
7. National Joint Replacement Registry. Analysis of State and Territory Health Data. All Arthroplasty. Supplementary Report 2017. Adelaide: AOA; 2017.
8. National Joint Registry. 14th Annual Report 2017. http://www.njrreports.org.uk/Portals/0/PDFdownloads/NJR%2014th%20Annual%20Report%202017.pdf. Accessed 3 July 2018.
9. Kurtz S, Ong K, Lau E, Mowat F, Halpern M. Projections of primary and revision hip and knee arthroplasty in the United States from 2005 to 2030. J Bone Joint Surg Am. 2007;89:780e5.
10. Coulter CL, Scarvell JM, Neeman TM, Smith PN. Physiotherapist directed rehabilitation exercises in the outpatient or home setting improve strength, gait speed, and cadence after elective total hip replacement: a systematic review. J Physiother. 2013;59:219–26.
11. Kramer JF, Speechley M, Bourne M, Rorabeck C. Comparison of clinic- and home-based rehabilitation programs after total knee arthroplasty. Clin Orthop Relat Res. 2003;410:225–34.
12. Mockford BJ, Thompson NW, Humphreys P, Beverland DE. Does a standard outpatient physiotherapy regime improve the range of knee motion after primary total knee arthroplasty? J Arthroplast. 2008;23:1110–4.
13. Han ASY, Nairn L, Harmer AR, Crosbie J, March L, Parker D, et al. Early rehabilitation after total knee replacement surgery: a multicenter, noninferiority, randomized clinical trial comparing a home exercise program with usual outpatient care. Arth Car Res. 2015;67:196–202.
14. Russell TG, Buttrum P, Wootton R, Jull GA. Internet-based outpatient telerehabilitation for patients following total knee arthroplasty: a randomized controlled trial. J Bone Joint Surg Am. 2011;93:113–20.
15. Ko V, Naylor J, Harris I, Crosbie J, Yeo A, Mittal R. One-to-one therapy is not superior to group or home-based therapy after total knee arthroplasty: a randomized, superiority trial. J Bone Joint Surg Am. 2013;95:1942–9.
16. Austin MS, Urbani BT, Fleischman AN, Fernando ND, Purtill JJ, Hozack WJ, et al. Formal physical therapy after total hip arthroplasty is not required: a randomized controlled trial. J Bone Joint Surg Am. 2017;99:648–55.
17. Coulter C, Perriman DM, Neeman TM, Smith PN, Scarvell JM. Supervised or unsupervised rehabilitation after total hip replacement provides similar improvements for patients: a randomised controlled trial. Arch Phys Med Rehabil. 2017;98:2253–64. https://doi.org/10.1016/j.apmr.2017.03.032
18. Bozic KJ, Ward L, Vail TP, Maze M. Bundled payments in total joint arthroplasty: targeting opportunities for quality improvement and cost reduction. Clin Orth Rel Res. 2014;472:188–93.
19. Soderstrom L, Tousignant P, Kaufman T. The health and cost effects of substituting home care for inpatient acute care: a review of the evidence. Can Med Ass J. 1999;160:1151–5.
20. Krummenauer F. The incremental cost effectiveness of in-patient versus outpatient rehabilitation after total hip arthroplasty. Results of a pilot investigation. Eur J Med Res. 2008;13:267–74.
21. RACS Surgical Practical Variation Report - Orthopaedic procedures. https://surgeons.org/news/surgical-variance-reports/. Accessed 3 July 2018.
22. Hart A, Bergeron SG, Epure L, Huk O, Zukor D, Antoniou J. Comparison of US and Canadian perioperative outcomes and hospital efficiency after total hip and knee arthroplasty. JAMA Surg. 2015;150:990–8.
23. Fu MC, Samuel AM, Sculco PK, MacLean CH, Padgett DE, McLawhorn AS. Discharge to inpatient facilities after total hip arthroplasty is associated with increased postdischarge morbidity. J Arthroplast. 2017;32:S144–9.
24. Waddell J, Johnson K, Hein W, Raabe J, Fitzgerald G, Turibio F. Orthopedic practice in total hip arthroplasty and total knee arthroplasty: results from the global Orthopaedic registry (GLORY). Am J Orthop. 2010;39(9 Suppl):5–13.
25. Mahomed NN, Davis AM, Hawker G, Badley E, Davey JR, Syed KA, et al. Inpatient compared with home-based rehabilitation following primary unilateral total hip or knee replacement: a randomized controlled trial. J Bone Joint Surg Am. 2008;90:1673–80.
26. Buhagiar MA, Naylor JM, Simpson G, Harris IA, Kohler F. Understanding consumer and clinician preferences and decision making for rehabilitation following arthroplasty in the private sector. BMC Health Serv Res. 2017;17(1): 415. https://doi.org/10.1186/s12913-017-2379-9.
27. Zuckerman JD. Inpatient rehabilitation after total joint replacement. JAMA. 1998;279:880.
28. Cushner F, Agnelli G, Fitzgerald G, Warwick D. Complications and functional outcomes after total hip arthroplasty and total knee arthroplasty: results from the global Orthopaedic registry (GLORY). Am J Orthop. 2010;39(9 Suppl):22–8.
29. Benz T, Angst F, Oesch P, Hilfiker R, Lehmann S, Mueller Mebes C, et al. Comparison of patients in three different rehabilitation settings after knee or hip arthroplasty: a natural observational, prospective study. BMC Musculoskel Dis. 2015;16:317.
30. Tribe KL, Lapsley HM, Cross MJ, Courtenay BG, Brooks PM, March LM. Selection of patients for inpatient rehabilitation or direct home discharge following total joint replacement surgery: a comparison of health status and out-of-pocket expenditure of patients undergoing hip and knee arthroplasty for osteoarthritis. Chronic Illness. 2005;1:289–302.
31. Chua M, Hart A, Harris IA, Mittal R, Xuan W, Naylor JM. Early mobilisation after total hip or knee arthroplasty: a multicentre prospective observational study. PLoS One. 2017;12(6):e0179820. https://doi.org/10.1371/journal.pone.0179820
32. Naylor JM, Hart A, Mittal R, Harris IA, Xuan W. The value of inpatient rehabilitation after uncomplicated total knee arthroplasty: a propensity score analysis. Med J Aust. 2017;207:250–5.
33. Austin PC. Balance diagnostics for comparing the distribution of baseline covariates between treatment groups in propensity-score matched samples. Stat Med. 2009;28:3083–107.
34. D'Agostino RB. Tutorial in biostatistics. Propensity score methods for bias reduction in the comparison of a treatment to a non-randomized control group. Stat Med. 1998;17:2265–81.
35. Stuart EA, Lee BK, Leacy FP. Prognostic score–based balance measures for propensity score methods in comparative effectiveness research. J Clin Epidemiol. 2013;66:S84–90.
36. Haukoos JS, Lewis RJ. The propensity score. JAMA. 2015;314:1637–8.
37. Caliendo M, Kopeinig S. Some practical guidance for the implementation of propensity score matching. IZA Discussion Paper No. 1588, 2005. http://ftp.iza.org/dp1588.pdf. Accessed 3 July 2018.
38. Rosenbaum PR. Sensitivity analysis in observational studies. In: Everitt BS, Howell DC, editors. Encyclopaedia of statistics in behavioral science. Chichester: Wiley; 2005.
39. Naylor JM, Descallar J, Grootemaat M, Badge H, Harris IA, Simpson G, et al. Is satisfaction with the acute-care experience higher amongst consumers treated in the private sector? A survey of public and private sector arthroplasty recipients. PLoS One. 2016;11(8):e0159799. https://doi.org/10.1371/ journal.pone.0159799 23.
40. Clavien PA, Barkun J, de Oliveira ML, Vauthey JN, Dindo D, Schulick RD, et al. The Clavien-Dindo classification of surgical complications. Ann Surg. 2009;250:187–96.
41. Beard DJ, Harris K, Dawson J, Doll H, Murray DW, Carr AJ, et al. Meaningful changes for the Oxford hip and knee scores after joint replacement surgery. J Clin Epidemiol. 2015;68:73–9.
42. Chatterji R, Naylor JM, Harris IA, Armstrong E, Davidson E, Ekmejian R, et al. An equivalence study: are patient-completed and telephone interview equivalent modes of administration for the EuroQol survey. Health Qual Life Outcomes. 2017;15(1):18. https://doi.org/10.1186/s12955-017-0596-x.
43. Paulsen A, Roos E, Pedersen A, Overgaard S. Minimal clinically important improvement (MCII) and patient acceptable symptom state (PASS) in total hip arthroplasty (THA) patients 1 year postoperatively. Acta Orthop. 2014; 85:39–48.

11

A ceramic bone substitute containing gentamicin gives good outcome in trochanteric hip fractures treated with dynamic hip screw and in revision of total hip arthroplasty

Mindaugas Stravinskas[1], Sarunas Tarasevicius[1], Simonas Laukaitis[1], Malin Nilsson[2*], Deepak Bushan Raina[2] and Lars Lidgren[2]

Abstract: Background: The primary objective was to investigate the clinical and radiological outcome in patients undergoing major hip surgery using a novel antibiotic containing bone substitute for local augmentation in trochanteric fracture fixation or revision of total hip arthroplasty (THA).

Methods: We implanted a novel biphasic bone substitute CERAMENT™|G consisting of hydroxyapatite, calcium sulphate and gentamicin for bone regeneration and local antibiotic delivery in 20 patients treated surgically for trochanteric femoral fracture or uncemented hip revision. Preoperative, postoperative, 3 months and 1 year clinical and radiological assessment were performed including registration of any complications. In one trochanteric fracture patient, histological analyses were performed of bone biopsies taken at removal of hardware.

Results: None of the trochanteric fractures or revision of THA showed any large migration. No local wound disturbances were seen and no infection was observed at one year follow-up. All trochanteric fractures healed at 3 months with a minimal sliding screw displacement on average 3 mm. Radiological analysis showed signs of bone remodeling and new bone formation in the substitute, illustrated also by histology in the biopsies taken from one trochanteric fracture at one year post-op.

Conclusions: Local CERAMENT™|G was shown to be safe in a limited prospective major hip surgery study. Remodeling of the bone graft substitute was observed in all patients.

Keywords: Hip surgery, Infection, Ceramic bone substitute, Antibiotics, Gentamicin, Bone remodeling

Background

Deep bone and joint infections after orthopaedic procedures are a devastating complication which may require revision surgery and longterm systemic antimicrobial treatment [1]. Conventional approaches used to treat acute infections may not work for chronic biofilm infections and in many cases promote antimicrobial resistance and further biofilm formation [2, 3]. Use of antibiotic-impregnated cement spacers is the standard method to provide direct local delivery of antibiotics which are mainly released from the surface of the cement and limited from the voids within the cement. The most extensively studied and commercially available implant for controlled local release of antibiotics is non-biodegradable polymethylmethacrylate (PMMA) bone cement [4].

CERAMENT™|G is an injectable biphasic bone substitute, composed of 60% calcium sulphate, which resorbs and provides gradual porosity for new bone ingrowth, supported by 40% hydroxyapatite that acts as matrix for bone cells. It also contains gentamicin

* Correspondence: malin@lalit.se
[2]Department of Orthopedics, Lund University Hospital, Lund, Sweden
Full list of author information is available at the end of the article

sulphate (175 mg/10 mL). Recent studies have shown promising results of CERAMENT™|G on bone regeneration, and prevention or eradication of infection [5]. Dvorzhinskiy et al. described where CERAMENT™|G was used for treating osteomyelitis in the tibias of rats [6]. The gentamicin containing bone substitute increased new bone growth as compared with empty control in a debrided osteomyelitic environment. Animals treated with CERAMENT™|G showed no evidence of infection and retained a higher bone mass compared to the contralateral (non-operated) side 6 months post-op.

In a previous study, we investigated local elution of gentamicin in patients treated for trochanteric fractures or revision of total hip arthroplasty (THA) when CERAMENT™|G was used for bone defect reconstruction [7]. A high level of gentamicin was initially detected in the wound drainage fluid, followed by a decreasing concentration, while in blood serum gentamicin concentration was below the recommended systemic level. However, we found no studies investigating the clinical and radiological outcomes of trochanteric fractures or revision of THA patients, when bone substitute containing antibiotics was used in major hip surgery. This study is a continuation of our previous work [7] and the aim was to investigate the clinical and radiological outcomes of patients undergoing trochanteric fracture fixation or revision of THA with CERAMENT™|G used for bone defect augmentation.

Methods

From June 2014 to September 2016, 20 patients with trochanteric fracture internal fixation surgery using a dynamic hip screw (DHS) and aseptic revision of THA with uncemented stem were included in a single center, prospective, observational study. Patients with systemic aminoglycoside usage before surgery, septic process in the hip joint, psychiatric or neurological disorders, renal failure, impaired hearing, and hypersensitivity to aminoglycosides were excluded.

Synthetic bone graft substitute (CERAMENT™|G, BONESUPPORT AB, Lund, Sweden) was used to augment the bone defects at implantation of either DHS or after implantation of cementless femoral component. For the fracture patients, CERAMENT™|G was injected into the bone defect in the trochanteric region after placing the dynamic screw but before plate implantation (Fig. 1). While in the revision of THA cases CERAMENT™|G was injected into visible bone defects around the proximal part of the prosthesis after distal fixation of the uncemented stem (Fig. 2). In cases where a cemented acetabular component was chosen, plain PMMA bone cement (without antibiotic) was used for component fixation.

X-ray examination of the operated site was performed the first day after surgery, and patients were mobilized and started to walk using crutches. Clinical and radiological outcome was performed at 3 months and at 1 year follow-up.

For the trochanteric fracture patients radiological analysis included anteroposterior (AP) and lateral views. We estimated postoperative fracture reposition and it was considered satisfactory if femoral neck angle was < 10° of varus or < 15° of valgus compared to the uninjured contralateral hip and the fracture displacement was < 5 mm on both AP and lateral post-operative radiographs [8].

The position of the lag screw was assessed from the mapping of the femoral head and the tip-apex distance (TAD). Fixation was deemed to be adequate if the lag screw was placed to central/central (AP/lateral view), inferior/central, or inferior/posterior Cleveland zones [9]. A TAD of less than 25 mm was considered optimal. Sliding was measured along the dynamic screw. The

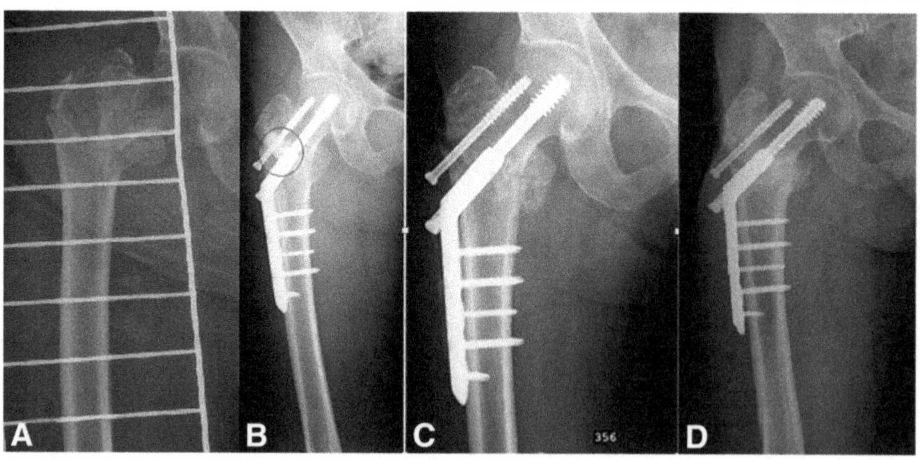

Fig. 1 DHS patient's proximal part of the femur healing. Preoperative image shows the trochanteric fracture (**a**). In the postoperative image (**b**) CERAMENT™|G is seen (circled in red). In the X-ray image after 3 months (**c**), the bone graft substitute is difficult to differentiate from bone. Image after 1 year (**d**) shows complete healing. This patient needed DHS removal because of local discomfort

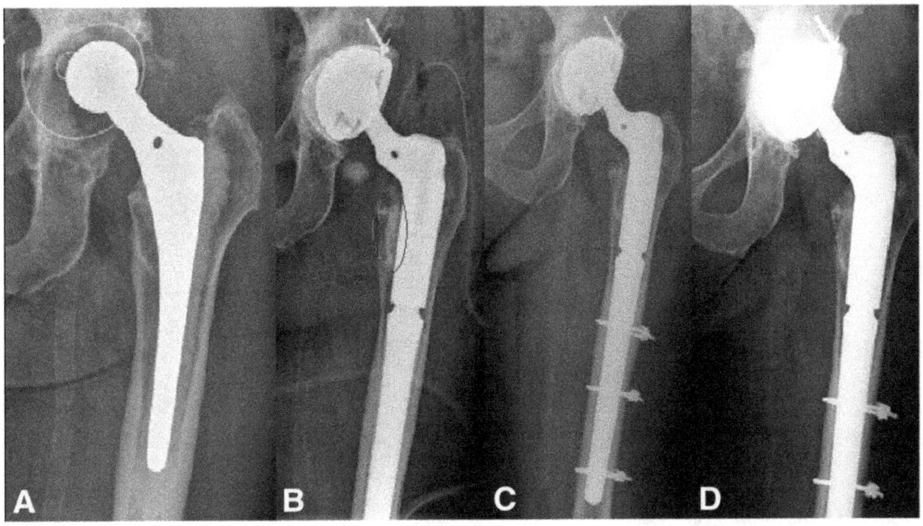

Fig. 2 Revision of THA using a cementless femoral component. Preoperative image shows unstable components (**a**). The proximal part of the femur postoperatively (**b**) shows CERAMENT™|G present (circled in red). In the X-ray after 3 months (**c**), the bone graft substitute is difficult to differentiate from bone. Image after 1 year (**d**) shows bone healing

fracture was considered as healed if bone trabeculae were visible across the fracture line. Absence of bridging bone at the line of the fracture after 3 months was considered as non-union [10].

For revision of THA patients, the radiological analysis was performed of the proximal part of the femur where the CERAMENT™|G had been injected. Bone density changes such as: new bone formation, cortical healing as well as subsidence of implant were analyzed.

To evaluate functional outcome at 3 months and 1 year follow-up, patients were asked if they had pain at the operated site and if they were able to bear weight on the operated leg. They were also asked to evaluate their quality of life (QoL) from 1 to 100 using VAS (Visual Analog Scale).

Additionally, all wound or systemic complications related to surgery were recorded.

One patient had hardware removal due to local discomfort of the DHS after 1 year. At the time of the surgery a bone biopsy from the CERAMENT™|G implantation site was taken for further histology analysis. The biopsy was fixed in 4% formalin in neutral buffered saline overnight followed by decalcification in 10% EDTA solution for 3 weeks. Routine paraffin embedding procedures were used before sectioning the specimen to a thickness of 5 μm using a semi-automaticmicrotome (Thermo Scientific, U.S.A). Sections were allowed to adhere to coated glass slides for 48 h prior to routine H&E staining.

Results

The prospective study consisted of 20 patients (3 men, 17 women) with a mean age of 74.8 years, (±SD 9.5 years, range 57–90 years) who underwent either trochanteric fracture fixation using DHS or aseptic revision of THA using uncemented distal fixation modular stem (10 for each group) (Tables 1 and 2). The distal stem used was tapered and the whole stem coated with Porous Plasma Spray (PPS®) (Arcos, ZimmerBiomet, USA). A mean of 7.28 mL (±SD 1.10 mL, range 5–9 mL) of CERAMENT™|G was implanted for patients with trochanteric hip fracture and mean of 7.61 mL (±SD 0.49 mL, range 7–9 mL) for revision of THA patients.

Out of 20 included patients, one trochanteric fracture patient died during follow-up unrelated to the implantation of CERAMENT™|G (myocardial infarction), and one refused follow-up, leaving 8 trochanteric fracture and 10 revision of THA patients for final analysis.

Radiological analysis of trochanteric fractures showed that reposition of bone fragments was satisfactory according to previously described criteria in all cases. AP view evaluation revealed that the dynamic screw was placed in the center of the femoral head for 9 patients while for one patient it was placed inferiorly, while in lateral view all dynamic screws were placed centrally. Mean TAD value was 19.7 mm (±SD 3.3 mm, range 14.3–25.2 mm) (Table 3).

Table shows the type of the fracture according to the AO classification, the placement of the lag screw in femoral head, tip-apex distance (TAD), caput-collum-diaphyseal (CCD) angles and femoral neck shortening after 3 months and 1 year follow-up.

The mean sliding distance of the screw (shortening of the femoral neck) was 3.1 mm (±SD 3.5 mm, range 0.7–11.8 mm) after 3 months and remained almost unchanged at 1 year follow-up (Table 3). Caput-collum-

Table 1 Trochanteric fracture patient data

Patient No.	Age	Gender	Pain in op leg	Clin function	VAS for QoL 3 months	VAS for QoL 1 year	Outcome	Complications
1	83	F	No	Full	85	90	Healed fr.	–
2	83	F	No	Can't walk	30[a]	No foll up	No foll up	–
3	62	F	No	Full	65	88	Healed fr.	–
4	75	F	No	Full	70	80	Healed fr.	–
5	85	F	Died	–	–	–	–	–
8	64	F	No	Difficult	80	80	Healed fr.	–
14	81	F	No	Full	60	80	Healed fr.	–
15	80	F	No	Full	80	90	Healed fr.	–
19	78	F	No	Full	80	80	Healed fr.	–
20	89	F	No	Full	50	90	Healed fr.	–
Mean	78.0				71.3	84.8		
S.D.	8.3				11.4	4.8		

[a]excluded from Mean and S.D. due to no follow-up at 1 year

diaphyseal (CCD) angles of the operated hips were in the range of 120°-134° (mean 129.9° ± SD 3.7°), and similar to the CDD angles of the healthy contralateral hip (mean 129.1° ± SD 2.5°) (Table 3), with no varus or valgus deformity after fracture fixation. Radiological bone healing was observed in all available trochanteric fracture patients for follow-up.

At 3 months follow-up, 7 patients were walking independently, with no need of walking aids, while one patient had some walking problems and used a cane for support. The same results were observed at 1 year follow-up (Table 1).

Radiological visualisation of CERAMENT™|G was possible on postoperative x-rays, however at 3 months and 1 year follow-up the material was difficult to differ from new bone growing into the apatite scaffold (Fig. 1).

One trochanteric fracture patient (No 3) had additional surgery after 1 year follow-up, the hardware was removed due to some discomfort in trochanteric region (Fig. 1). During the surgery, the extraction of the dynamic screw was extremely difficult, probably due to excessive bone ongrowth on the hardware. Bone biopsies were taken from the trochanteric region for subsequent analysis. Histological analysis showed viable and mature bone in all biopsies (Fig. 3). High magnification of one of the specimens showed the presence of a loose hydroxyapatite conglomerate (indicated by the black arrows in Fig. 4). A second specimen showed islands of viable trabecular bone and the space between the trabeculae was filled with marrow like tissue (Fig. 5).

All 10 revision of THA patients reported having full recovery at 3 months, which was unchanged at 1 year follow-up. Two complained of light pain in the

Table 2 Cementless hip revision patient data

Patient No.	Age	Gender	Pain in op leg	Leg function	VAS of QoL at 3 months	VAS of QoL at 1 year	Defect type (Paprovsky classification)		Graft healing	Complications
							acetabulum	femur		
6	67	F	No	Full	60	75	IIb	IIIa	yes	–
7	62	F	No	Full	75	80	IIa	IIIb	yes	–
9	67	M	No	Full	70	70	IIa	IIIb	yes	–
10	90	M	No	Full	90	100	IIIa	IIIa	yes	–
11	84	F	Yes	Full	60	85	IIIa	IIIb	yes	–
12	57	M	No	Full	40	78	IIb	IIIa	yes	–
13	68	F	No	Full	65	80	IIIa	II	yes	–
16	68	F	No	Full	85	95	IIb	II	yes	–
17	74	F	Yes	Full	50	65	IIa	IIIa	yes	–
18	78	F	No	Full	70	90	IIIa	IIIa	yes	–
Mean	71.5				66.5	81.8				
S.D.	9.6				14.3	10.4				

Table 3 Data of the trochanteric fractures - screw placement, angles and neck shortening

Patient No.	Fracture type	Screw position	TAD (mm)	CCD angle after op. (°)	CCD angle healthy leg (°)	CCD angle at 3 months (°)	CCD angle 1 year (°)	Neck shortening at 3 months (mm)	Total shortening at 1 year (mm)
1	A3.1	Central/Central	25.2	131	134	130	128	11.8	13.4
2	A1.2	Central/Inferior	14.3	133	130	–	–	–	–
3	A2.1	Central/ Central	22.2	130	128	127	127	4.7	6.5
4	A1.2	Central/ Central	17.8	129	130	129	128	2.4	2.7
5	A2.1	Central/ Central	16.2	120	130	died	–	–	–
8	A1.2	Central/ Central	19.7	134	131	133	133	2.0	2.2
14	A2.1	Central/ Central	17.6	132	127	128	128	0.7	1.1
15	A1.1	Central/ Central	18.6	129	130	126	126	0.8	0.9
19	A1.3	Central/ Central	20.3	132	126	130	130	1.0	1.2
20	A1.1	Central/ Central	24.6	129	125	129	–	1.2	
Mean			19.7	129.9	129.1	129.0	128.6	3.1	4.0
S.D.			3.3	3.7	2.5	2.0	2.1	3.5	4.2

operated hip (Table 2) but radiological analysis showed that the bone density had increased in the proximal part of the femurs, where the bone defect was filled with CERAMENT™|G. No bone resorption was observed. No signs of osteolysis or loosening were observed in the acetabular or femoral components (Table 2).

Mean value of VAS for quality of life for the hip revision patients after 3 months was 66.5 (±SD 14.3, range 40–90) and at 1 year 81.8 (±SD 10.4, range 65–100), while for DHS patients the mean value was 71.3 (±SD 11.4, range 50–80) at 3 months and 84.8 (±SD 4.8, range 80–90) at 1 year follow-up (Tables 1 and 2).

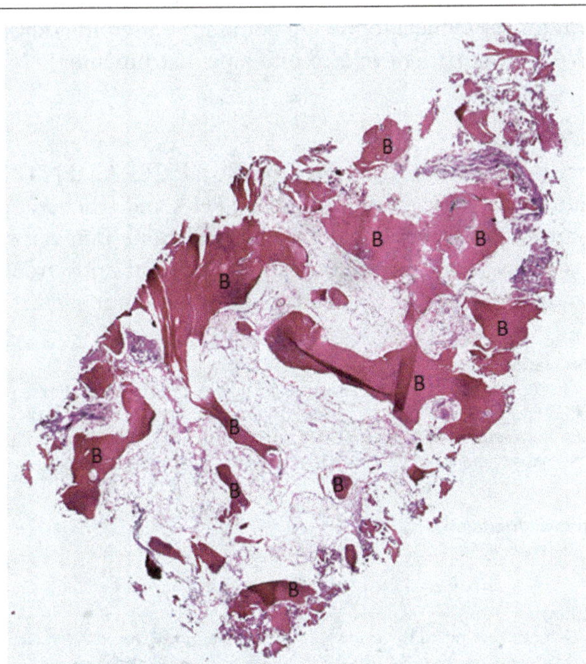

Fig. 3 Specimen of the tissue surrounding the removed lag screw shows viable and mature bone (B)

None of the patients had impaired hearing, kidney function or any allergic reactions to gentamicin. No wound complications or local infections were registered in any patient.

Discussion

To our knowledge, this is the first study investigating the local use of biodegradable bone graft substitute with antibiotics for bone defect reconstructions in aseptic revision of THA and trochanteric fracture patients.

A previous study showed that gentamicin from CERAMENT™|G elutes with a high burst rate through the first days after operation [7]. The local level of the concentration is sufficient not only to prevent infection, but also for eradication of recurrent bone

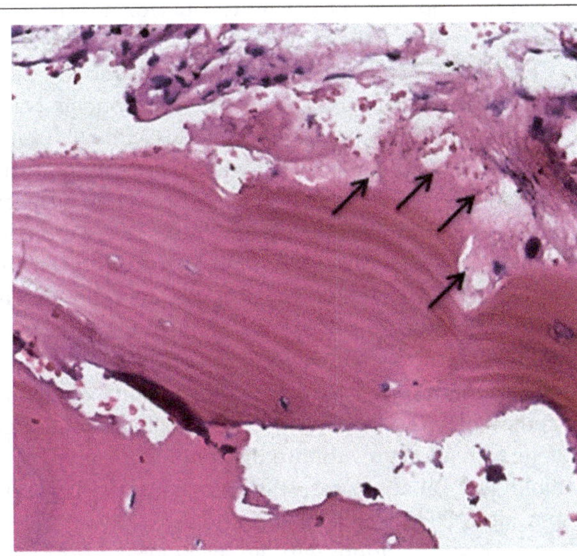

Fig. 4 Higher magnification shows the presence of hydroxyapatite conglomerate (indicated by the black arrows)

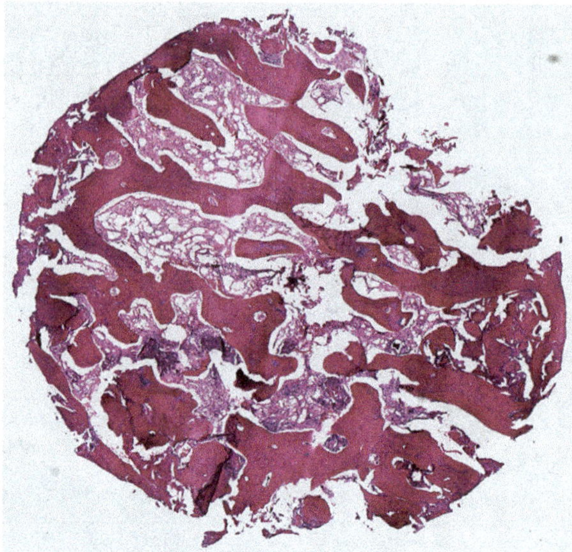

Fig. 5 A second biopsy of the tissue surrounding the removed lag screw. Islands of viable trabecular bone is seen and the space between trabeculae is filled with marrow-like tissue

or joint infections [11], thus is it not surprising that no signs of infection were observed in our investigated group.

The bone graft substitute does not improve immediate prosthesis-bone interface strength. In short term the use of a proximal bone graft substitute might not be necessary as a distally fixed stem would provide sufficient support. However, after remodeling, the proximal bone graft substitute gives mechanical support due to increased new bone formation around the prosthesis. The antibiotic elusion provided from the bone graft substitute protects the bone bed from infections. This is in concordance with findings reported in previously performed in vivo studies, where an uncemented knee joint prostheses and CERAMENT™|G were implanted in rabbits and showing better implant fixation in the host bone as compared to the control group without CERAMENT™|G [5]. Our experience of removing a dynamic hip screw from the trochanteric region where CERAMENT™|G had been implanted was that extremely high forces were needed. We assume that excessive new bone formation, probably related to CERAMENT™|G implantation and subsequent ongrowth into the sliding screw may explain the difficulties in hardware removal. However, no conclusions can be drawn from this limited case series and additional comparative studies need to be carried out. Histology confirmed new bone formation growth into the ceramic material.

Radiological analysis of the trochanteric fracture patients after DHS implantation showed a low level of dynamic screw migration, with an avarage of 3 mm at 3 months in our group with osteoprotic geriatric patients, while in a larger study by Platzer et al. a mean value of screw migration together with femoral neck shortening in non geriatric patients was reported to be 11 mm at 1 year follow-up [12]. Augmentation with a slow resorbing calcium phosphate (apatite) has not been shown to improve fixation in femoral neck fractures [10]. Since long term fixation is dependent on the amount and quality of new bone formed around the implant, we believe that the use of a biphasic material with part being replaced by ingrowing bone that surrounds the apatite may be beneficial for fracture stability and implant fixation. By adding antibiotics to the bone graft substitute, it is in addition possible to prevent surgical site infections in surgery carrying high risk [11]. The disadvantage of using antibiotics as standard in ceramic material may lead to over-use and not be necessary for all patients and even be harmful for patients suffering from renal insufficiency [13]. We suggest that CERAMENT™|G implantation at the fracture site could improve healing, bone formation and stabilization in the trochanteric fractures, thus preventing dynamic screw migration and shortening of the femoral neck.

There are several limitations in this study. The number of patients included is low and the study should be considered as a clinical feasibility study to show for the first time clinical outcome of an antibiotic eluting injectable bone substitute CERAMENT™|G used in major hip surgery. The prime objective was to extensively analyze the pharmacokinetics which has been reported elsewhere [7], but it contained no clinical follow-up. The study reports trochanteric fractures and revision THA, which are different conditions and with different outcome. The methods for clinical follow-up could have used in addition to VAS other patient related outcome instruments.

Conclusions

Our limited study indicates that local CERAMENT™|G could be safely used in revision of THA and trochanteric fractures, to prevent infection and fill bone defects. No local or systemic complications were found and circulation disturbances in the femoral head were not seen.

Abbreviations

AP: Anteroposterior; CCD: Caput-collum-diaphyseal; DHS: Dynamic hip screw; EDTA: Ethylenediaminetetraacetic acid; H&E: Haematoxylin and eosin stain; PMMA: Polymethylmethacrylate; PPS®: Porous Plasma Spray; QoL: Quality of Life; TAD: Tip-apex distance; THA: Total hip arthroplasty; VAS: Visual Analog Scale

Acknowledgements

The materials were provided by BONESUPPORT AB, Lund, Sweden.

Funding

The financial support to the researchers was granted by VINNOVA innovation agency in Sweden (grant 2017–00269), VR-Research funding agency in Sweden (grant 2015–06717) and the Foundation for Disabled people.
The funding bodies had no role in the design of the study, data collection, analysis, and interpretation of data or in writing the manuscript.

Authors' contributions

MS: Collected patient data and performed the surgeries, wrote Background, Methods and Results, read and approved the manuscript. ST: Supervised the collection of data and the surgeries and wrote Discussion and Conclusion, read and approved the manuscript. SL: did the biopsy for the histology study, read and approved the manuscript. MN: did statistics analyses and read and approved the manuscript. DBR: prepared the bone taken at revision and performed the histology and interpretation, gave valuable comments during writing as well as reviewed and approved the manuscript. LL: supervised and managed the collaboration between the two institutes, read and approved the manuscript.

Consent for publication

Written consent for publication was obtained from all participants as a paragraph included in the informed consent.

Competing interests

Prof Lars Lidgren is a member of the board of BONESUPPORT AB and Orthocell Ltd.

Author details

[1]Lithuanian University of Health, Kaunas, Lithuania. [2]Department of Orthopedics, Lund University Hospital, Lund, Sweden.

References

1. Koh CK, Zeng I, Ravi S, Zhu M, Vince KG, Young SW. Periprosthetic joint infection is the main cause of failure for modern knee arthroplasty: an analysis of 11,134 knees. Clin Orthop Relat Res. 2017;475:2194–201.
2. Gilbert P, Das J, Foley I. Biofilm susceptibility to antimicrobials. Adv Dent Res. 1997;11:160–7.
3. Rafiq I, Gambhir AK, Wroblewski BM, Kay PR. The microbiology of infected hip arthroplasty. Int Orthop. 2006;30:532–5.
4. Cancienne JM, Tyrrell Burrus M, Weiss DB, Yarboro SR. Applications of local antibiotics in orthopedic trauma. Orthop Clin North Am. 2015;46:495–510.
5. Zampelis V, Tägil M, Lidgren L, Isaksson H, Atroshil I, Wang J-S. The effect of a biphasic injectable bone substitute on the interface strength in a rabbit knee prosthesis model. J Orthop Surg Res. 2013. https://doi.org/10.1186/1749-799X-8-25.
6. Dvorzhinskiy A, Perino G, Chojnowski R, Van Der Meulen M, Ross F, Bostrom M, Yang N. Cerament bone void filler with gentamicin increases bone formation and decreases detectable infection in a rat model of debrided osteomyelitis. Bone Joint J. 2015;97B:9.
7. Stravinskas M, Horstmann P, Ferguson J, Hettwer W, Nilsson M, Tarasevicius S, Petersen MM, McNally MA, Lidgren L. Pharmacokinetics of gentamicin eluted from a regenerating bone graft substitute. Bone Joint Res. 2016;5:427–35.
8. Baumgaertner MR, Solberg BD. Awareness of tip-apex distance reduces failure of fixation of trochanteric fractures of the hip. J Bone Joint Surg Br. 1997;79:969–71.
9. Zirngibl B, Biber R, Bail HS. How to prevent cut-out and cut-through in biaxial proximal femoral nails: is there anything beyond lag screw positioning and tip–apex distance. Int Orthop. 2013;37:1363–8.
10. Mattsson P, Larsson S. Calcium phosphate cement for augmentation did not improve results after internal fixation of displaced femoral neck fractures: a randomized study of 118 patients. Acta Orthop. 2006;7:251–6.
11. McNally MA, Ferguson JY, Lau CK, Diefenbeck MD, Scarborough M, Ramsden AJ, Atkins BL. Single-stage treatment of chronic osteomyelitis with a new absorbable, gentamicin-loaded, calcium sulphate / hydroxyapatite biocomposite. A prospective series of 100 cases. Bone Joint J. 2016;98-B:1289–96.
12. Platzer P, Thalhammer G, Wozasek GE, Vécsei V. Femoral shortening after surgical treatment of trochanteric fractures in nongeriatric patients. J Trauma. 2008;64:982–9.
13. Nergelius G, Vinge E, Grubb A, Lidgren L. Renal impairment after hip or knee arthroplasty. Urinary excretion of protein markers studied in 59 patients. Acta Orthop Scand. 1997;68(1):34–40.

12

The influence of patient factors on femoral rotation after total hip arthroplasty

Taro Tezuka*, Yutaka Inaba, Naomi Kobayashi, Hyonmin Choe, Syota Higashihira and Tomoyuki Saito

Abstract

Background: A postoperative change in femoral rotation following total hip arthroplasty (THA) might be the cause of dislocation due to the change in combined anteversion. However, very few studies have evaluated the femoral rotation angle following THA, or the factors that influence femoral rotation. We aimed to evaluate changes in femoral rotation after THA, and to investigate preoperative patient factors that influence femoral rotation after THA.

Methods: This study involved 211 hips treated with primary THA. We used computed tomography to measure the femoral rotation angle before and one week after THA. In addition, multiple regression analysis was performed to evaluate preoperative patient factors that could influence femoral rotation after THA.

Results: The femoral rotation angle was 0.2 ± 14° externally before surgery and 4.4 ± 12° internally after surgery ($p < 0.001$). Multiple regression analysis revealed that sex ($\beta = 0.19$; $p = 0.003$), age ($\beta = 0.15$; $p = 0.017$), preoperative anatomical femoral anteversion ($\beta = -0.25$; $p = 0.002$), and preoperative femoral rotation angle ($\beta = 0.36$; $p < 0.001$) were significantly associated with the postoperative femoral rotation angle. The final model of the regression formula was described by the following equation: [*postoperative femoral rotation angle* = 5.41 × *sex* (female: 0, male: 1) + 0.15 × *age* - 0.22 × *preoperative anatomical femoral anteversion* + 0.33 × *preoperative femoral rotation angle* - 10.1].

Conclusion: The current study showed the mean internal change of 4.6° in the femoral rotation angle one week after THA. Sex, age, preoperative anatomical femoral anteversion and preoperative femoral rotation were associated with postoperative femoral rotation. The patients who were male, older, and who exhibited lesser preoperative anatomical femoral anteversion or greater preoperative femoral rotation angles, tended to demonstrate an externally rotated femur after THA. Conversely, patients who were female, younger, and who exhibited greater preoperative anatomical femoral anteversion or lesser preoperative femoral rotation angles, tended to demonstrate an internal rotation of the femur after THA.

Keywords: Total hip arthroplasty, Femoral rotation, Femoral anteversion, Multiple regression analysis

Background

Total hip arthroplasty (THA) is one of the most effective procedures for relieving arthritic pain caused by destructive hip diseases. However, despite improvements in prostheses, postoperative complications still occur. Among them, dislocation is a severe complication that sometimes leads to revision surgery [1, 2], and a meta-analysis has reported hip dislocation to be one of the common causes of THA failure [3]. Recently, postoperative changes in pelvic tilt have been reported, which cause angular changes of the acetabular components and dislocation [4–11]. A postoperative modification of the femoral rotation angle also might be the cause of dislocation due to the changes in combined anteversion; however, there were only three reports that investigated changes in femoral rotation after THA [12–14]. Uemura et al. reported that femurs rotated internally after THA [12, 14]. Akiyama et al. also found femoral internal rotation to occur after THA, and this rotation was associated with underlying disease, preoperative range of hip internal rotation, gender, surgical approach, leg lengthening, and a postoperative change in femoral anteversion [13]. Thus, the aims of the current study were to investigate the change of femoral rotation after THA and to investigate the preoperative patient factors that influenced femoral rotation after THA in our cohort.

* Correspondence: tettu59@hotmail.com
Department of Orthopedic Surgery, Yokohama City University, 3-9 Fukuura, Kanazawa-ku, Yokohama, Japan

Methods

The study was approved by the authors' institutional review board of Yokohama City University (B170100008), and informed consent was obtained from all patients. Inclusion criteria for the current study were as follows: hips treated with THA between 2008 and 2013, and patients whose hips were examined using with computed tomography (CT) before and one week after THA. In total, 299 hips met the inclusion criteria. Exclusion criteria included a hip flexion contracture of more than 10 °, and absence of CT imaging from the anterior superior iliac spine (ASIS) to the femoral condyles; 23 and 65 patients were excluded, respectively. Therefore, 211 hips of 179 patients were enrolled in the current study (Fig. 1). These patients included 137 females and 42 males, and the mean age at surgery was 62 ± 12 years (range: 34–89 years). The mean body mass index (BMI) was 24 ± 4.0 kg/m^2 (range: 14–35 kg/m^2). The diagnoses were osteoarthritis in 164 hips (78%), osteonecrosis of the femoral head in 34 (16%), rheumatoid arthritis in 11 (5.1%) and subchondral insufficiency fracture of the femoral head in 2 hips (0.9%).

All surgeries were performed by two surgeons (YI and NK), and there was no difference in surgical approach, operative method and postoperative rehabilitation. One hundred and fifty-five hips were treated with a mini-direct lateral approach, and 56 hips were treated with an anterolateral approach.

The femoral prostheses used in the current study included 43 SL-PLUS™ stems (Smith and Nephew, Memphis, TN, USA); 53 SL-PLUS™ MIA stems (Smith and Nephew); 74 Accolade stems (Stryker Orthopedics, Mahwah, NJ, USA) with a 132 or 127 neck-shaft angle; 5 CentPillar stems (Stryker Orthopedics); 6 Exeter stems (Stryker Orthopedics); 1 Supersecure Fit stem (Stryker Orthopedics); 11 Taperloc stems (Biomet, Warsaw, IN, USA); 15 VerSys Fiber Metal MidCoat stems (Zimmer, Warsaw, IN, USA); and 3 VerSys Heritage stems (Zimmer). Surgeons decided to use each type of prosthesis in an attempt to optimize each patient's kinematics based on preoperative radiographs and considering the proximal femoral bone quality or the presence of osteoporosis. More specifically, cemented stems were used for a patient with severe rheumatoid arthritis, severe osteoporosis, or a canal flare index < 3. Acetabular prostheses used in the current study included 96 Reflection cups (Smith and Nephew); 75 Trident Acetabular cups (Stryker Orthopedics); 6 ADEPT cups (Stryker Orthopedics); 5 Crossfire all polyethylene cups (Stryker Orthopedics); 11 M2a Magnum cups (Biomet); 15 Trilogy cups (Zimmer); and 3 ZCA natural spacer cups (Zimmer).

All acetabular components except for the cemented cup were implanted with the use of the Stryker Navigation System II Cart with CT-based Hip Navigation software, version 1.1 (Stryker Orthopedics) or the Stealth Station Navigation System Treon Plus with Universal HIP software (Medtronic Inc., Minneapolis, MN, USA). Forty-three femoral components were implanted with the use of the Stryker Navigation System.

For preoperative planning, a combined anteversion of 37.3 ° was planned as derived from the equation, [*combined anteversion = cup anteversion + anatomical stem anteversion* × 0.7] as reported by Widmer et al. [15] in the functional pelvic plane (FPP) as described in our previous report [16].

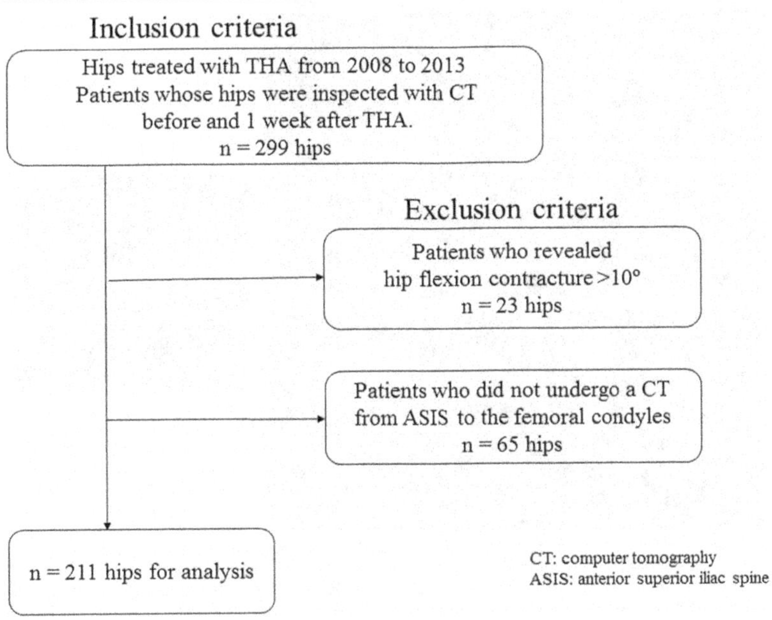

Fig. 1 Inclusion and exclusion criteria of the study participants

Clinical assessment

Each patient underwent careful visual assessment during gait and the evaluation for the presence of any discomfort or pain was performed during gait or physical examination of hip passive flexion, due to its association with hip impingement. This evaluation was performed at one week and at one year postoperatively. We also monitored the occurrence of hip dislocations during the study period.

Radiographic assessment

A CT from the pelvis to the distal femur was obtained before and one week postoperatively to make three-dimensional planning and to detect the presence of venous thromboembolism, and we evaluated the CT data for the current study. During the CT examination, the patient lay supine with the lower extremities in a relaxed position. In the CT evaluation, we defined the line between the anterior points of the bilateral ASISs as the ASIS line in the axial plane. The anterior pelvic plane included the ASIS line, and the ASIS line indicated the guidepost of pelvic rotation in the axial plane. Next, three angles were measured. Angle A was defined as the angle between the line of the CT berths and the ASIS line and was considered positive if the pelvis rotated towards the affected side, and negative if the pelvis rotated towards the healthy side. Angle B was defined as the angle between the line of the CT berths and the line connecting the femoral head center with the femoral neck center. Angle C was defined as the angle between the line of the CT berths and the posterior condylar line (PCL) (Fig. 2). The femoral rotation angle was defined as the angle between the PCL and the ASIS line and was calculated as Angle C - Angle A. The femoral rotation angle was positive if the femur rotated externally, and negative if the femur rotated internally. The anatomical femoral anteversion was defined as the angle between the PCL and the line connecting the femoral head and neck centers and was calculated as Angle B - Angle C. The functional femoral anteversion was the angle between the ASIS line and the line connecting the femoral head and neck centers and was calculated as Angle B - Angle A. From the postoperative CT images, we calculated the femoral rotation angle, the anatomical stem anteversion and the functional stem anteversion in the same manner. Among 211 hips, we also measured the femoral rotation angle at one year after surgery using CT images of 25 hips that were taken for other studies [17, 18]. We compared the values with those of one week after THA to evaluate the time-course change in rotation after the surgery. At one year after THA, anteroposterior and lateral radiographs of the hip were taken to detect any abnormal findings that indicated the femoral component loosening, such as progressive axial subsidence more than 3 mm or varus or valgus migration or the presence of a complete radiolucent line surrounding femoral components.

Radiographic measurements were taken two times after an interval of at least two weeks by a single author, and intra-observer reliabilities of the radiographic measurements were assessed using intra-class correlation coefficients. The average values of the radiographic measurements were

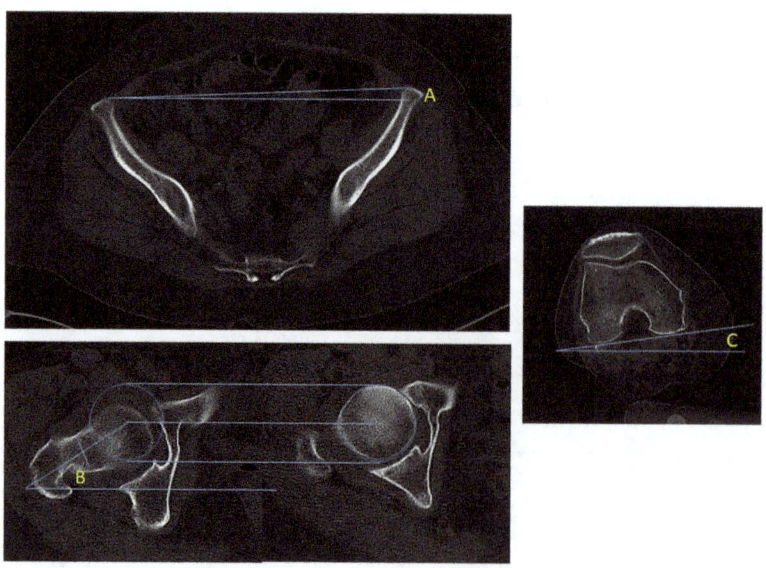

Fig. 2 Measurements on pelvic and lower extremity axial computer tomography (CT). Angle **a** is defined as the angle between the line of the CT berths and the line connecting both anterior superior iliac spines. Angle **b** is defined as the angle between the line of the CT berths and the line connecting the femoral head center with the neck center. Angel **c** is defined as the angle between the line of the CT berths and the posterior condylar line

calculated and analyzed. For the inter-observer reliability, TT and SH assessed each of the measurements using inter-class correlation coefficients, which can range from – 1 to 1, with 1 indicating perfect agreement. Table 1 shows the intra- and inter-class correlation coefficients for each measurement, which were considered excellent.

Statistical analysis

The paired *t*-test was used to evaluate the differences in each radiographic measurement (pre- and post- femoral rotation angle, anatomical femoral or stem anteversion, and functional femoral or stem anteversion). To evaluate differences in radiographic variables between groups treated by different surgeons, the unpaired *t*-test was performed. Analysis of variance (ANOVA) was performed to test the differences among groups with different types of stems.

To analyze the factors that influence the femoral rotation angle after THA, a regression analysis was performed. At first, a simple regression analysis was performed with the following factors as explanatory variables: sex, age, BMI, preoperative anatomical femoral anteversion and preoperative femoral rotation angle. Furthermore, variables with *p*-values < 0.05 were populated for regression analysis as a multivariate assessment and entered into the final equation. The adjusted coefficient of multiple determination (adjusted R^2) was used to indicate how much variability in the femoral rotation angle after THA was accounted for by the independent variables. Standardized regression coefficients (β) and associated *p*-values were determined to assess statistical significance ($p < 0.05$). All statistical analyses were performed using SPSS, version 21.0 (IBM Corp., Armonk, NY, USA).

Results

No patients had complaints one week after surgery except pain originating from the incision scar and there were no symptoms of impingement or gait abnormalities that could be clearly associated with excessive femoral rotation. All patients could walk independently with or without a cane and were discharged from the hospital at 10 days after THA. At one year after surgery, there were no complaints of gait abnormalities. No dislocations were observed throughout the study period.

Table 1 The intra- and interclass correlation coefficients for each radiographic measurement

	Angle A		Angle B		Angle C	
	Preop	Postop	Preop	Postop	Preop	Postop
Intraclass CC	0.92	0.93	0.90	0.97	0.95	0.98
Interclass CC	0.91	0.92	0.90	0.97	0.95	0.97

CC correlation coefficient, *Preop* preoperative, *Postop* postoperative

The mean preoperative femoral rotation was 0.2 ± 14° and the mean postoperative femoral rotation was – 4.4 ± 12° ($p < 0.001$) (Table 2). Among 211 hips, 88 hips (41.7%) had internally rotated femurs before and after THA, and 43 hips (20.4%) had femurs rotated externally before THA and internally after THA. Twenty hips (9.5%) showed femoral internal rotation before THA and external rotation after THA. Fifty-three hips (25.1%) demonstrated femurs rotated externally before and after THA. (Table 3). The mean preoperative femoral rotation angle of 110 hips showing internal rotation before THA was – 11 ± 7.9 ° and the mean femoral rotation angle of 97 hips that revealed an external rotation before THA was 12 ± 8.1 °. The mean femoral rotation angle of 134 hips that revealed internal rotation after THA was – 11.7 ± 7.5 ° and among the 134 hips, 17 hips showed the femoral rotation angle less than – 20 °. The mean femoral rotation angle of 74 hips showing external rotation after THA was 8.5 ± 7.3 ° and among the 74 hips, there were 6 hips revealed the femoral rotation angel more than 20 °. The preoperative anatomical femoral anteversion was 22 ± 14°, and the postoperative anatomical stem anteversion was 31 ± 14° ($p < 0.001$) (Table 2), which indicated the surgeons increased stem anteversion by 9° during THA. The preoperative functional femoral anteversion was 22 ± 12°, and the functional stem anteversion was 27 ± 13° ($p < 0.001$) (Table 2). These results indicated that functional stem anteversion increased by 5° after THA, while the surgeons increased anatomical stem anteversion by 9°. The difference between pre- and postoperative anatomical anteversion was larger than the difference between pre- and postoperative functional anteversion ($p < 0.001$); this was caused by changes in femoral rotation. There was no significant difference in radiographic variables between groups treated by different surgeons, and ANOVA testing showed that there was no significant difference in radiographic variables among groups with different types of femoral implants.

Table 4 shows the results of the univariate and multiple regression analyses. The simple regression analysis showed that sex, age, preoperative anatomical femoral anteversion and preoperative femoral rotation angle had a significant influence on the postoperative femoral rotation angle. Figure 3 shows a scatter plot of pre- and postoperative femoral rotation angles. There was a positive correlation between preoperative and postoperative femoral rotation angles ($r = 0.55$; $p < 0.001$). The final model of the multiple regression analyses revealed that sex ($\beta = 0.19$; $p = 0.003$), age ($\beta = 0.15$; $p = 0.017$), preoperative anatomical femoral anteversion ($\beta = -0.25$; $p = 0.002$), and preoperative femoral rotation angle ($\beta = 0.36$; $p < 0.001$) were significantly associated with the postoperative femoral rotation angle (Table 4). The results of multiple regression analyses indicated that patients who were male, older, and exhibited

Table 2 The results of the radiographic measurements

	Preop (range)	Postop (range)	*p*
Femoral rotation angle (°)	0.2 ± 14 (− 42–37)	−4.4 ± 12 (− 32–32)	< 0.001
Anatomical femoral (stem) anteversion (°)	22 ± 14 (− 14–63)	31 ± 14 (− 11–59)	< 0.001
Functional femoral (stem) anteversion (°)	22 ± 12 (− 11–66)	27 ± 13 (− 2–70)	< 0.001

Preop preoperative, *Postop* postoperative

lesser preoperative anatomical femoral anteversion or greater preoperative femoral rotation angles tended to show an externally rotated femur after THA. Conversely, the patients who were female, younger, and had greater preoperative anatomical femoral anteversion or lesser preoperative femoral rotation angles, tended to demonstrate an internal rotation of the femur after THA. The final model of the regression formula was obtained as the following equation: [*the postoperative femoral rotation angle* = 5.41 × *sex* (female: 0, male: 1) + 0.15 × *age* - 0.22 × *preoperative anatomical femoral anteversion* + 0.33 × *preoperative femoral rotation angle* - 10.1]. The final model accounted for 40% of the variation in postoperative femoral rotation angle (adjusted $R^2 = 0.40$).

The average femoral rotation angle of 25 hips whose CT images were available at one week and one year after THA was − 5.5 ± 12 ° and − 11 ± 12 ° respectively ($p < 0.001$). There was a strong positive correlation between measurements of femoral rotation angles taken one week and one year after surgery ($r = 0.80$; $p < 0.001$). There were no findings that could indicate the femoral component loosening.

Discussion

It is well-known that the orientation of acetabular and femoral components is one of the key factors affecting the THA success [19, 20]. From a historical aspect, the so-called "safe zone" of the acetabular cup angle is one of the crucial notions in reducing dislocation risk after THA [21]. Subsequently, the concept of "combined anteversion," which is the sum of the acetabular and femoral anteversion, has been proposed for the decreasing dislocations and increasing impingement-free range of motion [15, 22, 23].

Several studies have reported on the relation between pelvic tilt and acetabular component angles [11, 24–28]. In general, the pelvis tilts posteriorly from supine to standing and with time after THA, especially in older patients whose lumbo-lordotic angle is smaller [4]. Considering this change in pelvic tilt and angle of acetabular components, the usability of the FPP has been reported [16, 29, 30]. However, there are few studies regarding the femoral rotation angle after THA [12, 14], and a limited number of reports have evaluated which patient factors affect the femoral rotation angle after THA [13].

In the current study, there was no patient who had complaints, abnormal gait or dislocation clearly due to the femoral rotation, however, there were 17 hips showed the femoral rotation angle of femur less than − 20 ° and 6 hips showed external rotation more than 20 °. Until now, there were no reports about established methods to prevent excessive femoral rotation after THA. Akiyama et al. reported that the internal rotation of the hip after THA increased with posterolateral approach which damages short rotators [13]. To use posterior approach might be one of effective procedures to prevent the excessive external rotation for hips that were considered to have external rotation after THA.

Akiyama et al. also reported that the femoral internal rotation showed an average increase of 11° after THA, while the current study showed the mean change in the femoral internal rotation angle after THA was 4.6°. They performed 82% of their THAs using the posterior approach [13], and all THAs in the current study were performed with a mini-direct lateral approach or anterolateral approach. This might be the cause of difference in the femoral rotation angle compared to the report of Akiyama et al. Furthermore, this fact also might be the reason that the surgical approach did not influence femoral rotation after THA in the current study.

There was a strong positive correlation between the preoperative and postoperative femoral rotation angles, and regression analysis revealed that the preoperative

Table 3 The number of hips in each position pre- and post-surgery

		Preop			
		Internal rotation	Neutral	External rotation	Total
Postop	Internal rotation	88 (41.7%)	3 (1.4%)	43 (20.4%)	134
	Neutral	2 (0.9%)	0 (0%)	1 (0.5%)	3
	External rotation	20 (9.5%)	1 (0.5%)	53 (25.1%)	74
	Total	110	4	97	211

Preop: preoperative, Postop: postoperative

Table 4 The results of regression analysis

Univariate regression analysis				
		Regression coefficient	β	*p*
Sex (female:0, male:1)		5.35	0.19	0.006
Age		0.24	0.23	0.001
Body Mass Index		0.34	0.11	0.122
Surgical approach		0.73	0.03	0.697
Preoperative anatomical femoral anteversion		−0.46	−0.55	< 0.001
Preoperative femoral rotation angle		0.48	0.55	< 0.001
Multivariate regression analysis				
	Adjusted R^2	Regression coefficient	β	*p*
Sex (female:0, male:1)	0.40	5.41	0.19	0.003
Age		0.15	0.15	0.017
Preoperative anatomical femoral anteversion		−0.22	−0.25	0.002
Preoperative femoral rotation angle		0.33	0.36	< 0.001

femoral rotation angle was a significant factor in predicting postoperative femoral rotation. In addition to preoperative femoral rotation, sex, age and preoperative anatomical femoral anteversion displayed a significant effect on postoperative femoral rotation angle; therefore, a preoperative plan might be made with consideration of patient preoperative characteristics. In particular, patients who were male, older and had an externally rotated femur or smaller preoperative anatomical femoral anteversion tended to show an externally rotated femur after THA, which might cause the impingement that lead to anterior dislocation. In contrast, patients who were female, younger and had an internally rotated femur or larger preoperative anatomical femoral anteversion tended to show an internally rotated femur that might result in posterior dislocation. In such cases, the results of the current study suggest that femoral prostheses should be implanted with less or more degree of anteversion, derived from the following equation; [5.41 × *sex* (female: 0, male: 1) + 0.15 × *age* - 0.22 × *preoperative anatomical femoral anteversion* + 0.33 × *preoperative femoral rotation angle* - 10.1].

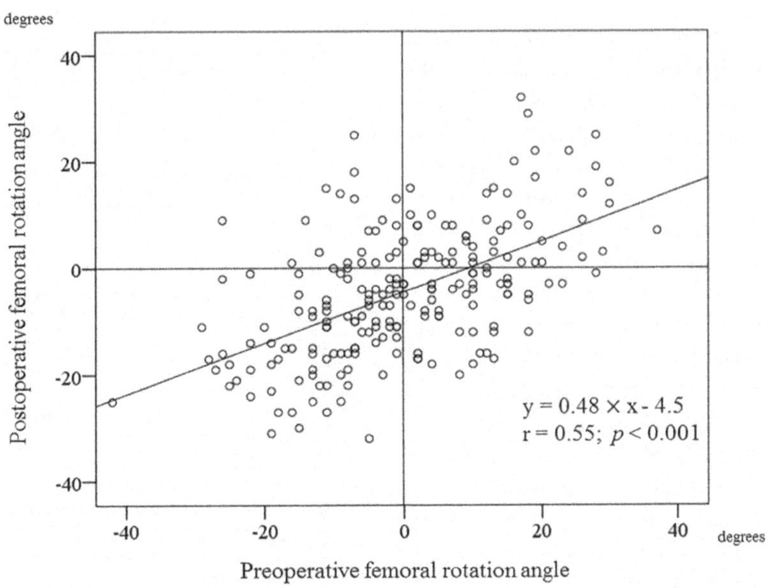

Fig. 3 The scatter chart of pre- and postoperative femoral rotation angles. The X axis is the preoperative femoral rotation angle, and the Y axis is the postoperative femoral rotation angle. There is a positive correlation between the preoperative femoral rotation angle and the postoperative femoral rotation angle (r = 0.55; $p < 0.001$)

Among the 211 hips, 25 hips underwent CT at one year after THA. The average femoral rotation angle was significantly different at one week and at one year after THA (− 5.5 ± 12° and − 11 ± 12°, respectively, $p < 0.001$) with a significant and strong correlation between them. The result of one year after THA was quite same as the result of Akiyama et al. [13]. Uemura et al. also reported that substantial variability was observed in the femoral rotation angle, especially during the postoperative period [14]. We could not identify what factors would affect the change in the femoral rotation angle between one week and one year after THA in the current study, but one of the reasons might be recovery of muscles around the hip joint after THA. The result of the current study indicated that the femoral rotation left the possibility of changing internally by a mean of 5 ° until one year after THA.

To the best of authors' knowledge, this is the first study to propose an equation to predict postoperative femoral rotation after THA using preoperative patient factors. However, there are several limitations to the current study. First, radiographic measurements were performed on the two-dimensional axial plane of a CT image, rather than via a three-dimensional reconstructed model. However, the measurement technique was consistent, and patients who showed any flexion contracture of more than 10° were excluded. Inter- and intraclass correlation coefficients were sufficiently high. Thus, we believe the data in the current study was reliable. Second, the evaluation was focused only on the supine position. Postural changes including standing or sitting were not considered, and further research should be address these factors.

From the results of the multiple regression analysis, we obtained an equation with which we could partially predict the postoperative femoral rotation using patient preoperative factors, and the equation might be helpful in determining femoral implant anteversion. The adjusted R^2 obtained from the multiple regression analysis was 0.40, which indicates there were other factors that significantly affected the femoral rotation. Akiyama et al. reported that the femoral rotation after THA was not only associated with certain pre- and perioperative factors, that is, underlying disease, pre-operative range of hip internal rotation, gender, surgical approach, but also with postoperative factors including leg lengthening and change of femoral anteversion [13]. Because the aim of the current study was to investigate the preoperative patient factors that influenced the femoral rotation after THA, we chose not to consider postoperative patient factors; however, these factors must have an influence on femoral rotation. Further investigation into the relationships between femoral rotation and other factors may be required.

Conclusions

The current study showed the mean internal change of 4.6° in the femoral rotation angle one week after THA. There was no significant difference in femoral rotation between groups treated with a mini-direct lateral approach and treated with an anterolateral approach. Sex, age, preoperative anatomical femoral anteversion, and preoperative femoral rotation angle were significant predictors for the postoperative femoral rotation angle in the supine position.

Abbreviations

adjusted R^2: Adjusted coefficient of multiple determination; ASIS: Anterior superior iliac spine; BMI: Body mass index; CT: Computed tomography; PCL: Posterior condylar line; THA: Total hip arthroplasty; β: Standardized regression coefficients

Acknowledgements

We thank all the patients involved in the study.

Authors' contributions

TT: study design, interpreting the data and writing the paper. YI: study design, critical revision. NK: data analysis and interpretation. HC: data analysis and interpretation. SH: data analysis and interpretation. TS: study design and critical revision. All authors read and approved the final manuscript.

Competing interests

The authors declare that they have no competing interests.

References

1. Morrey BF. Difficult complications after hip joint replacement. Dislocation. Clin Orthop Relat Res. 1997;344:179–87.
2. Brennan SA, et al. Dislocation of primary total hip arthroplasty and the risk of redislocation. Hip Int. 2012;22(5):500–4.
3. Bozic KJ, et al. The epidemiology of revision total hip arthroplasty in the United States. J Bone Joint Surg Am. 2009;91(1):128–33.
4. Suzuki H, et al. Postural and chronological change in pelvic tilt five years after Total hip arthroplasty in patients with developmental dysplasia of the hip: a three-dimensional analysis. J Arthroplast. 2016;31(1):317–22.
5. Siebenrock KA, Kalbermatten DF, Ganz R. Effect of pelvic tilt on acetabular retroversion: a study of pelves from cadavers. Clin Orthop Relat Res. 2003; 407:241–8.
6. Lazennec JY, et al. Hip-spine relationship: a radio-anatomical study for optimization in acetabular cup positioning. Surg Radiol Anat. 2004;26(2): 136–44.
7. Zhu J, Wan Z, Dorr LD. Quantification of pelvic tilt in total hip arthroplasty. Clin Orthop Relat Res. 2010;468(2):571–5.
8. Lembeck B, et al. Pelvic tilt makes acetabular cup navigation inaccurate. Acta Orthop. 2005;76(4):517–23.
9. Babisch JW, Layher F, Amiot LP. The rationale for tilt-adjusted acetabular cup navigation. J Bone Joint Surg Am. 2008;90(2):357–65.
10. Stefl M, et al. Spinopelvic mobility and acetabular component position for total hip arthroplasty. Bone Joint J. 2017;99-B(1 Supple A):37–45.
11. Tezuka T, et al. Influence of pelvic tilt on polyethylene wear after Total hip arthroplasty. Biomed Res Int. 2015;2015:327217.
12. Uemura K, et al. The validity of using the posterior condylar line as a rotational reference for the femur. J Arthroplast. 2016;31(1):302–6.

10. Stefl M, et al. Spinopelvic mobility and acetabular component position for total hip arthroplasty. Bone Joint J. 2017;99-B(1 Supple A):37–45.
11. Tezuka T, et al. Influence of pelvic tilt on polyethylene wear after Total hip arthroplasty. Biomed Res Int. 2015;2015:327217.
12. Uemura K, et al. The validity of using the posterior condylar line as a rotational reference for the femur. J Arthroplast. 2016;31(1):302–6.
13. Akiyama K, et al. Changes in axial alignment of the ipsilateral hip and knee after total hip arthroplasty. Bone Joint J. 2016;98-B(3):349–58.
14. Uemura K, et al. Can anatomic measurements of stem Anteversion angle be considered as the functional Anteversion angle? J Arthroplast. 2018;33(2):595–600.
15. Widmer KH, Zurfluh B. Compliant positioning of total hip components for optimal range of motion. J Orthop Res. 2004;22(4):815–21.
16. Inaba Y, et al. Preoperative planning for implant placement with consideration of pelvic tilt in total hip arthroplasty: postoperative efficacy evaluation. BMC Musculoskelet Disord. 2016;17:280.
17. Ike H, et al. Comparison between mechanical stress and bone mineral density in the femur after total hip arthroplasty by using subject-specific finite element analyses. Comput Methods Biomech Biomed Engin. 2015;18(10):1056–65.
18. Oba M, et al. Effect of femoral canal shape on mechanical stress distribution and adaptive bone remodelling around a cementless tapered-wedge stem. Bone Joint Res. 2016;5(9):362–9.
19. Charnley J. Total hip replacement by low-friction arthroplasty. Clin Orthop Relat Res. 1970;72:7–21.
20. Harris WH. Advances in surgical technique for total hip replacement: without and with osteotomy of the greater trochanter. Clin Orthop Relat Res. 1980;(146):188–204.
21. Lewinnek GE, et al. Dislocations after total hip-replacement arthroplasties. J Bone Joint Surg Am. 1978;60(2):217–20.
22. Dorr LD, et al. Combined anteversion technique for total hip arthroplasty. Clin Orthop Relat Res. 2009;467(1):119–27.
23. Nakashima Y, et al. Combined anteversion technique reduced the dislocation in cementless total hip arthroplasty. Int Orthop. 2014;38(1):27–32.
24. Blondel B, et al. Pelvic tilt measurement before and after total hip arthroplasty. Orthop Traumatol Surg Res. 2009;95(8):568–72.
25. Taki N, et al. Change in pelvic tilt angle 2 to 4 years after total hip arthroplasty. J Arthroplast. 2012;27(6):940–4.
26. Tannast M, et al. Anatomic referencing of cup orientation in total hip arthroplasty. Clin Orthop Relat Res. 2005;(436):144–50.
27. Haenle M, et al. Assessment of cup position from plain radiographs: impact of pelvic tilting. Surg Radiol Anat. 2007;29(1):29–35.
28. Kalteis TA, et al. In vitro investigation of the influence of pelvic tilt on acetabular cup alignment. J Arthroplast. 2009;24(1):152–7.
29. Nishihara S, et al. Measurements of pelvic flexion angle using three-dimensional computed tomography. Clin Orthop Relat Res. 2003;411:140–51.
30. Miki H, Kyo T, Sugano N. Anatomical hip range of motion after implantation during total hip arthroplasty with a large change in pelvic inclination. J Arthroplast. 2012;27(9):1641–50. e1

13

Multi-parametric muscle and fat correlation of computed tomography parameters to outcomes in a total hip arthroplasty population

Michael A. Heffler[1,2], Ryan Barlow[1,2], Yin Xi[2], Daichi Hayashi[3], Hayden Box[1], Michael Huo[1] and Avneesh Chhabra[1,2*]

Abstract

Background: Cross-sectional imaging is not currently used in planning Total Hip Arthroplasty (THA). The aim of our study is to determine correlations between CT parameters and outcomes following THA.

Methods: A prospective registry of patients who underwent total joint arthroplasty was reviewed for patients who: (1) underwent THA, (2) had a CT between 1 year before and 6 months after surgery, and (3) completed perioperative WOMAC and Harris Hip Score (HHS) questionnaires. Two readers measured CT parameters, yielding mean Hounsfield Units, area, average diameter, and perimeter of the psoas major, gluteus medius and minimus muscles. A segmentation algorithm determined visceral and subcutaneous fat area, and waist circumference. ICC was calculated for each measurement to examine inter-reader agreement. Regression analyses were performed to select measurements with most impact on outcome scores.

Results: Twenty-eight patients met inclusion criteria (17 female, 11 male), having mean (+/− standard deviation) age of 54.4 +/− 14.8 years and BMI 29.0 +/− 6.3 kg/m^2. Correlations were found between HHS and age (0.650, $p = 0.018$), height (−1.263, $p = 0.009$), visceral-to-subcutaneous fat area ratio at the psoas level (0.511, $p = 0.018$), and waist circumference at the psoas level (1.759, $p = 0.002$). Inter-reader analysis showed ICC > 0.850 for all measurements.

Conclusion: Age and height, as well as CT-derived visceral-to-subcutaneous fat area ratio and waist circumference significantly correlate with postsurgical HHS scores following THA. Our study suggests that parameters derived from cross-sectional CT imaging can be useful additional preoperative planning tool for THA.

Keywords: Computed tomography, Total hip arthroplasty, Segmentation, Harris hip score

Background

Almost 700,000 Total Joint Arthroplasties (TJA) are performed in the United States each year, which include over 230,000 Total Hip Arthroplasties (THA) [1]. It is estimated that 15.1% of the THAs performed each year are revision procedures rather than primary operations, the economic impact of which is profound [1]. From 1997 to 2003, 19% of all Medicare spending on THA was consumed by revision operations [2]. THA is a widely used procedure, and the prevalence is projected to increase to as many as 668,700 procedures in 2030, with 96,700 (14.4%) of those estimated to be revision THA [1]. Methods to identify patients who will most likely benefit and likewise identify patients who will fail THA are immensely important because they can potentially aid in optimizing healthcare spending.

Cross-sectional imaging modalities, such as Magnetic Resonance Imaging (MRI) and Computed Tomography (CT), are not commonly used in preoperative screening of prospective THA patients. In 2015, Wiater et al. retrospectively examined a registry of patients who underwent reverse total shoulder arthroplasty (RTSA) and found significant correlations between radiographic

* Correspondence: Avneesh.Chhabra@UTSouthwestern.edu
[1]Department of Orthopedic Surgery, University of Texas Southwestern Medical Center, Dallas, TX, USA
[2]Department of Radiology, University of Texas Southwestern Medical Center, 5323 Harry Hines Blvd, Dallas, TX 75390-8896, USA
Full list of author information is available at the end of the article

parameters from MRI and postoperative outcome assessments [3].

CT measurement of the psoas major muscle has been used as a surrogate measure of sarcopenia [4]. It has been shown in some surgical and trauma populations that increased rates of overall morbidity [4–6], mortality [7], and decreased quality-of-life [8] significantly correlate with decreased psoas major area, volume, and density. The gluteal (abductor) muscles are considered highly important for overall hip function, especially for function after THA [9]. Due to superior soft tissue contrast and spatial resolution, CT examination of the pelvis can be used to evaluate both the abductor and psoas major muscle groups. In addition, evaluation of muscle size, muscle density, and fat segmentation with an analysis of fat fractions can be performed using independent software in a reproducible fashion.

Overall, there is a knowledge gap as to how these CT parameters ultimately can be related to outcomes of THA. No previous study has evaluated multi-compartment tissue analysis in the same setting and its relationship to outcomes of THA. The aim of our exploratory study was therefore to determine correlations between CT parameters and outcomes following THA.

Methods

Subjects

Patients were selected from a prospectively constructed registry of TJA patients at our institution. A retrospective review of this registry was performed under a HIPPA waiver and as part of an Institutional Review Board-approved study. This review yielded 802 TJA patients, 318 of whom underwent THA between 2006 and 2014.

At their initial visit, 6 months postoperatively, and 12 months postoperatively, THA patients completed the Western Ontario and McMaster Universities Osteoarthritis Index (WOMAC) Hip Score and Harris Hip Score (HHS) questionnaires in addition to normal follow-up.

We included patients who [1]: underwent THA [2], had a pelvic CT study performed for any reason in the time 1 year before or 6 months after the surgery, and [3] completed at least one set of postoperative questionnaires in addition to the initial visit questionnaires.

Image analysis and reader training

All CT images were reconstructed as 3 mm slices in a soft tissue window for evaluation. Images were processed using an independent software program, Aquarius intuition (TeraRecon, Foster City, CA).

Two second-year medical students (MH, RB) served as readers, and independently measured parameters at two levels. Each reader was trained by a board-certified, fellowship trained radiologist (AC) to identify and analyze defined slices and measure selected regions of interest (ROIs) (See Slice and ROI Selection). This training consisted of two sessions, each two-hours in length, where the readers were taught to identify the defined slices and measure the selected ROIs on CT images from non-study patients. Readers then practiced this workflow under the supervision of the radiologist.

Additionally, 10% of the study sample (3 CTs) were used as a training set. These images were measured by the two readers using separate but identical workstations, working simultaneously and cooperatively to ensure a standardized workflow. Subsequently, the readers collected measurements using identical workstations, independent of one another on the remaining 90%, such that each CT was eventually measured twice, once by each reader.

Slice and ROI selection

Two slices of interest were defined, and on each slice ROIs were selected. The psoas slice was defined as the first axial slice superior to the sacroiliac joint, but which does not visualize the sacroiliac joint (Fig. 1a and b). The ROIs on the psoas slice included the psoas major muscles, both ipsilateral and contralateral to surgery. These muscles were selected as ROIs because cross-sectional psoas area measured from axial CT has been used as a marker for core muscle mass and sarcopenia, and has been shown to be correlated with postoperative functional outcomes after THA [4, 10]. The gluteal slice was defined as the axial slice demonstrating fully open S1 anterior foramina (Fig. 1c and d). The ROIs on the gluteal slice included the gluteus medius-minimus complex, again ipsilateral and contralateral to surgery. These muscles were identified as ROIs because they contribute to the overall musculature surrounding the hip and gluteus medius atrophy has been found to predict limping after THA at 6 months postoperatively [9, 11].

Measurement of ROIs

On the psoas slice, three functions were performed: measurement of the psoas major ROI ipsilateral and contralateral to surgery and an automated fat-analysis segmentation algorithm. On the gluteal slice, three functions were performed: measurement of the gluteus medius-minimus ROI ipsilateral and contralateral to surgery and the same fat-analysis segmentation algorithm.

Measurement of each muscle was accomplished by manually constructing a polygon around the indicated muscle, yielding four parameters: mean Hounsfield units (Mean), cross-sectional area (Area), mean diameter (Diameter), and Circumference (Fig. 1a and c).

The fat-analysis segmentation algorithm also yielded four parameters: visceral fat area, subcutaneous fat area, ratio of visceral fat to total fat areas (Area Ratio, i.e. visceral fat area divided by the sum of visceral fat and

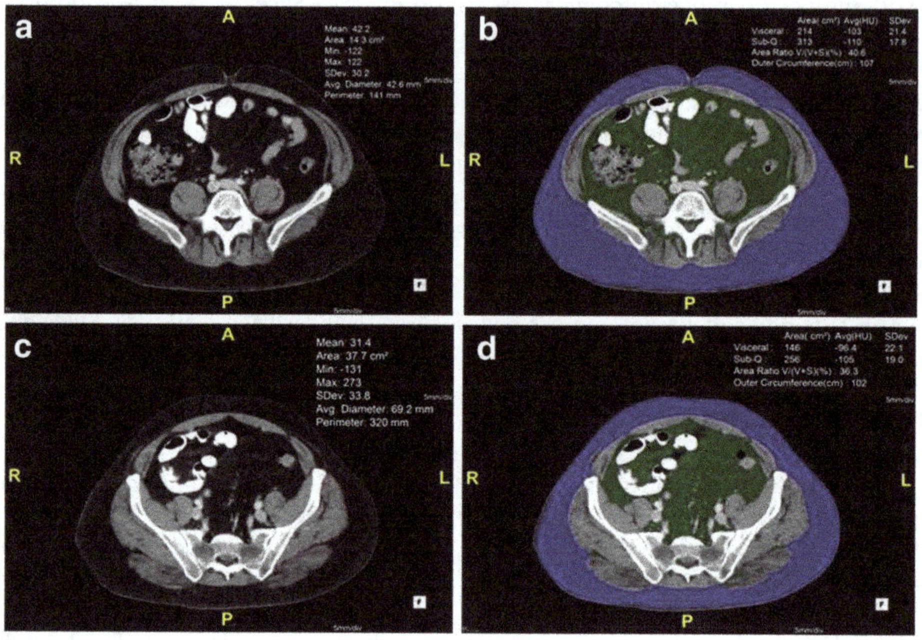

Fig. 1 Representations of the CT slices analyzed: (**a**) psoas slice with muscle polygon, (**b**) psoas slice with fat analysis algorithm, (**c**) gluteal slice with muscle polygon, and (**d**) gluteal slice with fat analysis algorithm

subcutaneous fat areas), and the waist circumference of the patient (Outer Circumference) (Fig. 1b and d).

Statistical analysis

A sensitivity analysis was performed between the study group and the overall THA group to determine whether the study sample differed significantly from the excluded registry population in demographic or clinical factors. Inter-reader agreement was assessed using the intraclass correlation coefficient (ICC) value for each measurement. Average measurements between the two readers were used for this analysis.

Additionally, univariate and multiple regression analyses were performed to determine the association between measurements and postsurgical outcome scores. The CT measurements and demographic data were used as independent variables and change in WOMAC and HHS were response variables. Change in WOMAC and HHS was defined as the difference between 12-month and initial scores.

In the multiple regression analysis, all CT measurements together with age, BMI, height, weight, and sex were initially included. A stepwise selection algorithm was then used to select the independent variables that most affected the response variables based on the F statistic. Using the selected independent variables, a multivariate model was constructed which was used to predict change in WOMAC and HHS.

All *p*-values of less than 0.05 were considered to be statistically significant. All statistical analysis was performed using Statistical Analysis Software (SAS Institute, Cary, NC).

Results

Subjects

Of the 318 THA patients in the registry, 13.2% (42/318) had a CT study performed in the indicated time frame. Of those 42 patients who underwent CT imaging, 66.7% (28/42, 17 females, 11 males) had a complete set of postoperative questionnaires (Fig. 2). Mean (+/− standard deviation) age was 54.4 +/− 14.8 years, height was 165.9 +/− 9.0 cm, weight was 80.0 +/− 19.3 kg, and mean BMI was 29.0 +/− 6.3 kg/m^2. Mean (+/− standard deviation) initial WOMAC score was 62.7 +/− 18.4 and initial HHS was 38.4 +/− 17.8.

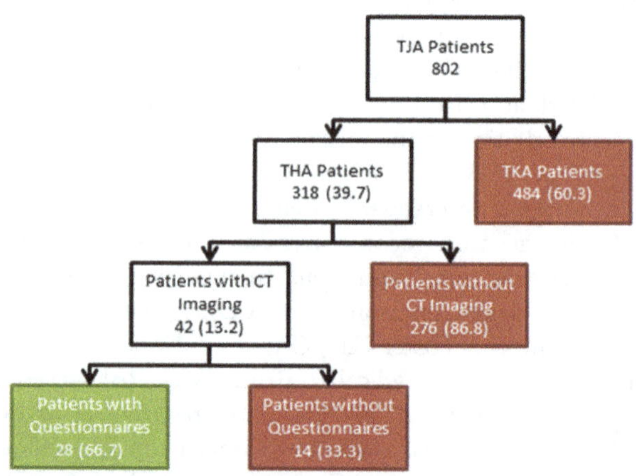

Fig. 2 Flowchart depicting patient inclusion and exclusion

Table 1 Sensitivity analysis between the study group and overall registry

Parameter	Excluded ($n = 290$)	Included ($n = 28$)	p-value	Registry THA Patients ($N = 318$)
Weight (kg)	86.38 ± 19.95	80.00 ± 19.25	0.089	85.88 ± 19.65
Height (cm)	170.2 ± 11.4	165.92 ± 8.98	0.042	170.2 ± 11.1
BMI	29.69 ± 5.73	28.96 ± 6.29	0.588	30.07 ± 11.87
Age	57.20 ± 12.57	54.43 ± 14.76	0.167	58.80 ± 12.71
Initial WOMAC Hip Score	58.74 ± 20.87	62.71 ± 18.37	0.519	59.16 ± 20.63
12 Month WOMAC Hip Score	–	30.04 ± 24.75	–	–
WOMAC Hip Score Change	–	−31.74 ± 27.05	–	–
Initial Harris Hip Score	41.75 ± 15.66	38.36 ± 17.77	0.225	41.45 ± 15.86
12 Month Harris Hip Score	–	67.08 ± 21.89	–	–
Harris Hip Score Change	–	27.56 ± 23.53	–	–
Females	141	17	–	158
Males	149	11	–	160
Right Sided Surgery	141	12	–	153
Left Sided Surgery	134	16	–	150
Bilateral Surgery	15	0	–	15

Statistical analysis

The study population was found to be similar to the overall THA group, with height being slightly different (Table 1). Analysis of agreement between the two readers showed an ICC > 0.85 for all measurements (Table 2). No significant correlation was found between any demographic or CT parameters and change in WOMAC Hip Score.

Significant univariate correlations were found between HHS and age (0.650, $p = 0.018$), height (−1.263, $p = 0.009$), Area Ratio at the psoas slice (Psoas Area Ratio, 0.511, $p = 0.018$), and Outer Circumference at the psoas slice (Psoas Outer Circumference, 1.759, $p = 0.002$) (Table 3, Fig. 3). Additionally, a non-significant trend was found between HHS and the mean Hounsfield units of the gluteus minimus-medius ipsilateral to surgery (Ipsilateral Gluteal Mean, 0.359, $p = 0.108$).

Correlations are reported such that a one unit increase in a given CT measurement is associated with the reported increase in HHS. For example, an increase in height of 1 cm is associated with a 1.263 decrease in HHS, and a one Hounsfield unit increase in Ipsilateral Gluteal Mean is associated with a 0.359 increase in HHS.

The resulting multivariate model that was produced was:

$$\begin{aligned} Predicted\ Change = {} & 0.42773 - 1.263 Height \\ & + 0.650 Age + 0.511 PAR \\ & + 1.759 POC + 0.359 IGM \end{aligned}$$

where PAR is Psoas Area Ratio, POC is Psoas Outer Circumference, and IGM is Ipsilateral Gluteal mean. When

Table 2 Results of inter-reader agreement analysis, with ICC shown for each measurement

Measurement	ICC Value	Measurement	ICC Value
Ipsilateral Iliopsoas Mean (HU)	0.978	Ipsilateral Gluteal Mean (HU)	0.914
Ipsilateral Iliopsoas Area (cm^2)	0.990	Ipsilateral Gluteal Area (cm^2)	0.895
Ipsilateral Iliopsoas Diameter (mm)	0.989	Ipsilateral Gluteal Diameter (mm)	0.905
Ipsilateral Iliopsoas Perimeter (mm)	0.946	Ipsilateral Gluteal Perimeter (mm)	0.957
Contralateral Iliopsoas Mean (HU)	0.959	Contralateral Gluteal Mean (HU)	0.991
Contralateral Iliopsoas Area (cm^2)	0.992	Contralateral Gluteal Area (cm^2)	0.930
Contralateral Iliopsoas Diameter (mm)	0.990	Contralateral Gluteal Diameter (mm)	0.940
Contralateral Iliopsoas Perimeter (mm)	0.858	Contralateral Gluteal Perimeter (mm)	0.959
Iliopsoas Visceral Fat Area (cm^2)	0.987	Gluteal Visceral Fat Area (cm^2)	0.980
Iliopsoas Subcutaneous Fat Area (cm^2)	0.965	Gluteal Subcutaneous Fat Area (cm^2)	0.976
Iliopsoas Area Ratio	0.904	Gluteal Area Ratio	0.921
Iliopsoas Outer Circumference (mm)	0.9995	Gluteal Outer Circumference (mm)	0.9999

Table 3 Significant results of univariate correlation between change in HHS and demographic and CT parameters

Parameter	Correlation Coefficient	*p*-value
Age	0.65033	0.018
Height	−1.2628	0.009
Iliopsoas Area Ratio	0.51126	0.018
Iliopsoas Outer Circumference	1.75897	0.002
Ipsilateral Gluteal Mean	0.35905	0.108

used to predict change in HHS for each patient, the model performed with $R^2 = 0.5858$ (Fig. 4).

Discussion

To the best of the authors' knowledge, this is the first attempt at evaluation of pelvis CT muscle and fat parameters and characterization of their bearing on THA outcomes. The software proved to be reliable in deriving muscle area, density, and circumference from CT images as confirmed by the inter-observer performance. The fat ratios are easily evaluated, yielding reproducible data regarding subcutaneous and visceral fat proportions. Outer waist circumference was also reproducibly measured.

While no significant correlation was found between any CT measurement and change in WOMAC Hip Score, it is apparent that some CT parameters correlated with the postoperative HHS assessment tool. However, some of the correlations we observed are not what would be expected. For instance, larger waist circumferences and higher visceral fat fractions, surrogate markers of obesity, have been shown to be associated with negative surgical outcomes [12, 13], but in this study, they were found to be associated with improved outcome after THA. We believe this anomaly may be due to the limitations of this study, such as its retrospective nature and relatively small sample size. However, a sensitivity analysis showed that the data adequately represented the overall THA study group.

Our data reflects a preliminary exploration of this topic and future studies should include prospective enrollment and a standardized multivariate statistical approach including intra-reader performance. Quantitative information obtained from preoperative imaging not only holds diagnostic value, it may also aid in prognostication. This information may prove beneficial in preoperative patient counseling and might aid preoperative and postoperative decision-making by identifying subpopulations of patients who may benefit by therapy aimed at improving muscle properties before undergoing THA. A follow-up study should involve prospective recruitment of patients with focus on uniform imaging procedures and consistent collection of outcome data in order to ensure a large sample size. While MRI is also a potential technique for the above measurements, in this retrospective evaluation CTs were available for these patients who uniformly had hip scoring performed prospectively. In addition, the Aquarius software used in this study is more useful for segmentation using CT data. Although MRI can provide fat fraction analysis with recent advanced Dixon techniques, it happens to be

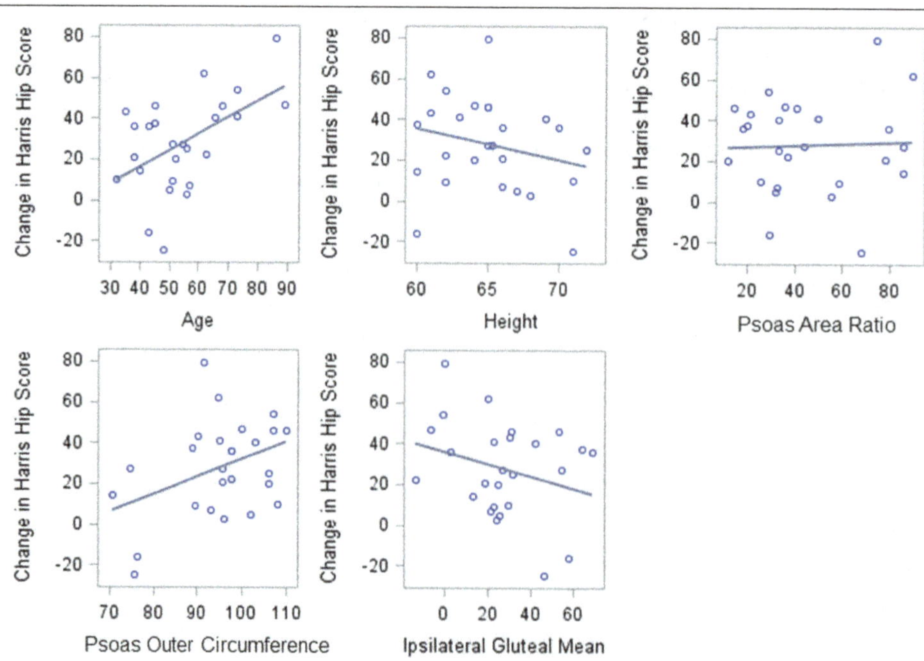

Fig. 3 Scatterplots of significant univariate correlations between change in HHS vs. demographic and CT parameters. The line shown is the linear, univariate correlation

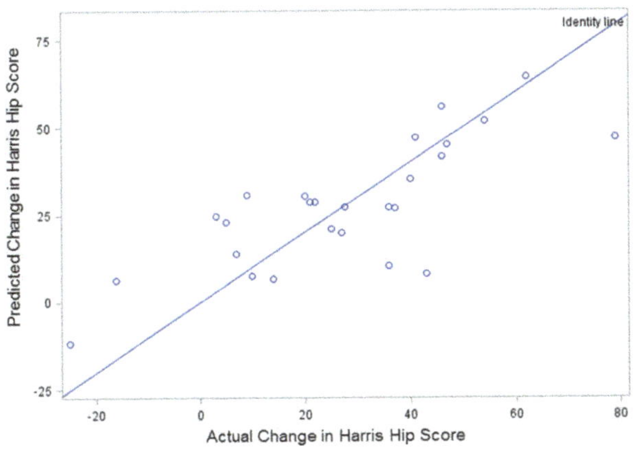

Fig. 4 Scatterplot of change in HHS as predicted by the multivariate regression vs. actual change in HHS. The line shown is a linear regression with $R^2 = 0.5858$

a more expensive study and the imaging may be limited by metal artifacts due to hip prosthesis. There has been recent encouraging work on muscle and fat composition using MRI with qualitative and quantitative muscle and fat fraction analyses yielding meaningful correlations of muscle volume and intramuscular steatosis with muscle power and post-surgical outcomes [14–17]. Similar work could be potentially performed in THA population using metal reduction techniques. Lastly, volumetric multi-slice evaluation is now available with recent software upgrades. In a future study, it could be employed using a similar dataset to determine whether correlations are markedly different from those presented in this study.

Conclusions

To conclude, multi-compartment tissue parameters derived from cross-sectional CT imaging can be useful as an additional preoperative planning tool for THA and establish a foundation for future prospective studies in this domain to expand validity of our preliminary results.

Abbreviations

CT: Computed Tomography; HHS: Harris Hip Score; ICC : Intra-class Correlation Coefficient; MRI: Magnetic Resonance Imaging; THA: Total Hip Arthroplasty; TJA : Total Joint Arthroplasty; WOMAC: Western Ontario and McMaster Universities Osteoarthritis Index

Acknowledgements

The authors acknowledge and thank Robert W. Bucholz, MD, who assembled the TJA registry over many years.

Funding

Only institutional sources of funding were used for this project.

Authors' contributions

The study was conceived by HB, AC, and MH. The study was designed by HB, AC, and MH. Data was acquired by MAH, RB, and HB. YX was responsible for the quality of the data, statistical data analysis, and data interpretation. The manuscript was prepared by MAH, RB, and AC. DH provided guidance for improvement of the manuscript content by revising it critically and advising inclusion of new, intellectually important content. The manuscript was edited by MAH, RB, AC, and DH. The manuscript was reviewed and approved for final publication by all authors.

Consent for publication

Not applicable.

Competing interests

AC is a consultant for Siemens regarding MSK CAD in areas not related to this study. DH and AC also serve on the editorial board of this journal, BMC Musculoskeletal Disorders. The authors declare no other competing interests.

Author details

[1]Department of Orthopedic Surgery, University of Texas Southwestern Medical Center, Dallas, TX, USA. [2]Department of Radiology, University of Texas Southwestern Medical Center, 5323 Harry Hines Blvd, Dallas, TX 75390-8896, USA. [3]Department of Radiology, Boston University Medical Center, Boston, MA, USA.

References

1. Kurtz S, Ong K, Lau E, Mowat F, Halpern M. Projections of primary and revision hip and knee arthroplasty in the United States from 2005 to 2030. J Bone Joint Surg Am. 2007;89:780–5.
2. Ong KL, Mowat FS, Chan N, Lau E, Halpern MT, Kurtz SM. Economic burden of revision hip and knee arthroplasty in Medicare enrollees. Clin Orthop Relat Res. 2006;446:22–8.
3. Wiater BP, Koueiter DM, Maerz T, et al. Preoperative deltoid size and fatty infiltration of the deltoid and rotator cuff correlate to outcomes after reverse total shoulder arthroplasty. Clin Orthop Relat Res. 2015;473:663–73.
4. Jones KI, Doleman B, Scott S, Lund JN, Williams JP. Simple psoas cross-sectional area measurement is a quick and easy method to assess sarcopenia and predicts major surgical complications. Color Dis. 2015; 17:O20–6.
5. Joglekar S, Asghar A, Mott SL, et al. Sarcopenia is an independent predictor of complications following pancreatectomy for adenocarcinoma. J Surg Oncol. 2015;111:771–5.
6. Cornet M, Lim C, Salloum C, et al. Prognostic value of sarcopenia in liver surgery. J Visc Surg. 2015;152:297–304.
7. Englesbe MJ, Patel SP, He K, et al. Sarcopenia and mortality after liver transplantation. J Am Coll Surg. 2010;211:271–8.
8. Fairchild B, Webb TP, Xiang Q, Tarima S, Brasel KJ. Sarcopenia and frailty in elderly trauma patients. World J Surg. 2015;39:373–9.
9. Lachiewicz PF. Abductor tendon tears of the hip: evaluation and management. J Am Acad Orthop Surg. 2011;19:385–91.
10. Wakabayashi H, Watanabe N, Anraku M, Oritsu H, Shimizu Y. Pre-operative psoas muscle mass and post-operative gait speed following total hip arthroplasty for osteoarthritis. J Cachexia Sarcopenia Muscle. 2016;7:95–6.
11. Nankaku MPP, Tsuboyama TPM, Aoyama TPM, Kuroda YPM, Ikeguchi RPM, Matsuda SPM. Preoperative gluteus medius muscle atrophy as a predictor of walking ability after total hip arthroplasty. Phys Ther Res. 2016;19:8–12.
12. Kovesdy CP, Czira ME, Rudas A, et al. Body mass index, waist circumference and mortality in kidney transplant recipients. Am J Transplant. 2010;10: 2644–51.

13. Aquina CT, Rickles AS, Probst CP, et al. Visceral obesity, not elevated BMI, is strongly associated with incisional hernia after colorectal surgery. Dis *Colon rectum* 2015;58:220-227.
14. Marcon M, Berger N, Manoliu A, et al. Normative values for volume and fat content of the hip abductor muscles and their dependence on side, age and gender in a healthy population. Skelet Radiol. 2016;45:465–74.
15. Lang T, Cauley JA, Tylavsky F, et al. Computed tomographic measurements of thigh muscle cross-sectional area and attenuation coefficient predict hip fracture: the health, aging, and body composition study. J Bone Miner Res. 2010;25:513–9.
16. Inacio M, Ryan AS, Bair WN, Prettyman M, Beamer BA, Rogers MW. Gluteal muscle composition differentiates fallers from non-fallers in community dwelling older adults. BMC Geriatr. 2014;14:37.
17. Lee S, Lucas RM, Lansdown DA, et al. Magnetic resonance rotator cuff fat fraction and its relationship with tendon tear severity and subject characteristics. J Shoulder Elb Surg. 2015;24:1442–51.

14

Hip stability after total hip arthroplasty predicted by intraoperative stability test and range of motion

Hiromasa Tanino*, Tatsuya Sato, Yasuhiro Nishida, Ryo Mitsutake and Hiroshi Ito

Abstract

Background: Dislocation continues to be a common complication following total hip arthroplasty (THA). A larger intraoperative range of motion (ROM) is believed to minimize dislocation risk, and intraoperative stability tests have been used to assess the ROM. However, it is not clear whether or not intraoperative stability tests can predict hip stability after THA. It is also unclear which angles are required in intraoperative stability tests. We investigated the usefulness of intraoperative stability tests, and other risk factors to predict hip stability after THA.

Methods: Patients operated by single surgeon at one hospital from June 2009 to December 2013 were evaluated. This study included 185 hips with 32 mm metal femoral head. The range of internal rotation with 90° hip flexion (IR angle) was measured as an intraoperative stability test. The variables studied as risk factors included age, height, weight, gender, cerebral dysfunction, preoperative diagnosis, history of previous hip surgery, and IR angle.

Results: Mean IR angle was statistically different between patients with dislocation and patients without dislocation (59.5° vs 69.6°: $p = 0.006$). Cerebral dysfunction and a history of previous hip surgery were statistically related with prevalence of dislocation ($p = 0.021$, and $p = 0.011$). The receiver-operating characteristic curve analysis suggested that the cutoff points for IR angle were 51° and 67°. Dislocation rate in larger IR angle group was significantly lower than the rate in smaller IR angle group when patients were divided by 51° ($p = 0.002$). Logistic regression analyses showed that significant risk factors were cerebral dysfunction (OR: 5.3 (95%CI 1.1–25.9); $p = 0.037$), history of previous hip surgery (OR: 8.6 (95%CI 1.2–63.0); $p = 0.035$), and IR angle (OR: 10.4 (95%CI 1.9–57.1); $p = 0.007$).

Conclusions: The results showed that intraoperative stability test, especially the IR angle, was a useful method to predict hip stability after THA, and a larger intraoperative ROM reduced the likelihood of dislocation. 51° and 67° were indicated as cutoff points for IR angle. Cerebral dysfunction and a history of previous hip surgery are also risk factors for the incidence of dislocation after THA.

Keywords: Dislocation, Total hip arthroplasty, Range of motion, Hip

* Correspondence: tanino@asahikawa-med.ac.jp
Department of Orthopaedic Surgery, Asahikawa Medical University, Midorigaoka-Higashi 2-1-1-1, Asahikawa 078-8510, Japan

Background

Dislocation continues to be a common complication following total hip arthroplasty (THA). In a recent study of 51,345 revision hip arthroplasties in the United States, dislocation was the most common cause of revision (22.5%), and was higher than both infection and aseptic loosening [1]. In the Australian Orthopaedic Association Registry, dislocation was reported as the reason for revision in 21.6% of cases, which was next after loosening [2]. Many factors affect the prevalence of dislocation after THA, including soft-tissue laxity, surgical approach, component position, patient factors, and component designs [3]. A larger intraoperative range of motion (ROM) is believed to minimize dislocation risk, and intraoperative stability tests have been used to assess the ROM [4]. Many in vitro studies have investigated the ROM of the hip, impingement, and dislocation mechanisms, and they reported the factors related to ROM, including component position, head diameter, and component design [5]. However, it is not clear whether or not intraoperative stability tests can predict hip stability after THA. It is also unclear which angles are required in intraoperative stability tests for a stable hip after THA because different angles have been indicated as an acceptable ROM [4, 6–9]. This study included patients with one metal femoral head diameter and evaluated the effect of intraoperative ROM on dislocation rates after THA. We also evaluated the combined effect of other risk factors in conjunction with intraoperative ROM. Our hypothesis was that intraoperative stability tests would be effective to indicate hip stability after THA, and that a large intraoperative ROM would reduce the likelihood of dislocation after THA.

Methods

Study population

Between June 2009 and December 2013, the senior surgeon performed primary THA in 274 consecutive patients (299 hips) at Asahikawa Medical University Hospital. For inclusion in the analysis, the following were required: primary THA, single surgeon at one hospital, intraoperative ROM data available, no second surgeries before the first dislocation event, follow-up longer than 6 months, and a 32 mm metal femoral head had been used. A 32 mm metal femoral head was used in 185 patients (199 hips) out of an initial 274 patients. Fourteen hips were excluded (ROM data availability 6 hips, second surgery before the first dislocation 1 hip, short follow-up 3 hips, and died within 6 months 4 hips), thus 185 hips (171 patients) were included and analyzed in this study (Fig. 1). The average age was 64 years (range, 20–87 years), and height and weight averaged 153 cm and 58 kg, respectively. There were 128 women and 43 men, with 81 left and 104 right THAs. The average length of follow-up was 14 months (range, 6–44 months). The preoperative diagnoses were osteoarthritis in 146, osteonecrosis of the femoral head in 23, rheumatoid arthritis in 9, and femoral neck fracture in 7. The project was approved by the Institutional Review Board at our hospital (AMU 800).

Surgery

All of the procedures were performed in the lateral decubitus position, using a posterolateral approach without posterior capsule or external rotator repair. All components were determined intraoperatively in a standard fashion based on preoperative templating, then

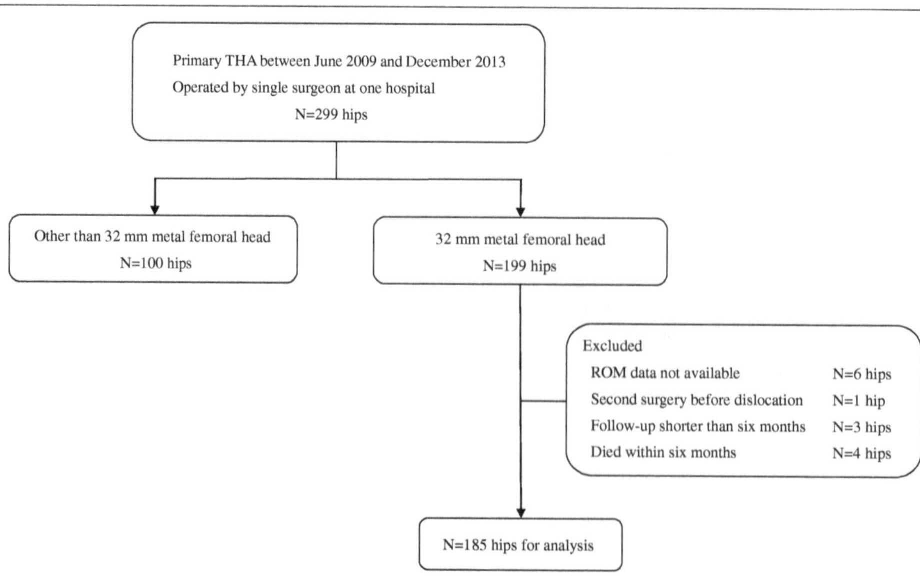

Fig. 1 Flowchart depicting patient inclusion and exclusion in the cross-sectional study

placed into position. In general, patients older than age 60 received cemented femoral fixation, and younger patients had cementless femoral prostheses. The femoral prostheses used in this series included 149 cemented 4-U prostheses (Nakashima Medical Co., Japan) [10, 11] and 36 cementless prostheses (S-ROM; Depuy, IN or 4-U CLS; Nakashima Medical Co.). All of the acetabular components were cementless, including a 146 4-U cup (Nakashima Medical Co.), a 25 Trilogy cup (Zimmer, IN), and a 14 4-U CLS cup (Nakashima Medical Co.). The diameter of the metal femoral head was 32 mm with a polyethylene liner in all hips. A standard flat liner was used in 5 hips and an elevated liner in 180.

Data collection

The variables studied as risk factors for dislocation after THA included age, height, weight, gender, cerebral dysfunction, preoperative diagnosis, and history of previous hip surgery. Cerebral dysfunction included mental confusion, dementia, and mental disorder at the time of surgery and dislocation; this was similar to another study [6]. Another category entitled *IR angle* was investigated as a measure of intraoperative stability. After all components were placed into position and removal of acetabular osteophytes and femoral neck remnants, the range of internal rotation with 90° hip flexion and 0° abduction/adduction (IR angle) was measured to determine the position of posterior dislocation, similar to Sultan et al. [12]. The femoral head was observed by the senior surgeon, while the hips were ranged by the assistant surgeon; the same assistant surgeon ranged all hips in this study. The point of instability was determined by direct visual inspection and was predefined as the point at which the head began riding out of the liner. A double-armed universal goniometer was used with one arm parallel to the floor and the other parallel to the tibia to determine hip rotation during measurement relative to the floor. The postoperative rehabilitation program was identical for all patients. Patients began ambulation on the first postoperative day and were allowed immediate full weight bearing using a walker or crutches. All patients included in this study were routinely followed-up at one clinic, and dislocation rates were obtained through clinic records.

Statistical analysis

For continuous variables, the normality of the data was assessed using Shapiro-Wilk test, and statistical analysis was done using a nonparametric Mann-Whitney U test. Statistical analysis was done using a chi-square test for nominal variables. Receiver-operating characteristic (ROC) curve was applied to determine the optimum cutoff point for IR angle. The cutoff point was determined by the Youden index [13]. The area under curve (AUC) was also calculated from ROC curve. Logistic regression was performed using all eight variables; age, height, weight, gender, cerebral dysfunction, preoperative diagnosis, history of previous hip surgery, and IR angle. A $p < 0.05$ was considered significant. Statistical analyses were performed using SPSS Version 24 (SPSS Inc., IL).

Results

Eleven patients (11 hips) sustained a hip dislocation resulting in a prevalence of 5.9%. Seven women and four men had 10 posterior dislocations and one anterior dislocation. Nine (82%) of the dislocations occurred during the first 3 months after surgery. Six patients had a single episode of dislocation and five had more than one dislocation. All dislocations were reduced without surgery. One of the 11 patients required revision of the cup, liner, and head because of instability.

Patient average age, height, weight and gender were not statistically different between patients with dislocation and patients without dislocation after THA ($p = 0.195$, $p = 0.298$, $p = 0.197$ and $p = 0.249$). There was a significant difference in the dislocation rates in the 29 patients (31 hips) classified as having cerebral dysfunction compared to the 142 patients (154 hips) with no cerebral dysfunction (16% vs 3.9%: $p = 0.021$). The preoperative diagnoses were categorized into 2 classes: 1) osteoarthritis, or 2) osteonecrosis of the femoral head, rheumatoid arthritis, and femoral neck fracture. Using this classification, there was no significant relationship between the class of diagnosis and the rate of dislocation ($p = 0.419$). A history of previous hip surgery was statistically related to prevalence of dislocation (33% vs 4.5%: $p = 0.011$) (Table 1).

The mean IR angle was 69.0° (range, 37–95°), and was statistically different between patients with dislocation and patients without dislocation after THA (59.5° vs 69.6°: $p = 0.006$) (Table 1). To investigate posterior stability, one patient with anterior dislocation was excluded from the subsequent analyses of IR angles. Mean IR angle was also statistically different between patients with posterior dislocation and patients who did not have a dislocation after THA (58.4° vs 69.6°: $p = 0.004$) (Fig. 2). The ROC curve analysis suggested the optimum cutoff point for IR angle was 51°, with a sensitivity of 0.5, a specificity of 1.0, a positive likelihood ratio of 9.7, and a negative likelihood ratio of 0.5. The AUC measured 0.8 (p = 0.004, 95%CI 0.6–0.9). When a sensitivity was 0.8, IR angle was 67°, with a specificity of 0.6, a positive likelihood ratio of 2.1, and a negative likelihood ratio of 0.3 (Fig. 3). Dislocation rate in larger IR angle group was significantly lower than the rate in smaller IR angle group when patients were divided by 51° (3.5% vs 33%: $p = 0.002$). For logistic regression analyses, all eight variables were used, and IR angle was used as a dichotomized variable (≥51° vs < 51°). Adjusting with age, height, weight, gender, and

Table 1 Studied Variables

Variables	Patients Without Dislocation (range)	Patients With Dislocation (range)	*p* Value
No. patients	160, 174 hips	11, 11 hips	
Average age (y)	64.4 (20–87)	59.1 (43–82)	0.195
Average height (cm)	152.7 (135.0–175.0)	156.8 (138.5–173.3)	0.298
Average weight (kg)	57.9 (34.0–91.0)	64.2 (36.0–93.0)	0.197
Gender			
Female	134	7	
Male	40	4	0.249
Cerebral dysfunction			
(+)	26	5	
(−)	148	6	0.021
Preoperative diagnosis			
OA	138	8	
ON, RA, Fx	36	3	0.419
History of previous hip surgery			
(+)	6	3	
(−)	168	8	0.011
IR angle	69.6° (37–95)	59.5° (45–75)	0.006

OA osteoarthritis, *ON* osteonecrosis of the femoral head, *RA* rheumatoid arthritis, *Fx* femoral neck fracture
No data missing

preoperative diagnosis, we observed that significant risk factors were the presence of cerebral dysfunction (OR: 5.3 (95%CI 1.1–25.9); $p = 0.037$), history of previous hip surgery (OR: 8.6 (95%CI 1.2–63.0); $p = 0.035$), and IR angle (OR: 10.4 (95%CI 1.9–57.1); $p = 0.007$) (Table 2).

Discussion

We investigated the usefulness of intraoperative stability tests, and other risk factors to predict hip stability after THA. Intraoperative stability testing, especially IR angle, was a useful method to predict hip stability after THA,

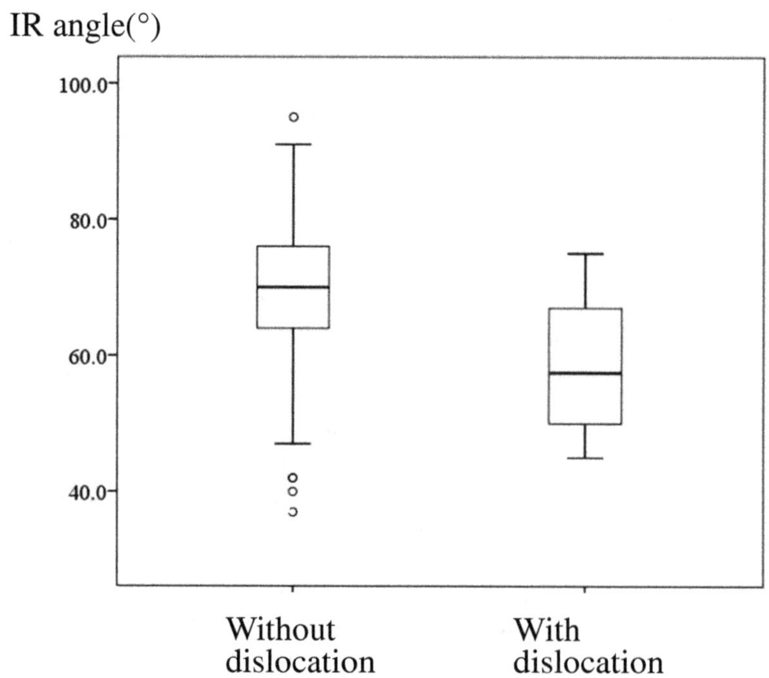

Fig. 2 Box-plots of IR angles without dislocation and with dislocation

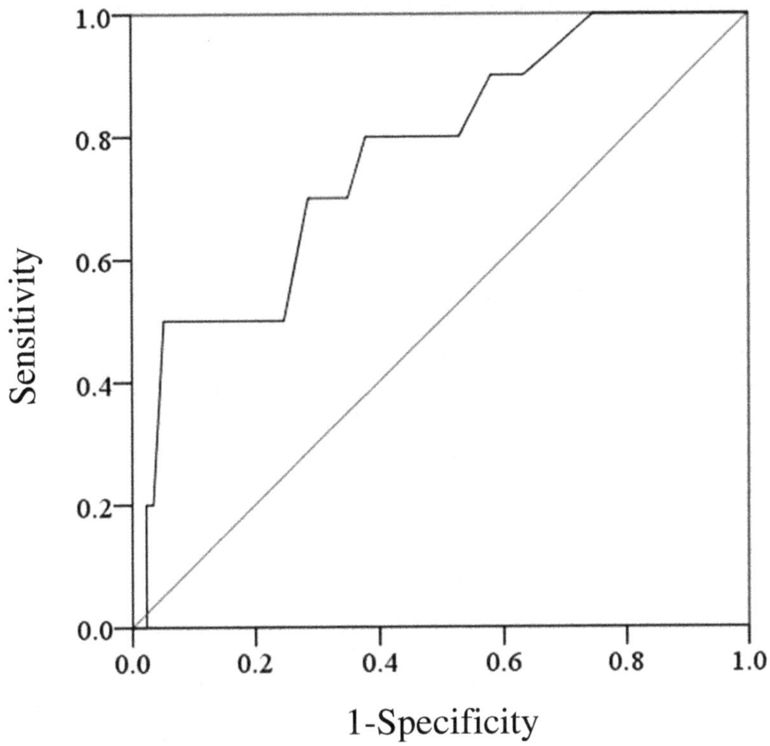

Fig. 3 ROC curve of IR angle. The ROC curve analysis suggested the optimum cutoff point for IR angle was 51°, with a sensitivity of 0.5, a specificity of 1.0, a positive likelihood ratio of 9.7, and a negative likelihood ratio of 0.5. The AUC measured 0.8 ($p = 0.004$, 95%CI 0.6–0.9). When a sensitivity was 0.8, IR angle was 67°, with a specificity of 0.6, a positive likelihood ratio of 2.1, and a negative likelihood ratio of 0.3

and a larger intraoperative ROM reduced the likelihood of dislocation after THA with a cutoff point of 51°. Cerebral dysfunction and a history of previous hip surgery are also risk factors for the incidence of dislocation after THA.

Robinson et al. reported IR angle was related to component position in their computational model, and Sultan et al. reported IR angle was related to the diameter of the prosthetic femoral head and the elevated liner intraoperatively [12, 14]. Recently, Bunn et al. investigated the relationship between intraoperative stability tests and high-risk activities for dislocation using computer modeling [15]. However, the validity of intraoperative stability tests in identifying risks for postoperative dislocation is unknown, as Bunn et al. stated [15]. Several different positions and tests have been used to investigate stability after THA. Harris described two critical positions to test the ROM: flexion plus internal rotation and extension plus external rotation [4]. The shuck test and drop kick test have been also used to test stability after THA [16]. The maximum flexion possible with the hip at 10° of adduction and 10° of internal rotation was used to test posterior stability in computational and experimental studies [17, 18]. Nadzadi et al. reported the kinematics of 5 positions associated with posterior dislocation and 2 positions associated with anterior dislocation [19]. It may be ideal to evaluate these 7 positions, but the authors feel it is too complex to implement during surgery. The results of this study showed that intraoperative stability test, especially the IR angle, was a useful method to predict posterior stability after THA. We found that cerebral dysfunction and history of previous hip surgery were also risk factors for the incidence of dislocation after THA, which is the same as in other studies [6].

Table 2 Association of Variables with the Incidence of Dislocation by Multiple Logistic Regression Analysis

Variables	Odds Ratio	95% Confidence Interval	*p* Value
Cerebral dysfunction	5.3	(1.1, 25.9)	0.037
History of previous hip surgery	8.6	(1.2, 63.0)	0.035
IR angle (ref. = ≥51°)	10.4	(1.9, 57.1)	0.007

It has not been clear which angles are required on intraoperative stability tests for stable hips after THA. Considerable variation in normal ROM exists among people and studies. The handbook of the American Academy of Orthopaedic Surgeons [20], which contains estimates of adult hip joint motion obtained from three referenced studies reported mean angles of internal rotation were 44°, 32°, and 33°. The prosthetic ROM must be larger than the normal ROM, as Widmer stated [21].

Harris reported that the limb after THA should flex to at least 110° and also go to 20° of internal rotation while at 90° of flexion without impingement [4]. Woolson et al. reported that hips after THA should have an intraoperative ROM of at least 90° of flexion combined with 30° of internal rotation without instability [6]. Sierra et al. reported 100° of flexion combined with 45° internal rotation as acceptable ROM [7]. Yoshimine used an IR angle of more than 30° as a moderate criteria of acceptable ROM conditions after THA in a computational study [8]. Recently, Lachiewicz and Soileau reported flexion past 90° and internal rotation of at least 60° as a stable hip using 36 mm or 40 mm femoral heads [9]. However, there were no explanations or reasons given for these acceptable ROMs. This study showed a larger intraoperative ROM reduced the likelihood of dislocation after THA, and 51° was indicated as a cutoff point for IR angle. Because it is important for surgeons to have an intraoperative stability test with a high sensitivity and our results showed IR angle was 67° when a sensitivity was 0.8, we also suggest 67° to be the severe criteria of cutoff point for IR angle. These cutoff points were larger than the normal ROM [20] and were also larger than the movements in commonplace maneuvers known to increase the risk for dislocation in THA [19]. Most modern THA systems provide the surgeon with a variety of options regarding neck lengths, head sizes, and acetabular liner configurations, allowing the surgeon to fine tune the components chosen for final implantation with the goal of providing the patient with optimum stability and ROM.

Many in vitro and computational studies have reported ROM at impingement [14, 17]. We measured the angle at dislocation. The angle at impingement and the angle at dislocation were not the same. Bartz et al. investigated the range of flexion of the hip joint from impingement to frank dislocation, and reported that it was between 2.1° to 7.3° [18]. Robinson et al. reported 12° of joint motion from the point of impingement until dislocation was simulated [14]. Thus, the IR angles we measured were slightly larger than the IR angles measured at impingement in computational and experimental studies.

This study has several limitations. The first limitation is related to the surgical approach and posterior capsule repair. It has been reported that the surgical technique of capsular and external rotator repair had a significant effect on reducing the dislocation rate when a posterolateral approach was used [7, 22]. The dislocation rate in this study was at the upper limit of dislocation rates among recent studies [22, 23], and the dislocation rate in this study may have been related to our use of a posterolateral approach without posterior capsular or external rotator repair.

The second limitation is that this study investigated only posterior instability. Although posterior dislocation is recognized as the most common instability mode and is reported to account for 75% to 90% of dislocations [24], this study did not investigate anterior instability. Although recent study reported the factors related with anterior instability [25], more studies are needed to investigate this limitation.

The third limitation of this study is that rigid orientation standards were not employed, in that the exact position of the pelvis in space relative to the operating room floor was not available. And the repeatability of IR angle measurements and accuracy test have not been reported. To investigate the repeatability of IR angle measurements, the IR angle was measured three times in three patients during surgery. The intraobserver reproducibility was calculated using interclass correlation coefficient. The intraobserver reproducibility was excellent with 1.0 (95%CI 0.8–1.0). Because the measurements of IR angle in this study were done by the single surgeon and the same assistant surgeon, the interobserver reliability was not investigated. And many clinical studies have stated IR angle as an intraoperative stability test [4, 6, 9], and in vivo, computational, and cadaver studies have measured IR angles [8, 12]. We investigated differences in intraoperative ROM in patients without dislocation compared to patients with dislocation. As a result, we believe the IR angle to be suitable for the objectives of this study.

The fourth limitation is related to the number of dislocations and the number of the variables in this study. Peduzzi et al. reported the validity of the logistic model became problematic when the ratio of the numbers of events per variable analysed became small [26]. We performed logistic regression using three variables that were statistically significant in a chi-square test or a nonparametric Mann-Whitney U test, and using all eight variables. Logistic regression analyses determined that significant risk factors were same in both analyses; the presence of cerebral dysfunction, history of previous hip surgery, and IR angle. So, we think logistic regression analyses in this study are robust.

Despite numerous case series in the literature documenting lower dislocation rates in association with enhanced soft- tissue repair techniques and the use of large diameter femoral heads, hip instability/dislocation was one of the most common causes of revision in large series reports [1, 2]. Additional research is necessary to understand the current causes of THA instability and to enhance stability following THA.

Conclusions

This study investigated the relationship between intraoperative stability tests and the incidence of dislocation after THA. Intraoperative stability testing, especially the IR angle, was a useful method to predict posterior stability after THA, and a larger intraoperative ROM reduced the likelihood of dislocation after THA. Cerebral dysfunction and a history of previous hip surgery are also risk factors for the incidence of dislocation after THA. Although different angles have been indicated as an acceptable ROM, 51° was indicated as a cutoff point for IR angle, and 67° was also indicated as the severe criteria of cutoff point for IR angle.

Abbreviations

95%CI: 95% Confidence interval; AUC: Area under curve; IR angle: The range of internal rotation with 90° hip flexion; OR: Odds ratio; ROC curve: Receiver-operating characteristic curve; ROM: Range of motion; THA: Total hip arthroplasty

Funding

No supporting grants for this study.

Authors' contributions

The study was conceived and designed by HT and HI. Data was acquired by HT, TS, YN, RM, and HI. HT performed the statistical analysis and drafted the manuscript. The manuscript was edited by TS, YN, RM, and HI. The manuscript was reviewed and approved for final publication by all authors.

Consent for publication

Not applicable.

Competing interests

The authors declare that they have no competing interests.

References

1. Bozic KJ, Kurtz SM, Lau E, Ong K, Vail TP, Berry DJ. The epidemiology of revision total hip arthroplasty in the United States. J Bone Joint Surg Am. 2009;91(1):128–33.
2. Australian Orthopaedic Association, National Joint Replacement Register. 2017. https://aoanjrr.sahmri.com/home Accessed 30 April 2018.
3. Tanino H, Harman MK, Banks SA, Hodge WA. Association between dislocation, impingement, and articular geometry in retrieved acetabular polyethylene cups. J Orthop Res. 2007;25(11):1401–7.
4. Harris WA. Advances in surgical technique for total hip replacement: without and with osteotomy of the greater trochanter. Clin Orthop Relat Res. 1980;146:188–204.
5. Amstutz HC, Lodwig RM, Schurman DJ, Hodgson AG. Range of motion studies for total hip replacements. A comparative study with a new experimental apparatus. Clin Orthop Relat Res. 1975;111:124–30.
6. Woolson ST, Rahimtoola ZO. Risk factors for dislocation during the first 3 months after primary total hip replacement. J Arthroplast. 1999;14(6):662–8.
7. Sierra RJ, Raposo JM, Trousdale RT, Cabanela ME. Dislocation of primary THA done through a posterolateral approach in the elderly. Clin Orthop Relat Res. 2005;441:262–7.
8. Yoshimine F. The influence of the oscillation angle and the neck anteversion of the prosthesis on the cup safe-zone that fulfills the criteria for range of motion in total hip replacements. The required oscillation angle for an acceptable cup safe-zone. J Biomech. 2005;38(1):125–32.
9. Lachiewicz PF, Soileau ES. Low early and late dislocation rates with 36- and 40-mm heads in patients at high risk for dislocation. Clin Orthop Relat Res. 2013;471:439–43.
10. Tanino H, Ito H, Higa M, Omizu N, Nishimura I, Matsuda K, Mitamura Y, Matsuno T. Three-dimensional computer-aided design based design sensitivity analysis and shape optimization of the stem using adaptive p-method. J Biomech. 2006;39(10):1948–53.
11. Ito H, Tanino H, Yamanaka Y, Nakamura T, Matsuno T. Hybrid total hip arthroplasty using specifically-designed stems for patients with developmental dysplasia of the hip. A minimum five-year follow-up study. Int Orthop. 2011;35(9):1289–94.
12. Sultan PG, Tan V, Lai M, Garino JP. Independent contribution of elevated-rim acetabular liner and femoral head size to the stability of total hip implants. J Arthroplast. 2002;17(3):289–92.
13. Imai N, Miyasaka D, Shimada H, Suda K, Ito T, Endo N. Usefulness of a novel method for the screening of deep vein thrombosis by using a combined d-dimer- and age-based index before total hip arthroplasty. PLoS One. 2017; 12(2):e0172849.
14. Robinson RP, Simonian PT, Gradisar IM, Ching RP. Joint motion and surface contact area related to component position in total hip arthroplasty. J Bone Joint Surg Br. 1997;79(1):140–6.
15. Bunn A, Colwell CW Jr, D'Lima DD. Effect of head diameter on passive and active dynamic hip dislocation. J Orthop Res. 2014;32(11):1525–31.
16. Charles MN, Bourne RB, Davey JR, Greenwald AS, Morrey BF, Rorabeck CH. Soft-tissue balance of the hip. The role of femoral offset restoration. J Bone Joint Surg Am. 2004;86(5):1078–88.
17. D'Lima DD, Urquhart AG, Buehler KO, Walker RH, Colwell CW Jr. The effect of the orientation of the acetabular and femoral components on the range of motion of the hip at different head-neck ratios. J Bone Joint Surg Am. 2000;82(3):315–21.
18. Bartz RL, Noble PC, Kadakia NR, Tullos HS. The effect of femoral component head size on posterior dislocation of the artificial hip joint. J Bone Joint Surg Am. 2000;82(9):1300–7.
19. Nadzadi ME, Pedersen DR, Yack HJ, Callaghan JJ, Brown TD. Kinematics, kinetics, and finite element analysis of commonplace maneuvers at risk for total hip dislocation. J Biomech. 2003;36(4):577–91.
20. Greene WB, Heckman JD, editors. The Hip. In: The clinical measurement of joint motion. Rosemont: American Academy of Orthopaedic Surgeons; 1994. p. 99–114.
21. Widmer KH, Zurfluh B. Compliant positioning of total hip components for optimal range of motion. J Orthop Res. 2004;22(4):815–21.
22. Kwon MS, Kuskowski M, Mulhall KJ, Macaulay WM, Brown TE, Saleh KJ. Does surgical approach affect total hip arthroplasty dislocation rates? Clin Orthop Relat Res. 2006;447:34–8.
23. Berry DJ, Knoch MV, Schleck CD, Harmsen WS. Effect of femoral head diameter and operative approach on risk of dislocation after primary total hip arthroplasty. J Bone Joint Surg Am. 2005;87(11):2456–63.
24. Sanchez-Sotelo J, Berry DJ. Epidemiology of instability after total hip replacement. Orthop Clin North Am. 2001;32(4):543–52.
25. Tanino H, Sato T, Nishida Y, Ito H. Anterior instability of total hip arthroplasty with posterolateral approach. Orthop Res Soc. 2016;1951. https://www.ors.org/abstract-search/.
26. Peduzzi P, Concato J, Kemper E, Holford TR, Feinstein AR. A simulation study of the number of events per variable in logistic regression analysis. J Clin Epidemiol. 1996;49(12):1373–9.

A prospective randomized comparison of the minimally invasive direct anterior and the transgluteal approach for primary total hip arthroplasty

Johannes C. Reichert[1,2*], Eberhard von Rottkay[2], Franz Roth[1], Tim Renz[1], Johannes Hausmann[1], Julius Kranz[1], Lars Rackwitz[2], Ulrich Nöth[1,2] and Maximilian Rudert[1]

Abstract

Background: The presented prospective randomized controlled single-centre study compares the clinical outcome up to 12 months after total hip arthroplasty using a minimally invasive single-incision direct anterior (DAA) and a direct transgluteal lateral approach.

Methods: A total of 123 arthroplasties were evaluated utilizing the Harris Hip Score (HHS), the extra short musculoskeletal functional assessment questionnaire (XSFMA), the Short Form 36 (SF-36) health survey, a Stepwatch™ Activity Monitor (SAM), and a timed 25 m foot walk (T25-FW). Postoperative x-ray images after THA were reviewed to determine inclination and stem positioning.

Results: At final follow-up, the XSFMA functional index scores were 10.3 (anterior) and 15.08 (lateral) while the bother index summed up to a score of 15.8 (anterior) and 21.66 (lateral) respectively, thus only differing significantly for the functional index ($p = 0.040$ and $p = 0.056$). The SF-36 physical component score (PCS) was 47.49 (anterior) and 42.91 (lateral) while the mental component score (MCS) summed up to 55.0 (anterior) and 56.23 (lateral) with a significant difference evident for the PCS ($p = 0.017$; $p = 0.714$). Patients undergoing THA through a DAA undertook a mean of 6402 cycles per day while those who had undergone THA through a transgluteal approach undertook a mean of 5340 cycles per day ($p = 0.012$). Furthermore, the obtained outcome for the T25-FW with 18.4 s (anterior) and 19.75 s (lateral) and the maximum walking distance (5932 m and 5125 m) differed significantly ($p = 0.046$ and $p = 0.045$). The average HHS showed no significant difference equaling 92.4 points in the anterior group and 91.43 in the lateral group ($p = 0.477$). The radiographic analysis revealed an average cup inclination of 38.6° (anterior) and 40.28° (lateral) without signs of migration.

Conclusion: In summary, our outcomes show that after 1 year THA through the direct anterior approach results in a higher patient activity compared to THA utilizing a transgluteal lateral approach while no differences regarding hip function are evident.

Keywords: Total hip arthroplasty, Direct anterior approach, Minimally invasive, Transgluteal approach, Prospective study

* Correspondence: johannes.c.reichert@googlemail.com
[1]Department of Orthopaedic Surgery, König-Ludwig-Haus, Center for Musculoskeletal Research, Julius-Maximilians-University, Brettreichstraße 11, 97074 Würzburg, Germany
[2]Department of Orthopaedic and Trauma Surgery, Evangelisches Waldkrankenhaus Spandau, Stadtrandstrasse 555, 13589 Berlin, Germany

Background

Total hip arthroplasty (THA) can generally be seen as a very successful procedure in the field of orthopaedics [1]. The demand for THA and especially minimally invasive surgeries (MIS) is continuously increasing [2] as successful THA results in pain relief and restored joint functionality allowing a higher degree of patient activity and therefore quality of life [3]. Minimally invasive THA is most commonly performed utilizing the direct anterior (DAA), the anterolateral and the posterior approach to the hip. MIS is associated with less blood loss [4], decreased perioperative pain levels, and faster recovery [3, 5]. However, there is still ample debate whether early functional outcomes differ using the DAA or a standard lateral approach [6].

Consequently, the primary aim of the present randomized controlled single-centre study was to prospectively compare the functional outcome, as measured by the HHS and SAM, between patients undergoing minimally invasive THA through a DAA with those undergoing THA through a conventional transgluteal approach. Secondary aims included comparison of the XSMFA (functional and bother index), a timed 25 m foot walk (T25-FW), and the short-form 36 questionnaire (SF-36 mental and physical).

Methods

The present investigator sponsored, prospective randomized controlled single-centre study was approved by the ethics committee of the medical faculty of the University of Würzburg (approval number 72/11) and compares two different surgical techniques, the minimally invasive DAA as described by Rachbauer [7] and the lateral transgluteal approach according to Bauer et al. [8]. The DAA was introduced in our orthopaedic department in 2008 as a routine approach for THA. Prior to 2008 the transgluteal approach was predominately used. An a priori power analysis using G*Power 3 was performed to determine the necessary sample size N for a two-sample t test of independent variables given an α error probability of 0.05, a desired power level of 0.8 (1-β), and a medium effect size of 0.5. The required N was calculated to be 60 per group. With a power level of 0.9 a total of 81 patients would have been required in each group. The study was powered to detect a 500 step difference in measurements obtained with the SAM at a single time point assuming an average of 5500 steps/day and a standard deviation of 1000. A significance level of 5% was chosen.

The SAM (StepWatch Activity Monitor, Orthocare Innovations, 6405 218th St SW, Suite 100, Mountlake Terrace, WA 98043–2180, US) is an example of an accelerometer based activity monitor that has been used widely in different population groups. The SAM is small (75 × 50 × 20 mm) and lightweight (38 g) and is worn at the ankle. The monitor contains a custom sensor that uses a combination of acceleration, position, and timing to detect steps. Thus the outputs of the SAM are based on the amount, rate, and pattern of walking. The SAM is calibrated based on each individual's height and gait pattern. Reported intraclass correlation coefficients (ICCs) for mean steps/day range from 0.86 to 0.99 representing an excellent test-retest reliability, and 95% limits of agreement of less than 40% [9].

Accounting for an expected drop out rate of 15% a number of 69 patients was planned to be recruited for each study arm. Between November 2011 and March 2014 148 consecutive patients were enrolled and allocated to the treatment groups by the principal investigator utilizing a computer generated block randomization list as described previously [10]. Block randomization is a commonly used technique to reduce bias and achieve balance in the allocation of participants to treatment arms. It increases the probability that each arm will contain an equal number of individuals by sequencing participant assignments by block. It was not possible to blind the patient for the allocated surgical technique, as the surgical incision site of the studied approaches was different.

Four patients were lost to follow up in the anterior group whereas 21 individuals dropped out of the lateral group leaving 73 (anterior) and 50 (lateral) complete data sets for analysis respectively. The main reason for dropout was a lack of time, 3 patients had moved away, two patients were diagnosed with a malignant disease and two patients had to be excluded by hindsight not meeting the radiologic inclusion criteria (Fig. 1).

A high rate of eligible patients declined trial participation as they explicitly asked for THA through a minimally invasive direct anterior approach.

Eight experienced, fellowship-trained surgeons performed the surgeries (Table 1).

Patients with primary osteoarthritis scheduled for cemented or non-cemented THA were enrolled following defined inclusion and exclusion criteria.

Exclusion criteria were an age < 40 or > 80 years, a Body-Mass-Index (BMI) > 35 kg/m^2; hip dysplasia or a congenital disorder of the hip, former osteotomies of hip, knee or pelvis; an impairment of the contralateral side or osteoarthritis of the ipsilateral knee, osteoporosis, degenerative spine disease, or a severe systemic disease (ASA-Score ≥ 4, malignant or cardiovascular disease).

The overall patient drop out and higher rate of patients lost to follow-up due to a lack of time and interest in the lateral group is considerable. However, both patient cohorts did not differ significantly after randomization regarding gender, age, BMI, educational and socioeconomic status, or any other specific patient

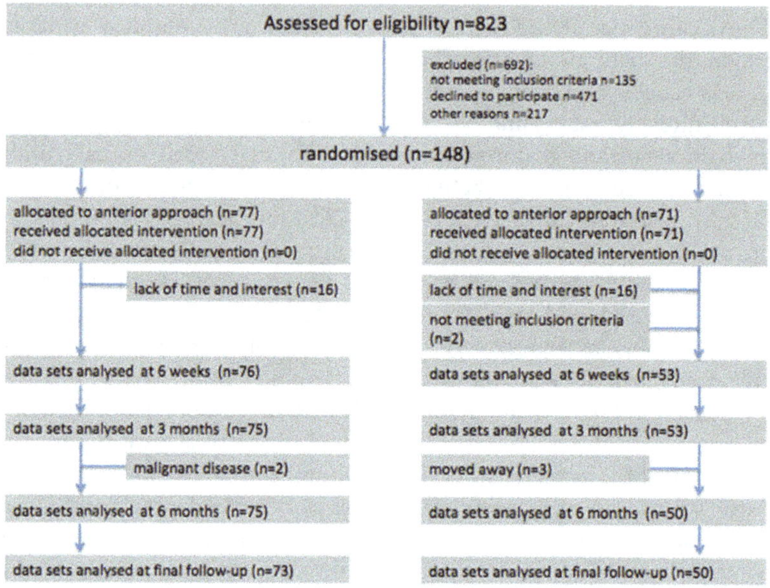

Fig. 1 Flow diagram of the progress through the phases of the randomised trial

characteristics thus contesting a general problem with randomization. As well, at baseline, completers did not differ from patients lost to follow-up.

The selected commercially available implants included Trilogy or Allofit cups (Trilogy® Acetabular Hip System; Allofit® Acetabular Cup System), the non-cemented M/L-Taper stem or the cemented M. E. Müller straight stem (all Zimmer). Overall, the anterior group included 4, the lateral group 5 cemented stems.

For all patients participating in the trial we applied established standardized treatment protocols, which included a multimodal pain management and rapid rehabilitation.

Patient examinations were carried out by a qualified physician 6 weeks prior to surgery and 6 weeks, 3, 6 and 12 months after surgery.

Activity was evaluated using the Stepwatch™ Activity Monitor (SAM) as the primary outcome measure (Orthocare Innovations, Oklahoma City, OK, USA) over a period of 7 days (preoperatively, 3 and 12 months after surgery) to calculate a daily average number of cycles [9].

Secondary outcome measures included the Harris hip score (HHS) [11] as an important clinical measure to evaluate hip function and the reciprocal extra short musculoskeletal functional assessment questionnaire

Table 1 Characteristics of evaluated patient collective preoperatively and at final follow-up

	Anterior		Lateral		
		Range		Range	*P* value
Preoperative					
Number of patients	77		71		
Age in years	63.2 (SD 8.2)	44-77	61.9 (SD 7.8)	50-78	0.193
Female	32 (42%)		32 (45%)		0.425
Body Mass Index (BMI)	28.1 (SD 3.7)	20.0-34.8	28.3 (SD 3.4)	20.9-42.2	0.869
Time of surgery	12/2011-3/2014		12/2011-3/2014		
Surgeons	8		8		
Final follow-up					
Number of patients	73		50		
Age in years	62.5 (SD 8.0)	44-77	62.2 (SD 8.5)	50-78	0.261
Female	32 (44%)		26 (52%)		0.195
Body Mass Index (BMI)	28.3 (SD 4.0)	20.0-34.8	28.7 (SD 3.2)	20.9-42.2	0.834

(XSMFA functional and bother index, 16 items) [12]. The domains covered by the HHS are pain, function, absence of deformity and range of motion. The HHS includes ten items and has a maximum score of 100 representing the best possible outcome. Additional secondary measures were a timed 25 m foot walk (T25-FW), and a visual analogue scale (VAS, range 1–10) to further characterize patient activity. The individual patient health status was monitored using the short-form 36 questionnaire (SF-36 mental and physical component summaries) [13].

Conventional x-ray projections of the pelvis (anterior--posterior, frog leg view) were used to assess bony implant integration, cup inclination, and stem orientation (valgus, neutral or varus) as described previously by Johnston et al. [14]. Two independent observers performed the assessment. At the time of follow-up, clinical examination was performed for all patients, respectively.

Source data verification was conducted by the study team. After regular trial termination, acquired data was tested for normal distribution using both the Kolmogorov-Smirnov and Shapiro-Wilk test. In case of normally distributed dependent variables the two-tailed t-test was used for between group comparisons, the Mann-Whitney-U test for non-parametric data.

The non-parametric Friedman test was chosen to analyse repeated measures within the two patient groups. As a post hoc test, the Wilcoxon signed-rank test was used and a Bonferroni adjustment made. Statistical analysis was carried out using SPSS 19.0 (IBM, Ehningen, Germany), and p-values < 0.05 were considered significant.

Results

In total, 77 arthroplasties were preformed through the minimally invasive DAA and 71 arthroplasties using the transgluteal lateral approach. The enrolment of more than 69 patients was allowed to possibly compensate for a drop out of more than nine patients per group.

Daily activity as determined by the StepWatch™ activity monitor resulted in an average of 4695 recorded load cycles per day preoperatively, 5992 (anterior) and 5239 (lateral) after 3 months, and 6402 and 5340 recorded load cycles after 1 year, respectively. The preoperatively recorded load cycles were pooled, as no statistical difference was determined between the groups ($p = 0.489$). Both 3 and 12 months after surgery, the patients operated using the direct anterior approach showed a significantly higher number of steps per day ($p = 0.035$ and $p = 0.012$) (Table 2). For the anterior group a significant increase was observed at final follow up ($p < 0.001$) compared to preoperative values and between month 3 and 12 ($p = 0.047$) while no significant change over time was seen for the lateral group (Table 3).

The average HHS revealed very good clinical results. Compared to preoperative scores a significant increase was seen 6 weeks postoperatively ($p \leq 0.001$) and again between 6 weeks and 3 months ($p = 0.039$, Table 4) for both groups. No significant difference between the two surgical approaches was determined at any time point equalling 92.4 points in the anterior group and 91.4 in the lateral group 12 months after surgery ($p = 0.477$)(Table 5). Moreover, no statistically significant differences were found for the different domains of the HHS.

In comparison to the preoperative scores (35.2, SD 16.1 and 40.5, SD 16.0, $p = 0.053$) the average functional index of the reciprocal XSFMA decreased significantly 6 weeks postoperatively. Again a significant decrease was seen between 6 weeks and 3 months for both groups and between month 3 and 6 for the lateral group to result in a score of 10.3 (SD 13.0) 12 months after THA using the anterior approach and 15.1 (SD 16.3) using the lateral approach (Table 6). After 6 weeks as well as 3 and 12 months postoperatively patients who had received THA over an anterior approach achieved significantly better XSMFA functional indices when compared to patients of the lateral group. No significant difference between the groups was determined at baseline and the 6 months time point (Table 7).

For the obtained bother indices no significant difference was found between the groups at any time point (Table 7). The preoperative bother index equalled 48.7 (SD 20.5, anterior) and 53.0 (SD 17.9, lateral) and significantly improved to 15.8 (SD 18.0, anterior) and 21.66 (SD 19.55, lateral) after 12 months. The increase after 6

Table 2 Comparison of StepWatch activity monitor outcomes at each time point

StepWatch Approach	Mean (SD)		95% CI		*P* value
	Anterior	Lateral	Anterior	Lateral	
Time points					
preoperative	4695 (1177)	4695 (1177)	4507-4887	4507-4887	n.a.
3 months	5992 (2170)	5239 (2309)	5501-6483	4617-5861	0.035[a]
12 months	6402 (2523)	5340 (1887)	5823-6981	4817-5863	0.012[a]

SD standard deviation, *CI* confidence interval
[a] Mann-Whitney-U test

Table 3 Within group comparison of StepWatch activity monitor outcomes over time

StepWatch	Mean (SD) Preoperative	3 months	*P* value	12 months	*P* value
Approach					
Anterior	4695 (1177)	5992 (2170)	0.078[a]	6402 (2523)	0.047[a]
Lateral	4695 (1177)	5239 (2309)	1.00[a]	5340 (1887)	1.00[a]

SD standard deviation
[a] Friedman test

Table 5 Between group comparison of the HHS at each time point

HHS	Mean (SD)		95% CI		*P* value
Approach	Anterior	Lateral	Anterior	Lateral	
Time points					
Preoperative	54.0 (14.2)	53.0 (15.7)	50.8-57.2	49.4-56.7	0.281[a]
6 weeks	81.6 (12.1)	82.4 (12.0)	78.3-83.7	78.8-85.2	0.068[a]
3 months	89.8 (9.3)	88.4 (9.9)	86.9-91.1	85.3-90.7	0.370[a]
6 months	90.3 (9.8)	89.1 (10.0)	87.8-92.2	86.2-91.8	0.556[a]
12 months	92.4 (8.6)	91.4 (9.1)	90.3-94.0	88.5-93.5	0.477[a]

SD standard deviation, *CI* confidence interval
[a] Mann-Whitney-U test

weeks compared to preoperative values was significant for both groups ($p < 0.001$), furthermore a significant increase was determined between 6 weeks and 3 months ($p = 0.005$ anterior; $p = 0.021$ lateral) (Table 6).

For the timed 25 m foot walk (T25-FW) the results after 6 weeks were significantly better compared to preoperative measurements in both groups ($p = 0.038$, anterior; $p = 0.041$, lateral), furthermore a significant increase was determined between 6 weeks and 3 months ($p = 0.043$ anterior; $p = 0.045$ lateral) (Table 6). The between group comparison showed no significant difference preoperatively and 6 and 12 weeks after intervention. However, 6 and 12 months after surgery, the patients in the anterior group showed significantly better results averaging 18.3 s (SD 4.1, anterior) compared to 19.9 s (SD 5.53, lateral, $p = 0.040$) and 18.1 s (SD 3.4, anterior) versus 19.8 (SD 4.6, lateral, $p = 0.046$) (Table 7).

Activity levels as assessed by the patients on a visual analogue scale (range 1–10) showed no significant difference preoperatively with 5.0 (SD 1.85, anterior) and 4.9 (SD 1.80, lateral) points ($p = 0.577$). Similar results were obtained after 6 weeks (6.9, SD 1.92 and 6.8, SD 2.90; $p = 0.75$). After 3 months, however, the patients of the anterior group described significantly higher activity levels (7.3, SD 1.65 and 6.8 SD 1.35; $p = 0.032$), which were confirmed at the final follow-up (7.5, SD 1.82 and 7.0, SD 1.57, $p = 0.016$) (Table 7). For both cohorts, the outcome 6 weeks after surgery was significantly better compared to preoperative measurements (each $p < 0.001$) (Table 6).

In addition the patients of the anterior group reported a significantly higher maximum walking distance before the onset of pain with an average of 6435 m (SD 4260) compared to 5125 m (SD 3868, $p = 0.045$, Table 7) at final follow-up.

The average scores obtained in the physical component of the SF-36 (PCS) were calculated to be 27.5 (SD 8.5, anterior) and 26.7 (SD 8.6, lateral) points preoperatively, significantly increasing to 39.7 (SD 9.7) and 37.8 (SD 9.99) 6 weeks after surgery ($p < 0.001$). Between weeks 6 and 12 after surgery again a significant increase to 44.6 (SD 9.16) and 43.1 (SD 9.72) was determined ($p < 0.001$, $p = 0.001$). The score after 6 months summed up to 46.0 (SD 10.0) and 44.8 (SD 9.95) finally resulting in 47.5 (SD 9.9) and 45.7 (SD 10.9) points 12 months postoperatively. The increase between the 3 and 12 month outcome was again statistically significant ($p = 0.041$ and $p = 0.043$) (Table 6). At each postoperative time point the patients in the anterior group achieved significantly higher scores ($p = 0.04$, $p = 0.031$, $p = 0.042$ and $p = 0.017$) (Table 7). The mental component (MCS) summed up to a score of 57.2 (SD 8.4, anterior) and 56.3 (SD 9.2, lateral) before surgery. The MCS did not change significantly over time (Tables 6 and 7).

Generally postoperative pain reduction was assessed to be good to very good. Pain intensity measurements revealed that as early as 6 months after surgery 94% (anterior) and 96% (lateral) of all patients were free of pain sensations.

The radiographic analysis revealed an average cup inclination of 38.6° (SD 5.7) in the anterior group compared to 40.3° (SD 6.2) in the lateral approach group (Table 8). None of the cups in either group presented with evidence of migration after 1 year.

Table 4 Within group comparison of the HHS over time

HHS	Mean (SD) preoperative	6 weeks	*P* value	3 months	*P* value	6 months	*P* value	12 months	*P* value
Approach									
Anterior	54.0 (14.2)	81.6 (12.1)	<0.001[a]	89.8 (9.3)	0.039[a]	90.3 (9.8)	1.000[a]	92.4 (8.6)	0.671[a]
Lateral	53.0 (15.7)	82.4 (12.0)	<0.001[a]	88.4 (9.9)	<0.001[a]	89.1 (10.0)	1.000[a]	91.4 (9.1)	0.526[a]

SD standard deviation
[a] Friedman test

Table 6 Within group comparison of the secondary outcome measures over time

	Mean (SD)		*P* value		*P* value		*P* value		*P* value
	Preoperative	6 weeks		3 months		6 months		12 months	
XSMFA fi									
Anterior	35.2 (16.1)	21.2 (14.2)	<0.001[a]	12.7 (12.5)	<0.001[a]	11.6 (12.1)	0.895[a]	10.3 (13.0)	1.000[a]
Lateral	40.5(16.0)	28.5(15.9)	<0.001[a]	18.8 (16.1)	<0.001[a]	15.8 (15.4)	0.037[a]	15.1 (16.3)	1.000[a]
XSMFA bi									
Anterior	48.7 (20.5)	26.6 (19.8)	<0.001[a]	19.8 (17.0)	0.005[a]	16.8 (15.8)	0.510[a]	15.8 (18.0)	1.000[a]
Lateral	53.0 (17.9)	33.0 (18.3)	<0.001[a]	33.0 (18.1)	0.021[a]	25.1 (17.9)	0.125[a]	21.7 (19.6)	1.000[a]
T25-FW									
Anterior	22.4 (5.2)	21.3(6.3)	0.743[a]	18.5 (3.7)	0.048[a]	18.3 (4.1)	1.000[a]	18.1 (3.4)	1.000[a]
Lateral	24.0 (3.9)	22.0 (4.2)	0.652[a]	19.4 (3.8)	0.049[a]	19.9 (5.5)	1.000[a]	19.8 (4.6)	1.000[a]
Activity VAS									
Anterior	5.0 (0.8)	6.9 (0.7)	<0.001[a]	7.3 (0.8)	1.000[a]	7.3 (0.7)	1.000[a]	7.5 (0.6)	1.000[a]
Lateral	4.9 (0.8)	6.8 (0.6)	<0.00[a]	6.9 (0.5)	1.000[a]	6.9 (0.7)	1.000[a]	7.0 (0.7)	1.000[a]
SF-36 PCS									
Anterior	27.4 (8.2)	39.1 (9.7)	<0.001[a]	44.6 (9.2)	<0.001[a]	46.0 (10.0)	1.000[a]	47.5 (9.9)	1.000[a]
Lateral	25.6 (8.7)	34.8 (9.8)	<0.001[a]	40.7 (10.1)	0.001[a]	42.7 (5.6)	0.277[a]	42.9 (11.9)	1.000[a]
SF-36 MCS									
Anterior	57.2 (8.5)	58.1 (8.7)	1,000[a]	56.0 (9.2)	1.000[a]	56.0 (10.0)	1.000[a]	55.0 (9.8)	1.000[a]
Lateral	56.3 (9.2)	59.3 (6.6)	0.931[a]	56.7 (8.3)	1.000[a]	55.8 (7.2)	1.000[a]	56.2 (6.9)	1.000[a]

SD standard deviation
[a] Friedman test

Stems positioning was assessed to be neutral in 92.5% (anterior) and 94% (lateral) of all cases while 5.5% (anterior) and 4% (lateral) were graded varus. A valgus stem orientation was found in 2% of cases in both groups.

In case of non-cemented THA, all implanted cups and stems showed radiographic evidence of osseointegration, regardless of the approach used.

Peri- and postoperative complications with THA trough the DAA were as follows: We observed three cases of lateral femoral cutaneous nerve (LFCN) palsy and performed one revision surgery due to aseptic loosening. All LFCN deficits had resolved spontaneously at final follow-up. Furthermore, a positive Trendelenburg sign indicative of gluteal insufficiency was observed in one patient. In addition, two leg length discrepancies > 1 cm occurred. These were clinically relevant and treated with orthopaedic insoles. In the lateral group one joint dislocation occurred, which was treated conservatively, moreover three leg length discrepancies compensated for with insoles, and one gluteal insufficiency.

Discussion

The demand for minimally invasive hip arthroplasty is continuously increasing [15]. Literature provides evidence for a decreased intra-operative blood loss, lower postoperative pain levels and a shorter recovery time in case of minimally invasive surgery [3–5]. The functional mid-term and long-term outcomes after THA using minimally invasive techniques are comparable with those of THA via standard approaches [16, 17]. The number of randomized trials to underline these findings, however, is still scarce. Consequently, we initiated a prospective randomized study comparing the minimally invasive DAA and standard transgluteal approach.

This study compared outcomes in 73 patients undergoing minimally invasive THA through a DAA with those in 50 patients undergoing THA through a direct lateral approach showed comparable or even superior functional outcomes and activity levels of the anterior approach group as evaluated by the HHS, XSFMA, SF-36, SAM, and T25-FW. The results obtained for both groups are within the expected range and similar to those reported in previous studies [18–20].

Functionality as represented by the HHS did not reveal a significant difference while obtained XSMFA functional indices differed significantly. Overall, our study results are in line with previous reports on minimal-invasive hip replacement [21, 22]. The differing outcome comparing the HHS and XSMFA, however, may find its reason in the different weightings of these scores. The subdivisions of the HHS are pain, functionality and deformities while the XSMFA is composed of two indices (functionality and bother) only. Moreover,

Table 7 Between group comparison of the secondary outcome measures at each time point

Approach	Mean (SD)		95% CI		*P* value
	Anterior	Lateral	Anterior	Lateral	
XSMFA functional index					
Preoperative	35.2 (16.1)	40.5(16.0)	31.4-38.6	36.3-43.7	0.053[a]
6 weeks	21.2 (14.2)	28.5(15.9)	17.8-24.2	23.7-32.3	0.026[a]
3 months	12.7(12.5)	18.8 (16.1)	9.2-14.8	13.7-22.3	0.023[a]
6 months	11.6(12.1)	15.8 (15.4)	8.3-13.7	10.7-19.3	0.094[a]
12 months	10.3(13.0)	15.1 (16.3)	7.3-13.3	10.5-19.5	0.040[a]
XSMFA bother index					
Preoperative	48.7 (20.5)	53.0 (17.9)	43.4-52.6	48.8-57.2	0.126[a]
6 weeks	26.6 (19.8)	33.0 (18.3)	21.6-30.5	28.1-37.9	0.055[a]
3 months	19.8 (17.0)	33.0 (18.1)	15.2-22.9	28.1-37.9	0.099[a]
6 months	16.8 (15.8)	25.1 (17.9)	12.4-19.6	20.0-30.0	0.149[a]
12 months	15.8 (18.0)	21.7 (19.6)	10.8-19.1	9.6-20.4	0.056[a]
T25-FW (s)					
Preoperative	22.4 (5.2)	24.0 (3.9)	20.8-23.2	23.1-24.9	0.193[a]
6 weeks	21.3(6.3)	22.0 (4.2)	19.6-22.4	20.0-23.1	0.385[a]
3 months	18.5 (3.7)	19.4 (3.8)	17.2-18.8	17.0-19.0	0.291[a]
6 months	18.3 (4.1)	19.9 (5.5)	17.1-18.9	17.5-20.5	0.040[a]
12 months	18.1 (3.4)	19.8 (4.6)	17.2-18.8	17.7-20.3	0.046[a]
Activity VAS					
Preoperative	5.0 (0.8)	4.9 (0.8)	4.8-5.2	3.8-4.2	0.461[a]
6 weeks	6.9 (0.7)	6.8 (0.6)	5.8-6.2	5.8-6.2	0.031[a]
3 months	7.3 (0.8)	6.9 (0.5)	6.8-7.2	5.9-6.1	0.080[a]
6 months	7.3 (0.7)	6.9 (0.7)	6.8-7.2	6.7-7.1	0.223[a]
12 months	7.5 (0.6)	7.0 (0.7)	6.9-7.1	6.8-7.2	<0.001[a]
Walking distance (m)					
12 months	6435 (4260)	5125 (3868)	5458-7412	4053-6197	0.045[a]
SF-36 PCS					
Preoperative	27.4 (8.2)	25.6 (8.7)	25.5-28.8	23.0-27.0	0.152[a]
6 weeks	39.1 (9.7)	34.8 (9.8)	36,8-41,2	31.4-36.6	0.004[a]
3 months	44.6 (9.2)	40.7 (10.1)	41.9-46.1	37.3-42.7	0.031[a]
6 months	46.0 (10.0)	42.7 (5.6)	43.7-48.3	40.5-43.6	0.042[a]
12 months	47.5 (9.9)	42.9 (11.9)	44.7-49.3	40.1-43.9	0.017[a]
SF-36 MCS					
Preoperative	57.2 (8.5)	56.3 (9.2)	55.1-58.9	53.9-58.1	0.405[a]
6 weeks	58.1 (8.7)	59.3 (6.6)	56.0-60.0	57.2-60.8	0.465[a]
3 months	56.0 (9.2)	56.7 (8.3)	53.9-58.1	53.8-58.2	0.774[a]
6 months	56.0 (10.0)	55.8 (7.2)	53.7-58.3	53.0-57.0	0.670[a]
12 months	55.0 (9.8)	56.2 (6.9)	52.8-57.3	54.1-57.9	0.714[a]

SD standard deviation, *CI* confidence interval
[a] Mann-Whitney-U test

the discriminative ability oft the HHS is impaired having a limited number of challenging items thus resulting in a ceiling effect [23]. Consequently, the patients who underwent THA by direct anterior MIS show a better functionality while the level of impairment is similar as in the lateral group 1 year after surgery. This is also reflected in the results of the SF-36 physical component score.

Table 8 Radiographic analysis of cup placement; surgery related complications

Measure	Anterior	Lateral
Mean inclination (°)	38.6 (SD 5.7)	40.28 (SD 6.2)
Exchange of parts	1 (aseptic loosening, 1.4%)	0
Persistent lateral femoral cutaneous nerve paraesthesia	3 (4.1%)	0
Joint dislocation	0	1
Leg length discrepancy >1cm	2 (2.7%)	3 (6%)
Trendelenburg	1 (1.4%)	1 (2%)

The StepWatch™ Activity Monitor represents an objective method of taking measurement. The results obtained with the SAM differed significantly between both cohorts. A comparison of these outcomes with previous literature reports proves difficult as a variety of devices were applied to record patient activity in the past. These include mechanical pedometers or traditional accelerometer-based step counting modalities. Furthermore, the periods of patient observation were greatly varying [24]. Nevertheless, the obtained study results correspond well with previously published patient activity levels after THA [25–27]. These outcomes are corroborated by the T25-FW measurements and the determined maximum walking distance at final follow up 12 months after surgery (Table 2).

We observed a higher incidence of varus positions in the DAA group, which was, however, not statistically significant but is a generally known phenomenon [28].

Moreover, a palsy rate of the lateral femoral cutaneous nerve (LCFN) of 4.1% was seen using the DAA although even higher incidences are described (14.8%) [29, 30]. The LCFN is a sensory nerve and supplies the anterior and lateral thigh. Its anatomic location varies greatly [31]. As a result, the LCFN is generally prone to injury utilizing a DAA. Persistent neuralgias were, however, not observed.

Joint dislocation after THA remains an unsolved problem. With the anterior approach rates of approximately 0.6–1.6% [32] are to be expected. In our study, one patient was diagnosed with a dislocated hip in the lateral group while no dislocation occurred in the DAA group.

Notably, one main advantage of the DAA over the lateral approach is that the gluteus tendons/muscles are left unharmed [33, 34]. With lateral approaches, on the other hand, gluteal insufficiency is observed regularly [35]. It was, however, observed in one study patient in each group.

Our study has several limitations. Only 21.5% of individuals found to be eligible for this study were enrolled. This could potentially lead to sampling bias. Due to patient loss to follow-up the possibility of an inadequate sample size must be considered, especially in regards to the lateral group. Another factor to criticise might be the strict set of exclusion criteria defined what might have influenced the results of both study groups.

Despite the above-mentioned limitations, we conclude that the minimally invasive DAA leads to similar or even superior clinical short and mid-term outcomes when compared to the lateral transgluteal approach.

Conclusions

THA in general significantly increases patients' activity, functionality and general physical health. After 1 year our outcomes show that THA through the direct anterior approach results in a higher patient activity compared to THA utilizing a transgluteal lateral approach while no differences regarding hip function as represented by the HHS are evident.

Abbreviations

ASA: American Society of Anesthesiologists; DAA: Direct anterior approach; HHS: Harris Hip Score; LFCN: Lateral femoral cutaneous nerve; MCS: Mental component score; PCS: Physical component score; SAM: Stepwatch™ Activity Monitor; SF-36: Short Form 36; T25-FW: Timed 25 m foot walk; THA: Total hip arthroplasty; VAS: Visual analogue scale; XSMFA: The extra short musculoskeletal functional assessment questionnaire

Acknowledgements

The authors thank Rolf Mickler-Strauch for his assistance with the statistical analysis of the generated data.

Funding

The study was financially supported by the Deutsche Arthrose-Hilfe (Grant P178-A49-Eulert-EP2nöth3-hüfte-opll-156 k-2008-12 and P235-A284-Rudert-EP2-nöth1-hüfte-op-II-67 k-2001-12). The funding body was not involved in collection, analysis, and interpretation of data and in writing the manuscript.

Authors' contributions

JCR was responsible for data collection, interpretation and manuscript preparation. EVR, FR, TR, JH and JK assisted with patient follow up after demission, data acquisition and analysis, and drafting the manuscript. LR, UN and MR were involved in hip replacement surgery, assisted with drafting the manuscript and figure preparation while MR was furthermore responsible for final proof reading. All authors read and approved the final manuscript.

Consent for publication

Not applicable.

Competing interests

The authors declare that they have no competing interests.

References

1. Khanduja V. Total hip arthroplasty in 2017 - current concepts and recent advances. Indian J Orthop. 2017;51:357–8.
2. Mjaaland KE, Svenningsen S, Fenstad AM, Havelin LI, Furnes O, Nordsletten L. Implant survival after minimally invasive anterior or anterolateral vs. conventional posterior or direct lateral approach: an analysis of 21,860 Total hip arthroplasties from the Norwegian arthroplasty register (2008 to 2013). J Bone Joint Surg Am. 2017;99:840–7.
3. Goebel S, Steinert AF, Schillinger J, Eulert J, Broscheit J, Rudert M, Noth U. Reduced postoperative pain in total hip arthroplasty after minimal-invasive anterior approach. Int Orthop. 2012;36:491–8.
4. Chimento GF, Pavone V, Sharrock N, Kahn B, Cahill J, Sculco TP. Minimally invasive total hip arthroplasty: a prospective randomized study. J Arthroplasty. 2005;20:139–44.
5. Noth U, Nedopil A, Holzapfel BM, Koppmair M, Rolf O, Goebel S, Eulert J, Rudert M. Minimally invasive anterior approach. Orthopade. 2012;41:390–8.
6. Eskelinen A. Minimally Invasive THA: Where are we now and where are we heading?: commentary on an article by Ciara Stevenson, FRCS, et al.: "minimal incision Total hip arthroplasty. A concise follow-up report on functional and radiographic outcomes at 10 years". J Bone Joint Surg Am. 2017;99:e109.
7. Rachbauer F. Minimally invasive total hip arthroplasty via direct anterior approach. Orthopade. 2005;34:1103–4. 1106–1108, 1110
8. Bauer R, Kerschbaumer F, Poisel S, Oberthaler W. The transgluteal approach to the hip joint. Arch Orthop Trauma Surg. 1979;95:47–9.
9. Mudge S, Taylor D, Chang O, Wong R. Test-retest reliability of the StepWatch activity monitor outputs in healthy adults. J Phys Act Health. 2010;7:671–6.
10. Efird J. Blocked randomization with randomly selected block sizes. Int J Environ Res Public Health. 2011;8:15–20.
11. Harris WH. Traumatic arthritis of the hip after dislocation and acetabular fractures: treatment by mold arthroplasty. An end-result study using a new method of result evaluation. J Bone Joint Surg Am. 1969;51:737–55.
12. Wollmerstedt N, Glatzel M, Kirschner S, Schneider J, Faller H, Konig A. Comparative analysis of patient-centered outcome of total hip and knee arthroplasty. Z Orthop Ihre Grenzgeb. 2006;144:464–71.
13. Garratt A, Schmidt L, Mackintosh A, Fitzpatrick R. Quality of life measurement: bibliographic study of patient assessed health outcome measures. BMJ. 2002;324:1417.
14. Johnston RC, Fitzgerald RH Jr, Harris WH, Poss R, Muller ME, Sledge CB. Clinical and radiographic evaluation of total hip replacement. A standard system of terminology for reporting results. J Bone Joint Surg Am. 1990;72:161–8.
15. Weber M, Benditz A, Woerner M, Weber D, Grifka J, Renkawitz T. Trainee surgeons affect operative time but not outcome in minimally invasive Total hip arthroplasty. Sci Rep. 2017;7:6152.
16. Stevenson C, Ogonda L, Blaney J, Dennison J, O'Brien S, Beverland D. Minimal incision Total hip arthroplasty: a concise follow-up report on functional and radiographic outcomes at 10 years. J Bone Joint Surg Am. 2017;99:1715–20.
17. Schwarze M, Budde S, von Lewinski G, Windhagen H, Keller MC, Seehaus F, Hurschler C, Floerkemeier T. No effect of conventional vs. minimally invasive surgical approach on clinical outcome and migration of a short stem total hip prosthesis at 2-year follow-up: a randomized controlled study. Clin Biomech. 2018;51:105–12.
18. Reichert JC, Volkmann MR, Koppmair M, Rackwitz L, Ludemann M, Rudert M, Noth U. Comparative retrospective study of the direct anterior and transgluteal approaches for primary total hip arthroplasty. Int Orthop. 2015; 39:2309–13.
19. Parvizi J, Restrepo C, Maltenfort MG. Total hip arthroplasty performed through direct anterior approach provides superior early outcome: Results of a Randomized, Prospective Study. Orthop Clin North Am. 2016;47:497–504.
20. Meermans G, Konan S, Das R, Volpin A, Haddad FS. The direct anterior approach in total hip arthroplasty: a systematic review of the literature. Bone Joint J. 2017;99-B:732–40.
21. Laffosse JM, Chiron P, Molinier F, Bensafi H, Puget J. Prospective and comparative study of the anterolateral mini-invasive approach versus minimally invasive posterior approach for primary total hip replacement. Early results. Int Orthop. 2007;31:597–603.
22. Wollmerstedt N, Faller H, Ackermann H, Schneider J, Glatzel M, Kirschner S, Konig A. Evaluation of the extra short musculoskeletal function assessment questionnaire XSMFA-D in patients with musculoskeletal disorders and surgical or medical in-patient treatment. Rehabilitation. 2006;45:78–87.
23. Wamper KE, Sierevelt IN, Poolman RW, Bhandari M, Haverkamp D. The Harris hip score: do ceiling effects limit its usefulness in orthopedics? Acta Orthop. 2010;81:703–7.
24. Shepherd EF, Toloza E, McClung CD, Schmalzried TP. Step activity monitor: increased accuracy in quantifying ambulatory activity. J Orthop Res. 1999;17: 703–8.
25. Wollmerstedt N, Noth U, Ince A, Ackermann H, Martell JM, Hendrich C. The daily activity questionnaire: a novel questionnaire to assess patient activity after total hip arthroplasty. J Arthroplasty. 2010;25:475–80. e471–473
26. Naal FD, Impellizzeri FM. How active are patients undergoing total joint arthroplasty?: a systematic review. Clin Orthop Relat Res. 2010;468:1891–904.
27. Silva M, McClung CD, Dela Rosa MA, Dorey FJ, Schmalzried TP. Activity sampling in the assessment of patients with total joint arthroplasty. J Arthroplast. 2005;20:487–91.
28. Beverland D. Approaches. In: Vidalain J-P, TAS S, Beverland D, et al., editors. The Corail® hip system. Berlin Heidelberg, Heidelberg: Springer; 2011. p. 193–216. https://doi.org/10.1007/978-3-642-18396-6_6.
29. Bhargava T, Goytia RN, Jones LC, Hungerford MW. Lateral femoral cutaneous nerve impairment after direct anterior approach for total hip arthroplasty. Orthopedics. 2010;33:472.
30. Smith TO, Blake V, Hing CB. Minimally invasive versus conventional exposure for total hip arthroplasty: a systematic review and meta-analysis of clinical and radiological outcomes. Int Orthop. 2011;35:173–84.
31. Hoberg M, Rudert M, Tillmann B. Minimally invasive hip arthroplasty - what must be spared? Orthopade. 2012;41:338–45.
32. Yi C, Agudelo JF, Dayton MR, Morgan SJ. Early complications of anterior supine intermuscular total hip arthroplasty. Orthopedics. 2013;36:e276–81.
33. Cadossi M, Sambri A, Tedesco G, Mazzotti A, Terrando S, Faldini C. Anterior approach in Total hip replacement. Orthopedics. 2017;40:e553–6.
34. Rykov K, Reininga IH, Knobben BA, Sietsma MS, Ten Have BL. The design of a randomised controlled trial to evaluate the (cost-) effectiveness of the posterolateral versus the direct anterior approach for THA (POLADA - trial). BMC Musculoskelet Disord. 2016;17:476.
35. Zahiri CA, Schmalzried TP, Szuszczewicz ES, Amstutz HC. Assessing activity in joint replacement patients. J Arthroplast. 1998;13:890–5.

Acetabular cup orientation and postoperative leg length discrepancy in patients undergoing elective total hip arthroplasty via a direct anterior and anterolateral approaches

Ronen Debi[1,4], Evyatar Slamowicz[1,4], Ornit Cohen[1,4], Avi Elbaz[2], Omri Lubovsky[1,4], Dror Lakstein[3], Zachary Tan[3] and Ehud Atoun[1,4*]

Abstract

Background: Total hip arthroplasty (THA) is considered a successful surgical procedure. It can be performed by several surgical approaches. Although the posterior and anterolateral approaches are the most common, there has been increased interest in the direct anterior approach. The goal of the present study is to compare postoperative leg length discrepancy and acetabular cup orientation among patients who underwent total hip arthroplasty through a direct anterior (DAA) and anterolateral (ALA) approaches.

Methods: The study included 172 patients undergoing an elective THA by a single surgeon at our institution within the study period. Ninety-eight arthroplasties were performed through the ALA and 74 arthroplasties through the DAA. Preoperative planning was performed for all patients. Assessment of the two groups included the following postoperative parameters: abduction angle, cup anteversion angle and leg length discrepancy (LLD). Additional analysis was done to evaluate component positioning by comparing deviation from the Lewinnek zone of safety in both approaches.

Results: For the DAA the absolute LLD was 11 mm, ranging from -6 mm to 5 mm. For the ALA, the absolute LLD was 36 mm, ranging from -22 mm to 14 mm. None of the DAA patients had an absolute LLD greater than 6 mm. Comparatively, 7.4% of the ALA group exceeded 6 mm of LLD in addition to 2.1% with LLD greater than 10 mm. 15% of the ALA group resided out of the Lewinnek abduction zone compared to 3% of the DAA group ($P = 0.016$). 17% of the ALA group were out of the Lewinnek anteversion zone as opposed to 8% of the DAA group ($P = 0.094$).

Conclusion: Our study demonstrates good component positioning outcomes and LLD values in patients following THA through the DAA compared to the ALA.

Keywords: THA, Approach, Anterolateral, Direct anterior, Anteversion, Abduction, Angle, Leg length discrepancy

* Correspondence: dratoun@gmail.com
[1]Department of Orthopedic Surgery, Barzilai Medical Center, 2 Hahistadrut Street, 78278 Ashkelon, Israel
[4]Affiliated to the Ben-Gurion University of the Negev, Beer sheva, Israel
Full list of author information is available at the end of the article

Background

Total hip arthroplasty (THA) is considered a successful surgical procedure for the treatment of end-stage hip osteoarthritis. It offers pain relief and significant improvement in patient function and quality of life [1]. The number of THA performed worldwide is expected to increase in the following decades due to increasing life expectancy [2].

THA is performed by several surgical approaches. Currently, the posterior and anterolateral approaches are the most commonly used worldwide. Data extracted from the global orthopedic registry in 2010 indicate that 55 and 33% of THA are performed using a posterior approach and anterolateral approach (ALA) respectively [3]. Since 2013, there has been a renewed interest in the direct anterior approach (DAA) - 10% of orthopedic arthroplasty surgeons consider it their preferred approach [4]. Reduced blood loss, rapid functional recovery, low dislocation rates and shorter hospital stays have been attributed to the muscle-sparing properties of the anterior approach [5].

Two recent systematic reviews and network meta-analysis aimed to evaluate the effectiveness of surgical approach for THA (posterior, posterior-2, anterolateral, direct lateral, and anterior). Outcome measures were the length of the incision, blood loss, operating time, length of stay, complications, gait analysis and post-operative clinical symptoms [6, 7]. However, both reviews did not compare the acetabular cup positioning and postoperative leg length discrepancy. The latter were found to correlate with pain, excessive wear and instability [8]. Some evidence suggests that both the anterolateral and anterior approaches were found to safely, reliably and accurately produce an optimal component positioning, as well as clinical leg length discrepancy [9–11].

The goal of our study was to further examine the effect of the surgical approach on postoperative leg length discrepancy and acetabular cup positioning in patients undergoing a total hip arthroplasty through either a DAA or ALA. We hypothesized that there would be no significant difference between these two groups.

Methods

Approval from Barzilay Medical Center Ethics Committee (IRB 0116–15-BRZ) was obtained.

A retrospective chart review was performed of patients undergoing an elective THR between January 2011 and December 2015 in our institute. The surgical approach was selected according to the availability of the dedicated DAA surgical table. Patients with extraarticular deformity, prior hip surgery, and contralateral THR were excluded from the study. One hundred fifty-eight patients were ultimately included, with 94 and 64 in the ALA and the DAA, respectively. All surgeries were performed by a single, fellowship trained orthopedic surgeon.

Surgical technique

Direct anterior approach

Surgery is performed in the supine position. Both patient's feet are secured into special boots connected to the DAA table. The skin incision starts approximately 3 cm lateral and 1 cm distal to the ipsilateral anterior superior iliac spine. Deep dissection is performed parallel to the fibers of the tensor fascia lata muscle. The fascia over the tensor muscle is incised and extended proximally and distally. The Smith-Peterson interval between the Tensor and the Sartorius muscles is used to access the joint. The ascending branch of the lateral femoral circumflex vessels are identified and cauterized. An L shaped hip capsulotomy is performed. The femoral neck is then osteotomized with the subsequent extrication of the femoral head. The neck cut is then verified in reference to the superior margins of the lesser trochanter. Intraoperative X-Ray imaging was utilized to ensure leg lengths and acetabular component positioning.

Anterolateral approach

Surgery is performed in the lateral decubitus position. A longitudinal skin incision is made over the lateral proximal thigh. The Tensor Fascia Lata is divided in line with the skin incision. Gluteus medius and Gluteus minimus are split in line with their fibers and a T shaped hip capsulotomy is performed. The soft tissue around the femoral neck is elevated and the hip is dislocated anteriorly. The lesser trochanter is then exposed. The femoral neck is osteotomized at the pre-planned level. Neck length is verified in reference to the superior margins of the lesser trochanter. Intraoperative XR or fluoroscopy was not used in the setting of the ALA approach.

Component implantation and closure

All patients received cementless Corail stems and Pinnacle cups (Depuy, Warsaw, Indiana). Intraoperatively, hip stability was assessed in several ways. Combined anteversion was assessed with the trial stem and adjusted as needed. Anterior and posterior stability was interrogated at extremes of range of motion and impingement was excluded. Stem offset was established during preoperative planning and verified using the palpable tension of the glutei and fascia lata after trial reduction. It is the surgical team's uniform preference to accept 3 to 5 mm of "push-pull" joint laxity unless hip stability is grossly compromised. The joint capsule is sutured back and the glutei are meticulously repaired. There were no enforced hip precaution protocols.

Post operatively

All patients underwent pre and postoperative pelvic digital radiography via a standard protocol. The pelvic AP views were taken with the patient supine, the XR beam centered over the pubic symphysis with both hips internally rotated 10 to 15 degrees to offset physiologic anteversion. Routine pre-operative planning was performed using dedicated software (TraumaCad, Voyant health, Petach-Tikva, Israel) [12].

The software was used to measure LLD, cup anteversion and cup abduction for each patient. The in situ prosthetic femoral head with its documented diameter was used for radiographic calibration. The LLD was measured as the difference of the perpendicular vertical displacement from the tangential ischial line to a consistent point of reference on the lesser trochanter when comparing both hips. The software extrapolates anteversion by measuring the area of the elliptical projection of the cup - the greater the area, the greater the magnitude of the anteversion. Cup abduction is calculated as the angle between the horizontal inter-teardrop line and the cup obliquity (Fig. 1). Lewinnek's standard safe-zone of abduction and anteversion angles range were considered (21). The range for anteversion angle is between 5 and 25 degrees, and for abduction angle is between 30 and 50 degrees.

The data distributions were examined using Kolmogorov-Smirnov tests for normality.

This study had 94 patients in the ALA group and 64 patients in the DAA group. In a previous study, the response within each subject group was normally distributed with a standard deviation of 6.5. If the true difference in the experimental and control means is 3.65, we will be able to reject the null hypothesis that the population means of the experimental and control groups are equal with a probability (power) of .932. The Type I error probability associated with this test of this null hypothesis is .05.

Statistical analysis was carried out with a one-way ANOVA test and the Enter method for correlation regression analysis (SPSS 21.0, SPSS Inc.) to examine the difference between digital radiographic measurements. P-values < 0.05 were considered significant.

Results

There was no statistically significant difference between the ALA group and the DAA group with regards to gender, age, and body mass index (BMI). (Table 1).

The LLD measurements in the DAA group was distributed within a total range of 11 mm from *-6 mm to 5 mm* compared to a total range of 36 mm from -22 mm to 14 mm for the ALA group. None of the DAA patients had an absolute LLD greater than 6 mm. Comparatively, 7.4% of the ALA group exceeded 6 mm of LLD in addition to 2.1% with LLD greater than 10 mm (Fig. 2).

Absolute LLD was found to be significantly lower ($P = 0.001$) in the DAA group. The average absolute LLD value of the DAA approach was 0.9 mm whereas the average discrepancy in the ALA was 2.4 mm (Table 2).

In 96.9% of the cases in the DAA group, the cup anteversion angle was within the Lewinnek zone as compared to 85.1% in the ALA group ($P = 0.016$). In 92.2% of the cases in the DAA group, the cup abduction angle was within the Lewinnek zone as compared to 83% in the AL approach ($P = 0.094$) (Table 3). The cup anteversion angle was significantly higher in the DAA group. There was no significant difference in cup abduction angle between two groups (Table 2).

Discussion

The use of the direct anterior approach for THA has become increasingly popular in recent years [4]. Its muscle sparing principles are suggested to be associated with shorter hospital stays, higher rates of patients discharged home and better short-term postoperative outcomes. Overall, complication rates in the available literature do not appear to exceed those of the conventional approaches for THA [13]. A meta-analysis performed by Higgins et al. comparing the clinical and surgical outcomes in patients undergoing THA via the DAA and

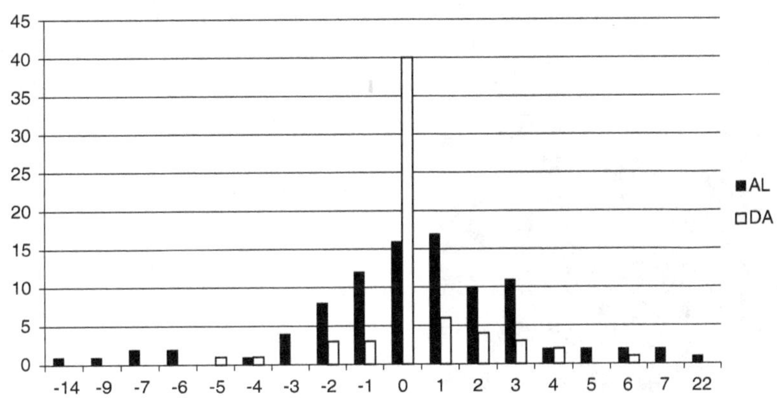

Fig. 1 Leg length discrepancy (mm) in the DAA and ALA approaches

Table 1 Population characteristics

	ALA	DAA	*p*-value
Mean age (SD)	64.8 (10.3)	64.5 (11)	0.875
Gender (F:M)	58:36	33:31	0.205
Mean BMI (SD)	29.2 (4.9)	28.7 (4.4)	0.501

ALA Anterolateral approach, *DAA* Direct anterior approach

Table 2 Acetabular component positioning and leg length discrepancy

	ALA ($n = 94$)	DAA ($n = 64$)	*p*-value
Mean anteversion Angle (°) (SD)	11.3 (6.6)	15 (5.5)	< 0.001
Mean Abduction Angle (°) (SD)	36.5 (5.9)	38.3 (6.1)	0. 069
Mean absolute LLD (mm) (SD)	2.4 (3.1)	0.9 (1.4)	0.001

ALA Anterolateral approach, *DAA* Direct anterior approach

posterior approaches favored the DAA in the metrics of post-operative pain, functional outcomes, length of hospitalization, hip stability and postoperative narcotic consumption [14]. The PRISMA meta-analysis comparing direct anterior and lateral approaches similarly suggested that DAA may be associated with improved early postoperative functional rehabilitation, lower levels of perceived pain, and shorter hospitalization time [15]. A recent network meta-analysis by Putananon et al. evaluated all surgical approaches for THA [6]. They suggest that a failure of fixation, instability, and damage to soft tissues, associated with the trauma of the surgical procedure are some of the reasons for post-operative pain, which prevent patients to return to full function and activity. However, in their report as well as another meta-analysis, less attention is given to the acetabular cup positioning and postoperative leg length discrepancy, which in our opinion are important when evaluating the effectiveness of the surgical approach.

Patient dissatisfaction due to LLD is common. Complications associated with LLD include gait disorders, nerve injury, lower back pain, hip instability and occasionally necessitating surgical revision. The amount of discrepancy that is clinically acceptable following THA is controversial. Several studies showed that most patients tolerated LLD up to 10 mm while others reported that even a small discrepancy could produce dissatisfaction [16]. The varied opinions in the literature can be attributed to having significant LLD increase both *technical* post-operative complications and cause *subjective* patient dissatisfaction, both of which may occur at a different length thresh-holds [17–19]. The results of our study showed that the LLD absolute range in the DAA group was 11 mm, ranging from *-6 mm to 5 mm* compared to a total range of 36 mm, ranging from -22 mm to 14 mm for the ALA group. None of the DAA patients had an absolute LLD greater than 6 mm. Comparatively, 7.4% of the ALA group exceeded 6 mm of LLD in addition to 2.1% with LLD greater than 10 mm (Fig. 1).

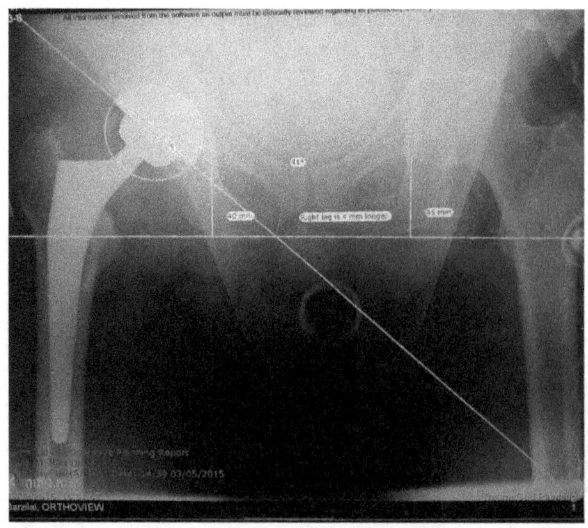

Fig. 2 AP view of cup position assessment

The orientation of the acetabular component greatly influences hip joint stability after THA. Postoperative radiological measurements of abduction and anteversion angle are a common method for evaluating acetabular component orientation [20]. A second method for evaluating acetabular component orientation is to assess cup placement in a target zone. Lewinnek et al. [21] defined a "safe zone" that minimizes instability after THA comprising of both cup abduction and anteversion within 40° ± 10° and 15° ± 10°, respectively. Dislocation rates are demonstrably higher with components residing outside the defined "safe zone". The Lewinnek concept of "safe zone" has to be a matter of recent controversy [22, 23], nevertheless, it remains an accessible method for confirming technical accuracy after THA [24]. In the current study, a higher percentage of the patients were within the defined "safe zone" in the DAA group compared to the ALA group (96.9% compared to 85.1% of cases, respectively, for cup anteversion angles and 92.2% compared to 83% of cases, for cup abduction angles). A possible explanation for the favorable accuracy of the DAA might be the intraoperative imaging that allows

Table 3 Comparison of the Lewinnek target zone

		ALA ($n = 94$)	DAA ($n = 64$)	*p*-value
Abduction (%) (n)	in zone	85.1 (80)	96.9 (62)	0.016
	out of zone	14.9 (14)	3.1 (2)	
Anterversion (%) (n)	in zone	83 (78)	92.2 (59)	0. 094
	out of zone	17 (16)	7.8 (5)	

Abduction zone: 30°-50°, Anteversion zone: 5°-25°
ALA Anterolateral approach, *DAA* Direct anterior approach

immediate feedback to the surgeon. The use of image intensification as verification of cup abduction and anteversion angles is technically easier in the supine position and allows components to be seated under sequential image guidance. This ensures acetabular component positioning and leg lengths [11]. In contrast, the ALA is performed in the lateral decubitus position, which complicates the acquisition of optimal and representative intraoperative imaging. The fact that only patients in the DAA had intraoperative x-ray may be a limitation to the current study, hence results and conclusions should be carefully considered. However, obtaining an intra-operative x-ray view of the component positioning in a lateral approach is more challenging and should be considered a limitation as well.

This study has several limitations. Firstly, although the DAA more frequently achieves better radiographic results than the ALA, both methods were found to be reasonably good in the setting of patient care. The differences, although statistically significant, are not enough to draw conclusions regarding clinical outcomes. Careful pre-operative templating and surgical experience may be the overriding factor regardless of approach [25]. Secondly, we acknowledge that missing information on intraoperative and postoperative complications, quality of life, and need for revision, is a limitation of the current study. However, Connolly and Kamath concluded that when surgeons have performed a modest number of procedures, the complication rates tend to markedly decrease in most studies to levels comparable to other approaches [13]. In the current study, all THAs were performed by a single, fellowship trained orthopedic surgeon, with > 100 cases experience in the DAA. Hence, it may be assumed that the frequency of complications rate did not differ between groups. Our purpose was to bring to the surgeon's attention the importance of evaluating intraoperative component positions and LLD to improve surgery success. From our experience, these two parameters are easier to control and achieve good outcomes when using the DAA approach, however, we cannot determine that these cannot be achieved in other approaches.

Conclusion

Our study demonstrates good component positioning outcomes and LLD values in patients following THA through the DAA compared to the ALA.

Abbreviations

ALA: Anterolateral approach; BMI: body mass index; DAA: Direct anterior approach; THA: Total hip arthroplasty

Authors' contributions

RD was responsible for the conception and design, and revising the article. SE was responsible for data collection, analysis and drafting the article. OC was responsible for data collection and analysis. AE was responsible for conception and design, and revising the article. OL was responsible for the conception and design, and revising the article. DL was responsible for analysis and drafting the article. ZT was responsible for conception and design, and for revising the article. EA was responsible for conception and design, analysis and drafting of the manuscript. All authors read and approved the final manuscript.

Competing interests

EA is a member of the editorial board of BMC Musculoskeletal disorders. The authors declare that they have no competing interests.

Author details

[1]Department of Orthopedic Surgery, Barzilai Medical Center, 2 Hahistadrut Street, 78278 Ashkelon, Israel. [2]AposTherapy Research Group, Herzelyia, Israel. [3]Department of Orthopaedic Surgery, Wolfson Medical Center , Holon, Israel. [4]Affiliated to the Ben-Gurion University of the Negev, Beer sheva, Israel.

References

1. Lavernia CJ, Alcerro JC. Quality of life and cost-effectiveness 1 year after total hip arthroplasty. J Arthroplast. 2011;26(5):705–9.
2. Kurtz S, et al. Projections of primary and revision hip and knee arthroplasty in the United States from 2005 to 2030. J Bone Joint Surg Am. 2007;89(4):780–5.
3. Waddell J, et al. Orthopaedic practice in total hip arthroplasty and total knee arthroplasty: results from the global Orthopaedic registry (GLORY). Am J Orthop (Belle Mead NJ). 2010;39(9 Suppl):5–13.
4. Chechik O, et al. Surgical approach and prosthesis fixation in hip arthroplasty world wide. Arch Orthop Trauma Surg. 2013;133(11):1595–600.
5. Petis S, et al. Surgical approach in primary total hip arthroplasty: anatomy, technique and clinical outcomes. Can J Surg. 2015;58(2):128–39.
6. Putananon C, et al. Comparison of direct anterior, lateral, posterior and posterior-2 approaches in total hip arthroplasty: network meta-analysis. Eur J Orthop Surg Traumatol. 2018;28(2):255–67.
7. Meermans G, et al. The direct anterior approach in total hip arthroplasty: a systematic review of the literature. Bone Joint J. 2017;99-B(6):732–40.
8. Knight JL, Atwater RD. Preoperative planning for total hip arthroplasty. Quantitating its utility and precision. J Arthroplasty. 1992;7(Suppl):403–9.
9. Jerosch J, Theising C, Fadel ME. Antero-lateral minimal invasive (ALMI) approach for total hip arthroplasty technique and early results. Arch Orthop Trauma Surg. 2006;126(3):164–73.
10. Tsai SW, et al. Modified anterolateral approach in minimally invasive total hip arthroplasty. Hip Int. 2015;25(3):245–50.
11. Matta JM, Shahrdar C, Ferguson T. Single-incision anterior approach for total hip arthroplasty on an orthopaedic table. Clin Orthop Relat Res. 2005;441:115–24.
12. Steinberg EL, et al. Preoperative planning of total hip replacement using the TraumaCad system. Arch Orthop Trauma Surg. 2010;130(12):1429–32.
13. Connolly KP, Kamath AF. Direct anterior total hip arthroplasty: comparative outcomes and contemporary results. World J Orthop. 2016;7(2):94–101.
14. Higgins BT, et al. Anterior vs. posterior approach for total hip arthroplasty, a systematic review and meta-analysis. J Arthroplast. 2015;30(3):419–34.
15. Yue C, Kang P, Pei F. Comparison of direct anterior and lateral approaches in Total hip arthroplasty: a systematic review and meta-analysis (PRISMA). Medicine (Baltimore). 2015;94(50):e2126.
16. Kersic M, et al. The impact of leg length discrepancy on clinical outcome of total hip arthroplasty: comparison of four measurement methods. J Arthroplast. 2014;29(1):137–41.
17. Benedetti MG, et al. To what extent does leg length discrepancy impair motor activity in patients after total hip arthroplasty? Int Orthop. 2010;34(8):1115–21.
18. Flecher X, Ollivier M, Argenson JN. Lower limb length and offset in total hip arthroplasty. Orthop Traumatol Surg Res. 2016;102(1 Suppl):S9–20.
19. White TO, Dougall TW. Arthroplasty of the hip. Leg length is not important. J Bone Joint Surg Br. 2002;84(3):335–8.
20. Fabeck L, et al. A method to measure acetabular cup anteversion after total hip replacement. Acta Orthop Belg. 1999;65(4):485–91.

21. Lewinnek GE, et al. Dislocations after total hip-replacement arthroplasties. J Bone Joint Surg Am. 1978;60(2):217–20.
22. Seagrave KG, et al. Acetabular cup position and risk of dislocation in primary total hip arthroplasty. Acta Orthop. 2017;88(1):10–7.
23. Abdel MP, et al. What safe zone? The vast majority of dislocated THAs are within the Lewinnek safe zone for acetabular component position. Clin Orthop Relat Res. 2016;474(2):386–91.
24. Sadhu A, et al. Acetabular component position and the risk of dislocation following primary and revision Total hip arthroplasty: a matched cohort analysis. J Arthroplast. 2017;32(3):987–91.
25. Lakstein D, et al. Radiographic templating of total hip arthroplasty for femoral neck fractures. Int Orthop. 2017;41(4):831–6.

Influence of surgical approach on heterotopic ossification after total hip arthroplasty – is minimal invasive better?

Maya Hürlimann[1,3†], Filippo-Franco Schiapparelli[1,3†], Niccolo Rotigliano[1,3], Enrique Testa[1], Felix Amsler[2] and Michael T. Hirschmann[1,3*]

Abstract

Background: Heterotopic ossification (HO) is a well-known complication after total hip arthroplasty (THA). Recently, the trend is to operate THA minimally invasive being less traumatic than standard approaches and promising a faster return to activity. The purpose of the study was to investigate if minimal invasive surgery (MIS), leads also to less HO after THA.

Methods: This retrospective study included 134 consecutive patients undergoing THA. In 42 (31.3%) patients a standard modified anterolateral (STD-Watson-Jones), in 28 (20.9%) patients a standard transgluteal Bauer approach (STD-Bauer), in 39 (29.1%) a MIS direct anterior approach (AMIS) and in 25 (18.7%) patients a MIS anterolateral (MIS-AL) approach was used. Standard preoperative anterior-posterior and lateral radiographs were assessed for occurrence of HO. HO was classified according to Brooker. In addition, short- and long-term adverse events were noted. Data was statistically analyzed using Chi-square tests, analysis of variance, multivariate data analysis and Pearson's correlation ($p < 0.05$).

Results: Overall, HO was found in 38 caucasian patients (28.4%) after THA. The STD-Watson-Jones group showed the highest HO rate (45.2% $n = 19$) with a significant difference to the AMIS (23.1% $n = 9$) and STD-Bauer approach (14.3% $n = 4$). No statistical difference was found to the MIS-AL approach (24.0% $n = 6$). Postoperative complications did not differ significantly except for a higher incidence of Trendelenburg`s sign in STD-Bauer.

Conclusions: The rate and degree of HO after THA were significantly different with regards to the surgical approach. The standard modified anterolateral approach resulted in the highest HO rate, however, MIS approaches showed higher HO rates than the STD-Bauer.

Keywords: Heterotopic ossification, Anterolateral minimal invasive approach, Watson-Jones, Periarticular ossification, Total hip arthroplasty, THA, Transgluteal Bauer, Direct anterior approach

* Correspondence: michael.hirschmann@ksbl.ch
[†]Equal contributors
[1]Department of Orthopaedic Surgery and Traumatology, Kantonsspital Baselland (Bruderholz, Liestal, Laufen), CH-4101 Bruderholz, Switzerland
[3]University of Basel, Basel, Switzerland
Full list of author information is available at the end of the article

Background

Heterotopic ossification (HO) is a well-known complication after total hip arthroplasty (THA) with a reported mean incidence of 24–32% [1–9]. There is only scarce evidence about the influence of the surgical approach on HO occurrence. Not more than two different approaches have yet been simultaneously compared in terms of HO [10, 11].

Although HO etiology remains unclear, it has been postulated that osteoinductive growth factors are released as consequence of soft tissue trauma inducing the formation of HO [12–14]. HO is believed to reach its complete formation after 6 to 12 weeks post-operative and not to progress anymore after this period [15]. Symptoms vary dependent on the severity of HO, and range from local pain to reduced range of hip motion [16, 17]. The Brooker's classification grades HO into four different grades [18]. Most of the cases of HO belong to grade I and II and generally run asymptomatic being a collateral finding in routine follow-up radiographs [19]. A less incidence of patients present severe HO classified as grade III and IV, with more hip pain and significantly reduced ROM, flexion, abduction, and external rotation of the hip when compared to grades 0, I and II [15, 20].

In modern THA a considerable number of surgical approaches are used. Besides the conventional standard approaches, minimally invasive surgery (MIS) approaches are increasingly used. These MIS approaches promise less gluteal insufficiency, a faster rehabilitation and a quicker return to normal daily life activities [1, 21].

The primary purpose of the present study was to investigate the influence of the following surgical approaches on HO: minimally invasive anterolateral (MIS-AL), minimally invasive anterior (MIS-AMIS), standard transgluteal (STD-Bauer), and the standard modified anterolateral (STD-Watson-Jones). The secondary purpose was to investigate if minimally invasive surgery (MIS) leads to less HO than standard THA approaches.

Methods

All patients who underwent primary THA in the period 2012–2013 in a university affiliated hospital with a minimum follow-up of 12 months and a signed informed consent were included in the present study. Patients without a preoperative and postoperative (at a least of 12 months) radiological control on radiographs and patients who did not sign the informed consent were not included. Indications for surgery were end-stage osteoarthritis and traumatic neck fractures. In this period the standard THA done was an uncemented Zweymüller type stem and a pressfit cup (Smith&Nephew, Switzerland).

In this period, four consultant surgeons of the same department performed a total of four different surgical approaches. Patients have been divided according to the performed surgical approach, standard modified anterolateral (STD-Watson-Jones) (group A), standard transgluteal Bauer approach (STD-Bauer) (group B), direct anterior minimally invasive (AMIS) (group C) and anterolateral minimally invasive (MIS-AL) (group D) (Table 1). The choice of the surgical approach was based on the preference of each surgeon.

In order to evaluate the HO onset and compare its incidence across the groups, pre-operative and 1-year post-operative radiological images (antero-posterior and lateral) were compared using a radiological display monitor (Fig. 1). The Brooker's classification system was used (Table 1) [18].

Patients' demographics including age, gender, relevant comorbidities (e.g. diabetes mellitus, cardiovascular diseases, osteoporosis, previous hip surgery) were noted. Intraoperative, early and late complications were obtained from the hospital archives system (KIS, Erne, Switzerland). The average time of hospital stay was calculated from hospital archives data.

Early mobilisation with full weight bearing was initiated under physiotherapeutic supervision on the first postoperative day. The postoperative protocol was identical for all groups.

Statistical analysis

All data were analyzed by an independent statistician (F.A.) using SPSS version 17.0 (SPSS Inc., Chicago, IL, USA). Continuous variables were described using means and standard deviations or medians and ranges. Categorical variables were tabulated with absolute and relative frequencies. In the groups A-D no significant differences were seen in terms of gender, age and relevant comorbidities ($p < 0.05$). Univariate analysis was performed using Pearson´s correlation to identify any correlations between the type of approach, demographic and outcome variables. ANOVA analysis was also done for each variable. Multivariate analysis (MVA) was performed for HO incidence, occurred complications and time of hospital stay. To analyze a direct relationship between surgical approach and HO, all influencing additional factors were excluded (osteoporosis, fractures, dislocations, Trendelenburg`s sign/muscular deficit, muscular deficits, urinary tract infection) and a MVA was performed including all the results that showed univariate significance. Multivariate analysis used a stepwise linear regression of all variables on the dependent variable surgical approach. $p < 0.05$ was considered statistically significant and $p < 0.1$ as a statistical tendency.

Table 1 Patient demographics as well as HO and complications divided by the type of THA approach used

		Approach				Total
		Standard		Minimally invasive		
		STD Watson-Jones	STD Bauer	AMIS	MIS-AL	
Gender						
Men		21	16	22	10	69
Women		21	12	17	15	65
Mean age		42	28	39	25	
Comorbidities						
Previous THA		14	12	12	7	45
Diabetes mellitus		5	5	7	5	22
Cardiovascular diseases		24	15	22	15	76
Osteoporosis		5	1	1	3	10
HO						
Grade 0	Count	23	24	30	19	96
	%	19,0%	3,6%	7,7%	12,0%	
Grade 1	Count	8	1	3	3	15
	%	19,0%	3,6%	7,7%	12,0%	
Grade 2	Count	5	2	4	1	12
	%	11,9%	7,1%	10,3%	4,0%	
Grade 3	Count	3	0	2	1	6
	%	7,1%	0,0%	5,1%	4,0%	
Grade 4	Count	3	1	0	1	5
	%	7,1%	3,6%	0,0%	4,0%	
Total	Count	42	28	39	25	134
	%	31,3%	20,9%	29,1%	18,7%	
Mean Stay in hospital		42	28	39	25	
Intraoperative complications		4	3	1	0	8
Early complications						
Bleeding		1	2	0	0	3
Wound healing problems/infection		4	1	1	4	10
Cardiovascular events		1	1	4	0	6
Pulmonary embolism		0	0	1	0	1
Postoperative anemia		42	28	39	25	134
Urinary tract infection		5	1	0	0	6
Late complications						
Fracture		3	1	1	1	6
Dislocation		0	2	1	0	3
Loosening		1	0	0	0	1
Leg length discrepancy		9	9	14	7	39
Trendelenburg sign/muscular deficits		10	10	3	2	25
Local sensory disturbances/pain		7	5	9	6	27
Revision surgery		2	2	1	3	8

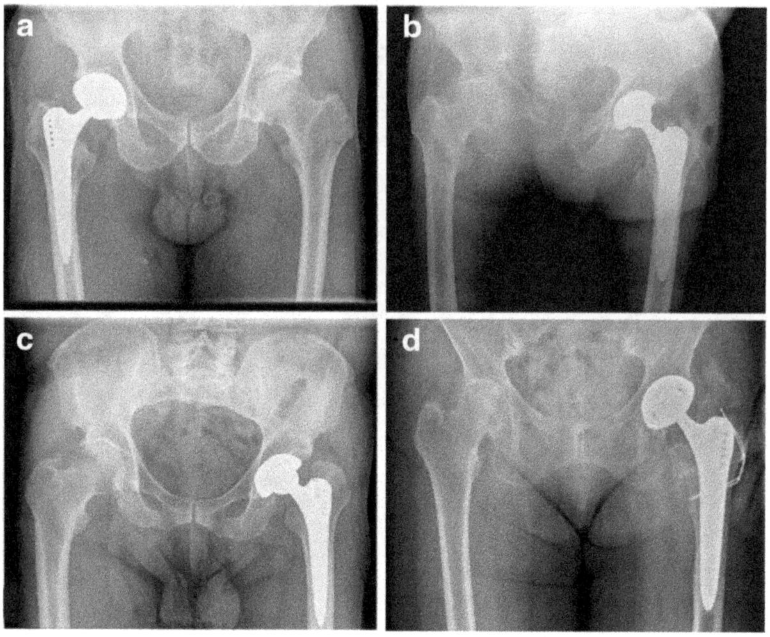

Fig. 1 One year follow-up standard radiographic control, examples of heterotopic ossification according to Brooker grade 1 (**a**), grade 2 (**b**), grade 3 (**c**) and grade 4 (**d**)

Results

One hundred thirty-four consecutive caucasian patients fulfilled the inclusion criteria. Forty-two patients (31.3%) were included in group A, 28 patients (20.9%) in group B, 39 patients (29.1%) in group C and 25 patients (18.7%) in group D (Table 1). HO was found in 28.4% of the patients with the highest incidence in group A (45.2%) followed by group D, (24.0%), group C (23.1%) and group B (14.3%) (Table 1). According to the Brooker's classification, among the 28.4% patients who developed HO, 11.2% had a grade I, 9.0% a grade II, 4.5% a grade III and 3.7% a grade IV (Table 1) (Fig. 1a-d). Focusing on grade III and IV since they are the ones with clinical relevance: group A showed the highest HO rate, 14.2% (7.1% each for grade III and grade IV) followed by group D, 8.0% (4% each for grade III and grade IV); group C, 5.1% (5.1% grade III) and group B with an 3.6% incidence (3.6% grade IV) (Table 1). Group A developed significantly more HO than group B ($p = 0.020$) and group C ($p = 0.038$). Group A and group D showed no significant difference in terms of HO rate ($p = 0.095$). Multivariate analysis showed that group A explained 5.0% of the factor "HO". In addition, the presence of osteoporosis explained 3.8% of the factor "HO". Overall, these two factors explained unadjusted 8.8% of the HO. Data about intraoperative, early and late complications are presented in Table 1. Urinary tract infection was significantly higher in group A (11.9%, $n = 5$) in comparison to group C (0.0%, $n = 0$; $p = 0.022$) and group D (0.0%, $n = 0$; $p = 0.009$). No statistical significant difference was seen in comparison to group B. (3.6%, $n = 1$, $p = 0.095$). The most frequent late complication was leg length discrepancy with an incidence of 29.1% in the overall study cohort. There was a significant difference between the groups ($p < 0.01$) for Trendelenburg`s sign indicating gluteal muscle insufficiency. It was seen in 35.7% of group B, 23.8% in of group A, 7.7% of group C and 8.0% of group D (Table 1). The average stay in hospital was 11.1 days (range 4–56 days) (Table 1). Patients in group C had a mean stay in hospital of 9.1 days, which was significantly shorter than group A (12.1 days), group B (11.5 days) and group D (12.1 days) (Table 1). The univariate Pearson's correlation of all variables is shown in Table 2.

Discussion

This is the first study comparing four different THA approaches in terms of HO. So far, only two types of surgical approaches were simultaneously compared. The overall incidence of HO in this study was 28.4%. Toom et al reported an HO incidence of 32% in 178 patients who underwent THA using a posterolateral approach [5]. Pavlou et al. noted an incidence of 24% in 39 patients who underwent THA using a STD-Watson-Jones approach [2]. Yanbin Zhu et al. reported a similar HO rate (30%) in a metanalysis involving 14 studies with a total of 6468 patients. However, the type of THA approach was not specified [4]. In summary, the overall HO incidence in the present study is in line with the previously reported HO rates in the published literature.

Table 2 Pearson correlation of demographic and outcome criteria (* = 0.05 ** = 0.01 *** = 0.001)

Pearson r	N	STD-Watson-Jones	STD-Bauer	AMIS	MIS-AL	MIS	Revision surgery	HO	Gender	Age	Previous THA
STD-Watson-Jones	134	1***	−0.35***	−0.43***	−0.32***	−0.65***	−0.03	0.22**	0.02	0.03	0
STD-Bauer	134	−0.35***	1***	−0.33***	−0.25**	−0.49***	0.03	−0.12	−0.06	0.01	0.1
AMIS	134	−0.43***	−0.33***	1***	−0.31***	0.67***	−0.09	−0.08	−0.06	0.07	−0.04
MIS-AL	134	−0.32***	−0.25**	−0.31***	1***	0.5***	0.12	−0.04	0.11	−0.12	−0.06
MIS	134	−0.65***	−0.49***	0.67***	0.5***	1***	0.01	−0.11	0.03	−0.03	−0.08
Revision surgery	134	−0.03	0.03	−0.09	0.12	0.01	1***	0.04	0.13	0.11	0.02
HO	134	0.22**	−0.12	−0.08	−0.04	−0.11	0.04	1***	0.11	0.14	0.16
Gender	134	0.02	−0.06	−0.06	0.11	0.03	0.13	0.11	1***	0.02	0.04
Age	134	0.03	0.01	0.07	−0.12	−0.03	0.11	0.14	0.02	1***	−0.07
Previous THA	134	0	0.1	−0.04	−0.06	−0.08	0.02	0.16	0.04	−0.07	1***
Diabetes	134	−0.08	0.02	0.03	0.05	0.06	−0.03	−0.05	0.09	0.09	−0.02
Cardiovascular diseases	134	0.01	−0.03	0	0.03	0.02	0.16	0.03	−0.24**	0.48***	−0.18*
Osteoporosis	134	0.11	−0.08	−0.12	0.08	−0.04	0.05	0.22*	0.24**	0.05	0.1
Hospital stay	134	0.13	0.04	−0.24**	0.09	−0.15	0.39***	0.17	0.2*	0.22*	0.12
Intraoperative complications	134	0.1	0.1	−0.09	−0.12	−0.18*	0.2*	0.07	0.13	0.16	0.02
Bleeding	134	0.01	0.17*	−0.1	−0.07	−0.14	−0.04	−0.08	0.05	0.03	0
Wound healing problems/ infections	134	0.05	−0.08	−0.12	0.16	0.01	0.41***	0.03	0.07	−0.06	−0.02
Cardiovascular events	134	−0.07	−0.02	0.18*	−0.1	0.08	0.1	−0.02	0.01	0.04	−0.15
Pulmonary embolism	134	−0.06	−0.04	0.14	−0.04	0.09	−0.02	−0.05	−0.08	0.05	0.12
Postoperative anemia	134	0.15	−0.05	−0.04	−0.07	−0.1	0.21*	0.06	0.17*	0.1	0
Urinary tract infections	134	0.24**	−0.02	−0.14	−0.1	−0.21*	0.1	0.15	0.15	0.07	0
Other neurological deficits/ delirium	134	−0.01	0.13	−0.12	0.01	−0.1	−0.07	−0.07	−0.05	0.18*	0.04
Fractures	134	0.09	−0.02	−0.06	−0.01	−0.06	0.25**	0.19*	0.15	0.24**	0.08
Dislocation	134	−0.1	0.17*	0.01	−0.07	−0.04	0.17*	0.01	0.05	0.09	−0.11
Loosening	134	0.13	−0.04	−0.06	−0.04	−0.08	0.34***	0.12	−0.08	0	−0.06
Leg length discrepancy	134	−0.11	0.03	0.1	−0.01	0.08	−0.09	−0.1	0	−0.03	−0.04
Trendelenburg sign/muscular deficits	134	0.09	0.23**	−0.18*	−0.13	−0.27**	0.04	0.07	0.07	0.06	0.07
Local sensory disturbances/pain	134	−0.06	−0.03	0.05	0.05	0.08	0.19*	0.1	0.03	−0.12	0

Table 2 Pearson correlation of demographic and outcome criteria (* = 0.05 ** = 0.01 *** = 0.001) *(Continued)*

Pearson r	*N*	Diabetes	Cardiovasc. diseases	Osteoporosis	Hospital stay	Intraoperative complications	Bleeding	Wound healing problems/ infections	Cardiovascular events	Pulmonary embolism	Postoperative anemia
STD-Watson-Jones	134	−0.08	0.01	0.11	0.13	0.1	0.01	0.05	−0.07	−0.06	0.15
STD-Bauer	134	0.02	−0.03	−0.08	0.04	0.1	0.17*	−0.08	−0.02	−0.04	−0.05
AMIS	134	0.03	0	−0.12	−0.24**	−0.09	−0.1	−0.12	0.18*	0.14	−0.04
MIS-AL	134	0.05	0.03	0.08	0.09	−0.12	−0.07	0.16	−0.1	−0.04	−0.07
MIS	134	0.06	0.02	−0.04	−0.15	−0.18*	−0.14	0.01	0.08	0.09	−0.1
Revision surgery	134	−0.03	0.16	0.05	0.39***	0.2*	−0.04	0.41***	0.1	−0.02	0.21*
HO	134	−0.05	0.03	0.22*	0.17	0.07	−0.08	0.03	−0.02	−0.05	0.06
Gender	134	0.09	−0.24**	0.24**	0.2*	0.13	0.05	0.07	0.01	−0.08	0.17*
Age	134	0.09	0.48***	0.05	0.22*	0.16	0.03	−0.06	0.04	0.05	0.1
Previous THA	134	−0.02	−0.18*	0.1	0.12	0.02	0	−0.02	−0.15	0.12	0
Diabetes	134	1***	0.27**	0.03	−0.03	−0.03	−0.07	−0.05	0	0.2*	0.16
Cardiovasc. diseases	134	0.27**	1***	−0.15	0.1	0.09	0.03	0.08	−0.03	0.08	0.17*
Osteoporosis	134	0.03	−0.15	1***	0.12	0.05	−0.04	0.03	−0.06	−0.02	0.02
Hospital stay	134	−0.03	0.1	0.12	1***	0.19*	0.15	0.29***	−0.06	−0.07	0.12
Intraoperative complications	134	−0.03	0.09	0.05	0.19*	1***	0.39***	0.17	−0.05	−0.02	0.29***
Bleeding	134	−0.07	0.03	−0.04	0.15	0.39***	1***	−0.04	−0.03	−0.01	0.06
Wound healing problems/ infections	134	−0.05	0.08	0.03	0.29***	0.17	−0.04	1***	−0.06	−0.02	0.16
Cardiovasc. events	134	0	−0.03	−0.06	−0.06	−0.05	−0.03	−0.06	1***	−0.02	−0.1
Pulmonary embolism	134	0.2*	0.08	−0.02	−0.07	−0.02	−0.01	−0.02	−0.02	1***	0.19*
Postoperative anemia	134	0.16	0.17*	0.02	0.12	0.29***	0.06	0.16	−0.1	0.19*	1***
Urinary tract infections	134	0.1	0.04	0.08	0.12	0.1	−0.03	0.35***	−0.05	−0.02	0.18*
Other neurological deficits/ delirium	134	−0.05	0.02	0.14	0.1	0.05	0.15	−0.08	−0.06	−0.02	0.09
Fractures	134	0.06	0.16	0.06	0.33***	0.58***	0.32***	0.52***	0.12	0.15	0.67***
Dislocation	134	0	0.12	0.08	0.21*	0.55***	−0.03	0.21*	−0.05	−0.02	0.28**
Loosening	134	−0.07	0.13	−0.04	−0.04	0.17*	0.32***	0.15	−0.03	−0.01	0.06
Leg length discrepancy	134	−0.04	0.08	−0.02	−0.02	−0.02	−0.01	−0.02	−0.02	−0.01	0.19*
Trendelenburg sign/muscular deficits	134	−0.02	−0.07	−0.12	−0.15	−0.02	0.01	0.07	0.18*	0.14	0.04
Local sensory disturbances/pain	134	−0.06	−0.01	0.16	0.07	0.04	0.06	0.01	−0.01	−0.04	0.08

Table 2 Pearson correlation of demographic and outcome criteria (* = 0.05 ** = 0.01 *** = 0.001) *(Continued)*

Pearson r	N	Urinary tract infections	Other neurological Deficits/delirium	Fractures	Dislocation	Loosening	Leg length discrepancy	Trendelenburg sign/muscular deficits	Local sensory disturbances/ pain
STD-Watson-Jones	134	0.24**	−0.01	0.09	−0.1	0.13	−0.11	0.09	−0.06
STD-Bauer	134	−0.02	0.13	−0.02	0.17*	−0.04	0.03	0.23**	−0.03
AMIS	134	−0.14	−0.12	−0.06	0.01	−0.06	0.1	−0.18*	0.05
MIS-AL	134	−0.1	0.01	−0.01	−0.07	−0.04	−0.01	−0.13	0.05
MIS	134	−0.21*	−0.16	−0.06	−0.04	−0.08	0.08	−0.27**	0.08
Revision surgery	134	0.1	0.36***	0.25**	0.17*	0.34***	−0.09	0.04	0.19*
HO	134	0.15	0.04	0.19*	0.01	0.12	−0.1	0.07	0.1
Gender	134	0.15	0.17*	0.15	0.05	−0.08	0	0.07	0.03
Age	134	0.07	0.16	0.24**	0.09	0	−0.03	0.06	−0.12
Previous THA	134	0	−0.01	0.08	−0.11	−0.06	−0.04	0.07	0
Diabetes	134	0.1	0.06	0	−0.07	−0.04	−0.02	−0.06	−0.02
Cardiovasc. diseases	134	0.04	0.16	0.12	0.13	0.08	−0.07	−0.01	−0.05
Osteoporosis	134	0.08	0.06	0.08	−0.04	−0.02	−0.12	0.16	−0.07
Hospital stay	134	0.12	0.33***	0.21*	−0.04	−0.02	−0.15	0.07	−0.09
Intraoperative complications	134	0.1	0.58***	0.55***	0.17*	−0.02	−0.02	0.04	0.03
Bleeding	134	−0.03	0.32***	−0.03	0.32***	−0.01	0.01	0.06	−0.08
Wound healing problems/ infections	134	0.35***	0.52***	0.21*	0.15	−0.02	0.07	0.01	0.14
Cardiovascular events	134	−0.05	0.12	−0.05	−0.03	−0.02	0.18*	−0.01	0.07
Pulmonary embolism	134	−0.02	0.15	−0.02	−0.01	−0.01	0.14	−0.04	−0.04
Postoperative anemia	134	0.18*	0.67***	0.28**	0.06	0.19*	0.04	0.08	0.01
Urinary tract infection	134	1***	0.5***	0.3***	−0.03	−0.02	0.1	0.08	0.16
Other neurological deficits/ delirium	134	0.21*	0.39***	−0.06	−0.04	−0.02	−0.06	0.01	−0.07
Fractures	134	0.5***	1***	0.37***	0.2*	0.05	0.11	0.07	0.08
Dislocation	134	0.3***	0.37***	1***	−0.03	−0.02	−0.06	0.17*	0.07
Loosening	134	−0.03	0.2*	−0.03	1***	−0.01	0.13	0.06	0.18*
Leg length discrepancy	134	−0.02	0.05	−0.02	−0.01	1***	−0.06	−0.04	0.17*
Trendelenburg sign/muscular deficits	134	0.1	0.11	−0.06	0.13	−0.06	1***	0.03	0.05
Local sensory disturbances/pain	134	0.08	0.07	0.17*	0.06	−0.04	0.03	1***	−0.05

The most important finding of the present study was that the rate and degree of HO after THA was significantly dependent from the surgical approach used. The STD-Watson-Jones approach showed a significantly higher HO rate than the STD-Bauer and AMIS approaches. This was also higher than the MIS-AL approach but without any statistical significance. This last finding has been also noted by Repantis et al. [10]. In contrast to the present study Biz et al. found a higher HO rate for the STD-Bauer approach ($p = 0.0163$) when compared to the STD-Watson-Jones [11]. These different results could be related to the different type of used implants that included also patients who underwent a hemiprothesis. To date, there is not a single study comparing the HO rate of patients who underwent THA using the STD-Watson-Jones and AMIS approach. With regards to HO rates in patients after THA using the AMIS approach, the results are conflicting. Whereas Tippets et al. reported a HO rate of 41.5%, [22] which is higher than in the present study, Newman et al. reported a HO rate of 24.3% [6], which is comparable with this study. It could be speculated if the reason for the highest HO rate in the STD-Watson-Jones group lies in the more traumatic dissection, which is clearly less invasive using a MIS approach. A recent study of Unger et al. [23] found that the AMIS approach for THA comes along with less muscle damage and hematoma, shorter operative and exposure time, less bleeding and faster rehabilitation time. Although the highest HO rate was seen in the STD-Watson-Jones group, it was not possible to state that minimally invasive approaches lead to less HO. Indeed, both AMIS and MIS-AL had a higher HO incidence than the STD-Bauer. This finding remained unexplained.

In this study the lower complications' rate with MIS (MIS-AL, AMIS) than with the standard techniques (STD-Bauer, STD-Watson-Jones) reflects the current knowledge and are considered as advantages of MIS as shown by Unger et al. [23]. However, among the complications, only the Trendelenburg sign was statistically significant for which the MVA showed an increased risk in the STD-Bauer group.

Another important finding of this study was the direct comparison of the stay in hospital among the four approaches. Patients who underwent THA using an AMIS approach had the shortest mean hospital stay. However, the average stay in hospital of the MIS-AL group was probably distorted by a patient, who developed an early infection, has been three times operated and remained in the hospital 56.0 days. The stay in hospital difference between AMIS and the STD-Watson-Jones was the only statistically significant difference.

So far, no study compared four surgical approaches for a THA with regards to the hospital stay. Ilchmann et. al. [24] noted a significantly shorter stay in hospital after the AMIS approach compared to the STD-Bauer approach. Yue et. al. found similar results in a meta-analysis [25]. However, the average stay in hospital was 9.1 days for the AMIS and 11.5 days for the STD-Bauer approach (Table 1). All together MIS approaches for THA appear to be beneficial in terms of HO as well as adverse events. Hence, if possible MIS approaches should be used. In conclusion, this study has proven the general superiority of MIS approaches in terms of HO and adverse events.

A considerable number of limitations need to be considered. The most important one is the retrospective study design. The possible selection bias was however limited by the consecutive patient selection.

Four different orthopedic surgeon operated on the patients reported and choose the approach with regards to their own preference, which might have influenced the outcome in each group. However, all surgeons were capable to perform all four different approaches. As it was the aim to focus on HO after THA no clinical outcome data was assessed. Furthermore, only patients with HO grades 3 and 4 were included. Patients, who developed complications during couse of treatment were also included, which could have led to a longer stay in hospital as well as increased HO development.

The major strength of the study presented is that it is the first study investigating HO onset in four different THA approaches. In addition, it represents a consecutive patient series with a good and balanced sample size.

Conclusion

This is the first study comparing the STD-Watson-Jones, STD-Bauer, AMIS and MIS-AL approaches in terms of HO. The rate and degree of HO after THA was significantly dependent from the surgical approach used. The STD-Watson-Jones presented the highest HO rate. A lower complications' rate was seen after minimally invasive approaches. Hence, if possible MIS approaches should be used. In conclusion, this study has proven the general superiority of MIS approaches in terms of HO and adverse events.

Abbreviations

AMIS: Minimally invasive direct anterior approach; HO: Heterotopic ossifications; MIS: Minimal invasive surgery; MIS-AL: Minimally invasive anterolateral; MVA: Multivariate analysis; STD-Bauer: Standard transgluteal Bauer approach; STD-Watson-Jones: Standard modified anterolateral Watson-Jones approach; THA: Total hip arthroplasty

Funding

This study received no funding.

Authors' contributions
Study conduct: MH, FFS, MTH. Data collection: MH, ET, NR. Data analysis: FA. Data interpretation: MH, FFS. MTH. Drafting manuscript: FFS. Revising manuscript content: FFS MTH. Approving final version of manuscript: MH, FFS, NR, ET, FA, MTH takes responsibility for the integrity of the data analysis.

Competing interests
The authors declare that they have no competing interests.

Consent for publication
Not applicable.

Author details
[1]Department of Orthopaedic Surgery and Traumatology, Kantonsspital Baselland (Bruderholz, Liestal, Laufen), CH-4101 Bruderholz, Switzerland. [2]Amsler Consulting, CH-4059 Basel, Switzerland. [3]University of Basel, Basel, Switzerland.

References
1. Spinarelli A, Patella V, Petrera M, Abate A, Pesce V, Patella S. Heterotopic ossification after total hip arthroplasty: our experience. Musculoskelet Surg. 2011;95(1):1–5.
2. Pavlou G, Salhab M, Murugesan L, Jallad S, Petsatodis G, West R, Tsiridis E. Risk factors for heterotopic ossification in primary total hip arthroplasty. Hip Int. 2012;22(1):50–5.
3. Schara K, Herman S. Heterotopic bone formation in total hip arthroplasty: predisposing factors, classification and the significance for clinical outcome. Acta Chir Orthop Traumatol Cech. 2001;68(2):105–8.
4. Zhu Y, Zhang F, Chen W, Zhang Q, Liu S, Zhang Y. Incidence and risk factors for heterotopic ossification after total hip arthroplasty: a meta-analysis. Arch Orthop Trauma Surg. 2015;135(9):1307–14.
5. Toom A, Haviko T, Rips L. Heterotopic ossification after total hip arthroplasty. Int Orthop. 2001;24(5):323–6.
6. Newman EA, Holst DC, Bracey DN, Russell GB, Lang JE. Incidence of heterotopic ossification in direct anterior vs posterior approach to total hip arthroplasty: a retrospective radiographic review. Int Orthop. 2015;40(9):1967–73.
7. Aljurayyan A, Tanzer D, Tanzer M. Acute revision hip arthroplasty: a previously unrecognized risk factor for heterotopic ossification. Eur J Orthop Surg Traumatol. 2016;26(2):183–8.
8. Harwin SF. Trochanteric heterotopic ossification after total hip arthroplasty performed using a direct lateral approach. J Arthroplasty. 2005;20(4):467–72.
9. Bal BS, Lowe JA, Gietler A, Aleto TJ. Heterotopic ossification after 2-incision total hip arthroplasty. J Arthroplasty. 2010;25(4):538–40.
10. Repantis T, Bouras T, Korovessis P. Comparison of minimally invasive approach versus conventional anterolateral approach for total hip arthroplasty: a randomized controlled trial. Eur J Orthop Surg Traumatol. 2015;25(1):111–6.
11. Biz C, Pavan D, Frizziero A, Baban A, Iacobellis C. Heterotopic ossification following hip arthroplasty: a comparative radiographic study about its development with the use of three different kinds of implants. J Orthop Surg Res. 2015;10(1):176.
12. Sneath RJ, Bindi FD, Davies J, Parnell EJ. The effect of pulsed irrigation on the incidence of heterotopic ossificiation after total hip arthroplasty. J Arthroplasty. 2001;16(5):547–51.
13. Nilsson OS, Persson PE. Heterotopic bone formation after joint replacement. Curr Opin Rheumatol. 1999;11(2):127–31.
14. Chalmers J, Gray DH, Rush J. Observation on the induction of bone in soft tissue. J Bone Joint Surg Br. 1975;57(1):36–45.
15. Board TN, Karva A, Board RE, Gambhir AK, Porter LM. The prophylaxis and treatment of heterotopic ossification following lower limb arthroplasty. J Bone Joint Surg Br. 2007;89(4):434–40.
16. Engelhardt Lexikon Orthopädie und Unfallchirurgie. http://www.lexikon-orthopaedie.com/pdx.pl?dv=0&id=01559.
17. Neal B. Effects of heterotopic bone formation on outcome after hip arthroplasty. ANZ J Surg. 2003;73(6):422–6.
18. Brooker AF, Bowerman JW, Robinson RA, Riley LHJ. Ectopic ossification following total hip replacement. Incidence and a method of classification. J Bone Joint Surg Am. 1973;55(8):1629–32.
19. Kocic M, Lazovic M, Mitkovic M, Djokic B. Clinical significance of the heterotopic ossification after total hip arthroplasty. Orthopedics. 2010;33(1):16.
20. OECD. Health at a Glance 2013: OECD Indicators. In. OECD Publishing; 2013. http://dx.doi.org/10.1787/health_glance-2013-en.
21. Alecci V, Valente M, Crucil M, Minerva M, Pellegrino CM, Sabbadini DD. Comparison of primary total hip replacements performed with a direct anterior approach versus the standard lateral approach: perioperative findings. J Orthop Traumatol. 2011;12(3):123–9.
22. Tippets DM, Zaryanov AV, Burke WV, Patel PD, Suarez JC, Ely EE, Figueroa NM. Incidence of heterotopic ossification in direct anterior total hip arthroplasty: a retrospective radiographic review. J Arthroplasty. 2014;29(9):1835–38.
23. Unger AC, Schulz AP, Paech A, Jürgens CH, Renken FG. Modified direct anterior approach in minimally invasive hip hemiarthroplasty in a geriatric population: a feasibility study and description of the technique. Arch Orthop Trauma Surg. 2013;133(11):1509–16.
24. Ilchmann T, Gersbach S, Zwicky L, Clauss M. Standard transgluteal versus minimal invasive anterior approach in hip arthroplasty: a prospective, consecutive cohort study. Orthop Rev. 2013;5(4):e31.
25. Yue C, Kang P, Pei F. Comparison of direct anterior and lateral approaches in total hip arthroplasty: a systematic review and meta-analysis (PRISMA). Medicine (Baltimore). 2015;94(50):e2126.

18

Monobloc implants in cementless total hip arthroplasty in patients with Legg-Calve-Perthes disease

Ze-Yu Luo[1], Hao-Yang Wang[1], Duan Wang[1], Hui Pan[2], Fu-Xing Pei[1] and Zong-Ke Zhou[1*]

Abstract

Background: The purpose of this study was to evaluate 10-year outcomes in cementless monobloc total hip arthroplasty (THA) in a group of hips with Legg-Calve-Perthes disease (LCPD).

Methods: We reviewed 71 patients (88 hips) who underwent cementless THA with a diagnosis of LCPD from 2003 to 2009. From the total of 71 patients, 34 men and 37 women with an average age of 49.94 years were included. The mean follow-up period was 10 years.

Results: The mean Harris Hip Score improved significantly from 46.42 to 89.70. Similarly, the postoperative range of motion, hip dysfunction and osteoarthritis outcome score and SF-12 score also significantly improved. The mean leg lengthening was 22.1 mm. During the follow-up, eight complications were noted, including two cases of intraoperative femoral fractures, two cases of sciatic nerve paralysis, two cases of heterotrophic ossifications, one case of thigh pain and one case of dislocation. One revision was conducted for a periprosthetic fracture, and the survivorship at 10 years was 98.3%.

Conclusions: These data suggest that the monobloc stem can lead to satisfactory outcomes for clinical function, radiological evaluation, restoration of the normal limb lengths, complications, and survivorship among LCPD patients undergoing total hip arthroplasty.

Keywords: Legg-calve-Perthes disease, Monobloc stem, Hip, Arthroplasty

Background

Legg-Calve-Perthes disease(LCPD) is characterized by osteonecrosis of the femoral head during childhood [1, 2]. Similar to other childhood hip disorders, LCPD has the development of degenerative coxarthrosis as its natural history [3]. Total hip arthroplasty (THA) is recommended for patients with end-stage hip disease [4]. Nevertheless, there are limited data available in the literature regarding the characteristics and complications of THA in patients with a history of LCPD [5–13].

THA for patients with LCPD is known to be technically demanding because of the flattens and widens of the femoral head, excessive anteversion of the femoral neck, a straight and narrow medullary canal of the femur, a shallow and retroverted acetabulum, and the abnormality caused by previous operations [5]. Coxa breva, a typical residual deformity of LCPD, consists of a short femoral neck, a large oval-shaped femoral head, a relatively overgrown greater trochanter, and a decreased femoral neck-shaft angle [3]. The acetabulum is also deformed, becomes flat, and loses its concavity to accommodate the deformed femoral head. Frequently, the femoral head is subluxated laterally and incompletely covered by the acetabulum [3]. In 1984, the S-ROM system (DePuy, Warsaw, IN) was developed as a stem for patients with these various types of anatomic deformities. This stem has a modular mechanism with a high degree of freedom. It consists of two parts, the sleeve and stem body. In addition, the stem and sleeve have various combinations, and independent reaming in the proximal metaphyseal region of the femur and the diaphyseal region enables robust fixation with respect to various intramedullary canal shapes. Using the S-ROM

* Correspondence: zongke@126.com
[1]Department of Orthopedics, West China Hospital/West China School of Medicine, Sichuan University, 37# Wuhou Guoxue Road, Chengdu 610041, People's Republic of China
Full list of author information is available at the end of the article

prosthesis to treat LCPD has been reported to provide excellent results [8]. However, in with respect to modular femoral components, some risk factors need to be considered, such as fretting, corrosion, and mechanical failure, which may affect the stability of the stem and result in osteolysis and loosening. A recent series has documented the eight-year outcomes of 68 THAs with the use of a monobloc stem for LCPD [5]. However, monobloc cementless stems for patients with a history of Perthes' disease raises several concerns: an increased risk of intraoperative femoral fracture, excessive anteversion of the femoral stem, malposition of the acetabular component, an increased risk of dislocation, unsatisfactory clinical and radiological results, and poor survivorship [5].

To address these concerns, we conducted this study to evaluate the 10-year outcomes of cementless monobloc THAs in a group of consecutive hips with LCPD.

Methods

This was a retrospective study conducted at West China Hospital, Sichuan University, which serves as a tertiary level center in China. The retrospective study protocol was approved by the Institutional Review Board of West China Hospital, and informed consent was obtained from all of the patients. Between June 2003 and December 2009, a total of 82 consecutive patients who underwent THA with a diagnosis of LCPD were included in our study. Eleven patients were excluded from the study for different reasons. Six patients were lost to follow-up after surgery and could not be contacted due to incorrect telephone numbers and addresses. Three patients with incomplete chart records were excluded. Two patients died of chronic medical problems which were unrelated to the THA. Therefore, 71 patients (88 hips) were included. The clinical data of our patients were evaluated retrospectively after receiving approval from the Institutional Review Board of West China Hospital.

Clinical data

There were 34 men and 37 women with an average age of 49.94 years (range, 25–73), and the average body-mass index (BMI) was 23.64 kg/m^2 (range, 15.8–30.9). At our institution, patients undergoing arthroplasty are followed-up prospectively at regular intervals (at 3 weeks, 6 weeks, 12 weeks, and 6 months after surgery and annually thereafter). The time to follow-up is calculated as the time from surgery to the most recent visit. A clinical evaluation was conducted by two independent observers (ZY-L and HY-W) with the use of the Harris Hip Score (HHS), hip dysfunction and osteoarthritis outcome score (covering pain, symptoms, daily living, sports and recreational activities, and quality of life) and the SF-12 scale (physical component summary and mental component summary). The preoperative or postoperative hip range of motion (ROM) and visual analog scale for pain or satisfaction (VAS, pain/satisfaction) were also recorded. All complications were noted.

Surgical technique

Before the operation, to restore the anatomical hip rotation center for monobloc prosthesis, an evaluation of the abnormal anatomy of the proximal femur and acetabulum, soft-tissue contracture, leg-length discrepancy and previous operations were routinely conducted. In patients with LCPD, the pelvis should be evaluated with special care to determine the amount of bone stock present for fixation of the cup. A three-dimensional CT scan is also helpful in evaluating the acetabulum. The width of the medullary canal is also noted because it may be narrow, especially in patients with LCPD. In these instances, a careful templating before surgery should be conducted. Templating aids in selecting the size of the implant that would restore the center of rotation of the hip and provide the best femoral fit.

All operations were performed via a posterolateral approach with the patient in the lateral decubitus position. In cases with remarkable LLD with coxa breva deformity, neck cutting was performed at the middle level of the femoral head, which is a more proximal location than that used in usual cases of THA for the restoration of LLD. The target position of the acetabular component was 40° to 45° abduction and 20° anteversion [5]. From small to large diameter, acetabular reaming was performed. The porous-coated acetabular component (DePuy, Pinnacle, Warsaw, IN) was inserted in the acetabular position with the use of a press-fit technique and fixed. Two screws were used to improve acetabular cup stability in one hip. The mean outer diameter of the acetabular cup was 52 mm (range 46 mm–58 mm). The mean head diameters were 34 mm (range 28 mm–36 mm), and three hips were 28 mm, 45 hips were 32 mm, and 40 hips were 36 mm. A ceramic-on-ceramic bearing was used in 78 hips (89%), a metal-on-polyethylene bearing was used in two hips (2%), and a ceramic-on-polyethylene bearing was used in eight hips (9%). After insertion of the acetabular cup, we focused on the femoral preparation. When preparing the femoral canal, restoration of the appropriate anteversion of the femur is necessary. The broach is aligned to match precisely the axis of the patient's femoral neck. It is important to not attempt to place the broach in additional anteversion because this would lead to under sizing of the stem and insufficient rotational stability. The monobloc stems were inserted along the endosteal geometry of the proximal femur without manipulation to adjust the stem version, and a Corail stem (DePuy) was conducted in 61 hips and a Trilock stem (DePuy) was inserted in the other hips. Femoral fractures were defined and treated according to the Vancouver classification [14].

All of the patients had an antibiotic prophylaxis with a third-generation cephalosporin for a day. Low-molecular-weight heparin (0.2 mL, or 2000 AxaIU, of Clexane [enoxaparin sodium]) was first administered 8 h after surgery and then every 24 h until hospital discharge. The patients were allowed full weight-bearing on the day after surgery.

Radiographic analysis

Radiographic evaluations were performed by two independent observers (ZY-L and HY-W) preoperatively and every time of follow-up with use of anteroposterior and lateral radiographs of the affected hip. The degree of deformity was defined by the classification system of Stulberg et al. [15] (Table 1). For determining the leg-length discrepancy, a line between the inferior edge of the acetabular teardrop (inter-teardrop line) can be used as the reference line. Perpendicular measurements to the tip of the greater trochanter are compared to compute the leg-length discrepancy. A radiographic evaluation was conducted by assessing the cup and femoral stem orientation and osteolysis at the times of follow-up.

The cup orientation was measured on the postoperative radiograph [8, 16]. While measuring the cup orientation on the anteroposterior radiographs, inclination is the angle between the face of the cup and the transverse axis (the inter-teardrop line); cup anteversion is calculated from the relative size of the major and minor diameters of the ellipse [16] (Fig. 1). Osteolysis around the cup was defined as a scalloped erosion exceeding 2 mm in diameter at the bone-prosthesis interface; the progressive widening of radiolucent lines >2 mm, migration of >2 mm, or 5° of cup tilting were defined as cup loosening [17]. Seven zones around the femoral component were described by Gruen et al. [18]. Anteversion of the femoral stem was calculated using the method described by Weber et al. [19] (Fig. 1). Stem fixation was classified as bony ingrowth and fibrously stable or being unstable according to the Engh classification [20–22]. Subsidence of the femoral component was defined by the method described by Loudon et al. [23]. Heterotopic ossification was graded according to Brooker et al. [24].

Table 1 The Criteria Define of Stulberg Classifications

Classification	Criteria Define
Class I	A completely normal hip joint
Class II	A spherical femoral head (same concentric circle on anteroposterior and frog-leg lateral radiographs), but with one or more of the following abnormal characteristics of the femoral head, neck, or acetabulum:
	(1) Larger than normal (although spherical) femoral head (coxa magna);
	(2) Shorter-than-normal femoral neck;
	(3) Abnormally steep acetabulum
Class III	A non-spherical (ovoid, mushroom-shaped, or umbrella-shaped) but not flat femoral head. Abnormal characteristics of the femoral head, neck, and acetabulum (as described for Class II) are present also.
Class IV	A flat femoral head and abnormalities of the femoral head, femoral neck, and acetabulum
Class V	A flat femoral head and a normal femoral neck and normal acetabulum

Statistical analysis

We assessed the means and standard deviations for quantitative data, the frequencies, and the percentages for the qualitative data. The continuous variables were compared with independent exponent t- tests. The Pearson chi-square test or Fisher exact test was used to analyze the qualitative comparative parameters. Kaplan-Meier was utilized in the analysis of survivorship with the end points as a revision for any component. All of the data analyses were performed using SPSS for Windows, Version 19.0 (IBM Corp, Armonk, NY, USA). The significance was set at $P < 0.05$.

Results

Clinical data

The mean duration of the follow-up was 10.09 ± 1.84 years (range 7.5–13.9), as shown in Table 2. The outcomes regarding hip function are listed in Table 3. The mean HHS improved significantly from 46.42 ± 6.11 points (range 35–56) preoperatively to 89.70 ± 5.46 points (range 77–97) postoperatively. For the range of motion (ROM), the flexion improved from 90.13 ± 11.24° (range 30°-110°) preoperatively to 120.32 ± 4.94° (range 102°-125°), and the abduction improved from 29.28 ± 5.50° (range 10°-40°) preoperatively to 41.26 ± 3.73° (range 30°-45°). In addition, the hip dysfunction and osteoarthritis outcome score and the SF-12 score improved postoperatively compared with those preoperatively, and this difference was significant (Table 3).

Radiographic outcomes

The mean cup anteversion and abduction were 25.95 ± 6.00° (range 15°-36°) and 39.01 ± 5.51° (range 27°-50°), respectively. The mean stem anteversion was 13.63 ± 4.10° (range 5° to 27°). Preoperative and postoperative LLD were 24.3 ± 7.8 mm (range 8 mm–36 mm) and 2.4 ± 2.8 mm (range – 2 mm-9 mm), respectively. The mean leg lengthening was 22.1 ± 7.8 mm (range 4 mm–36 mm) postoperatively. Although no cases with >10 mm of LLD were identified, three slightly limp patients were noted by the final follow-up.

No case noted radiolucent lines or migration around the acetabular cup. For the stems, we did not note a

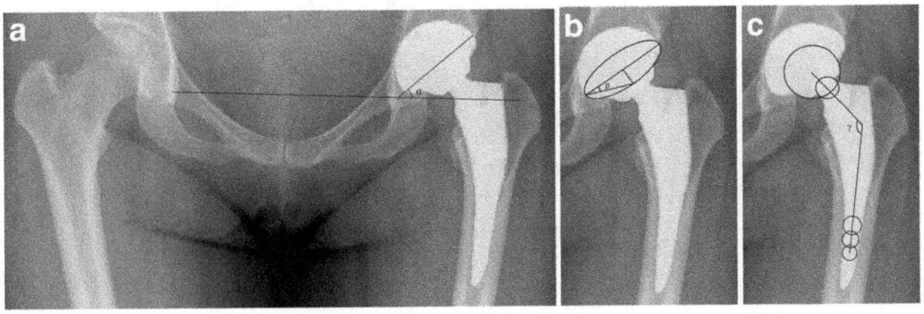

Fig. 1 The cup orientation and stem version were measured in an anteroposterior pelvic radiograph. **a** Postoperative acetabular inclination: α. **b** Postoperative acetabular anteversion: β. **c** The angle between the axes of the neck and stem was regarded as the neck–shaft angle: γ. The stem version was assessed by the γ

loosening or subsidence at the latest follow-up. One hip was detected with a radiolucent line around the proximal femoral, which was not progressed during the follow-up. Other femoral stems achieved either bony ingrowth or and fibrous ingrowth at the final follow-up (Fig. 2). Peri-articular heterotrophic ossification was present in two hips and each of the two cases was defined as class II with Brooker classification system and didn't require excision before the final follow-up.

Complications

Of the 88 hips, seven hips sustained a total of 8 complications (Table 2). Two cases experienced an intraoperative femoral fracture. All of the three cases were type A2 according to the Vancouver classification [14] were cured with cerclage cable. Two patients sustained a sciatic nerve paralysis with a leg lengthening of 31 mm and 36 mm. Both were resolved at the final follow-up. One patient complained of thigh pain at the last follow-up. One patient presented a dislocation at the first day after the operation and was treated with a closed reduction with no further sequelae. No evidence of deep venous thrombosis, calf muscular venous thrombosis and infection were noted during the follow-up.

Survivorship analysis

During the follow-up period, one revision was conducted for a periprosthetic fracture at 8 years. Using revision for any reason as an end point, the Kaplan-Meier survival estimate at 10 years was 98.3% (95% confidence interval [CI], 94.9%–99.9%) (Fig. 3).

Discussion

THA in a patient with Legg-Calve-Perthes disease can be a technically challenging procedure because of the high complication and the complex features of the bone, soft tissue contractures and the relatively young age of the patients [10]. The prior studies validated the benefits of THA in patients with severe arthritis associated with LCPD [5–13] (Table 4). However, most prior reports of LCPD included mixed groups of different types of components in a small number of patients [6, 10, 12]. To our knowledge, this is the largest reported series in which the results of a monobloc stem for the treatment of LCPD were evaluated, including (1) complications; (2) clinical and radiographic outcomes; and (3) survivorship.

LCPD is osteonecrosis of the juvenile hip, which was first described by Arthur Thornton Legg in 1909 as "An Obscure Affection of the Hip Joint", shortly after Roentgen technology was discovered in 1895. Some longitudinal studies have also shown that in some cases, Legg-Calve-Perthes disease that had begun as a purely femoral abnormality (producing a pistol grip deformity) could then secondarily lead to acetabular deformity [15]. Although the acetabulum can accommodate a deformed femoral head and restore what may seem like reasonable congruence on an AP radiograph, this cannot be achieved for all movements of the hip. This results in an 'incongruous incongruity', which could lead to subsequent osteoarthritis [25].

Resurfacing arthroplasty for LCPD is an alternative to conventional THA. Two authors have advocated the use of hip resurfacing for patients with LCPD because of the usually young age and high activity level of these patients [26, 27]. Although, it has advantages of preservation of the proximal femur, a wider range of motion, and low wear rate of its metal-on-metal bearing surface, it is difficult to gain leg length, and the greater trochanter causes impingement. In addition, the thick mantle cement is also known to be a possible cause of early failure [3].

The LCPD patient group has well-known negative prognostic factors for THA, such as young age and abnormality. The outcomes of the present series demonstrate that standard total hip replacement with a monobloc stem can be a feasible option for patients with osteoarthritis of the hip secondary to LCPD.

Increased anteversion of the femoral neck is a common finding for LCPD [28]. Accordingly, the stem may

Table 2 Baseline Characteristics, Radiographic Information, and Complications

Variables	Patients (*N* = 71)
Age, mean ± SD	49.94 ± 11.40
Gender[no.[%]of patients]	
Male	34(47.89%)
Female	37(52.11%)
Height(cm),mean ± SD	159.60 ± 6.59
Weight(Kg),mean ± SD	60.91 ± 11.54
BMI,mean ± SD	23.64 ± 3.62
Followup(year),mean ± SD	10.09 ± 1.84
Bilateral or unilateral[no.[%]of patients]	
Bilateral	17(23.94%)
Unilateral	54(76.06%)
Side[no.[%]of hips]	
Left	41(46.59%)
Right	47(53.41%)
Radiographic Information,mean ± SD	
Cup anteversion, °	25.95 ± 6.00
Cup abduction, °	39.01 ± 5.51
Femoral stem version, °	13.63 ± 4.10
Stulberg classifications [no.[%]of hips]	
Class II	1(1.14%)
Class III	30(34.09%)
Class IV	55(62.5%)
Class V	2(2.27%)
VAS Satisfaction, mean ± SD	9.82 ± 0.52
10	62(87.32%)
9	6(8.45%)
8	2(2.82%)
7	1(1.41%)
Complications[no.[%]of hips]	
Intraoperative femoral fracture	2(2.27%)
Postoperative temporary sciatic nerve paralysis	2(2.27%)
Heterotopic ossification	2(2.27%)
Thigh pain	1(1.14%)
Postoperative dislocation	1(1.14%)
Aseptic loosening	0
Deep vein thrombosis	0
Calf muscular venous thrombosis	0
Infection	0

BMI body mass index, *ONFH* Osteonecrosis of Femoral Head, *ASA* American Society of Anesthesiologists, *VAS* Visual Analogue Scale

Table 3 Outcomes Regarding Hip Function

Variables, mean ± SD	Patients (N = 71)		*P*
	Preoperative	Postoperative	
HHS			
Mean in points	46.42 ± 6.11	89.70 ± 5.46	0.01
Rating [no.[%]of patients]			
Excellent (90–100 points)	0	45(64.38%)	
Good (80–89 points)	0	23(32.39%)	
Fair (70–79 points)	0	3(4.23%)	
Poor (<70)	71(100%)	0	
VAS Pain	5.11 ± 1.30	0.30 ± 0.54	0.01
ROM			
Flexion	90.13 ± 11.24	120.32 ± 4.94	0.01
Abduction	29.28 ± 5.50	41.26 ± 3.73	0.01
HOOS			
Symptoms	11.37 ± 2.40	17.19 ± 1.45	0.01
Pain	19.39 ± 5.90	37.32 ± 2.05	0.01
Daily living	34.80 ± 3.78	65.77 ± 1.17	0.01
Sports and recreational activities	8.07 ± 1.77	14.55 ± 1.96	0.01
Quality of life	6.62 ± 1.21	13.42 ± 1.31	0.01
SF-12			
PCS	15.80 ± 2.69	23.11 ± 2.78	0.01
MCS	16.63 ± 2.80	24.55 ± 3.13	0.01
Limp [no.[%]of patients]			0.01
Severe	0	0	
Moderate	34(47.89%)	0	
Slight	20(28.17%)	3(4.23%)	
None	17(23.94%)	68(95.77%)	
Limb length discrepancy			
Mean in mm	24.3 ± 7.8	2.4 ± 2.8	0.01
Rating [no.[%]of hips]			
< 10	5(5.68%)	87(98.86%)	
10–20	21(23.86%)	1(1.14%)	
20–30	36(40.91%)	0	
30–40	26(29.55%)	0	

HHS Harris Hip Score, *VAS* Visual Analogue Scale, *HOOS* Hip dysfunction and Osteoarthritis Outcome Score, *ROM* range of motion; SF-12: 12-item short-form health survey questionnaire, *PCS* physical component summary, *MCS* mental component summary

be excessively anteverted and may result in dislocation. Therefore, choosing the femoral component is rather important. For this reason, custom-made versions have been preferred. Al-Khateeb reviewed 15 THAs with an average follow-up of 10 years [10]. Although, only one patient sustained a dislocation and was treated with a closed reduction with no further sequelae, the amount of revision arthroplasty was 21%. In addition, custom-made stems were rather expensive. Seufert et al. preferred the use of modular stem for the appropriate contact and restoration of appropriate anteversion [8]. However, concerns over taper fretting, corrosion and

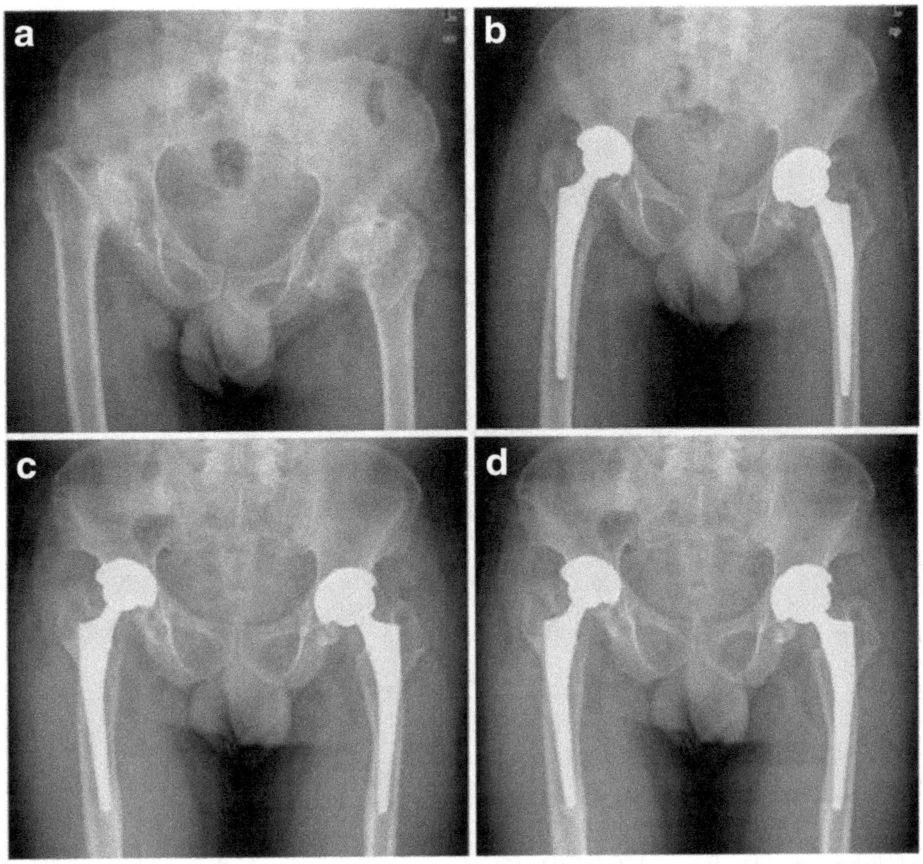

Fig. 2 The radiographs illustrated a 41-year-old man with bilateral Legg-Calve-Perthes disease (LCPD) treated by total hip arthroplasty (THA) with the monobloc stem. **a** Preoperative anteroposterior view. **b**: Postoperative radiographic image. The hip was reconstructed at the level of the anatomic hip center by total hip arthroplasty. No complication occurred during the operation. **c** At 4-year follow-up, no radiolucent lines were found. **d** At the 11-year follow-up, no migration, osteolysis, or subsidence was detected. The femoral and acetabular components were considered stable

even stem fracture with modular stems continue to be important factors when choosing this type of stem for a patient. Lee et al. assessed implant position and the medium-term results of monobloc cementless THA [5]. The mean stem version was 14.6° (range- 2.3° to 30°) with no hip dislocation. In the present study, the mean stem version was 13.63 ± 4.10° (range 5° to 27°), and one dislocation occurred. The dislocation was rare in Lee et al. and the present study, which demonstrated that the monobloc stem can achieve satisfactory results regarding the LCPD. However, Lee et al. only utilized the middle-length stem, and we chose both short and middle-length monobloc stem in this series, which could have affected the result.

Prior studies have demonstrated that standard total hip replacement could restore excellent clinical function for the LCPD patients [11, 12, 29]. In our series, we evaluated the clinical function of the patients with HHS, hip dysfunction and osteoarthritis outcome score (covering pain, symptoms, daily living, sports, and quality of life), the SF-12 scale (physical component summary and mental component summary) and the visual analog scale for pain or satisfaction (VAS, pain/satisfaction). We confirmed that the monobloc stem could improve hip function. In addition, the quality of life and mental condition also improved after the operation. Traina et al. demonstrated in a 10-year follow-up that the average Harris hip score improved from 50.1 to 87.5 for LCPD [12]. Seufert et al. confirmed that Harris hip scores, on average, improved from 49.8 (26–73) to 93.9 (82–100) ($P < 0.05$) after a minimum of 2 years of follow-up [8]. Thus, our series compares favorably with other reports of THA in LCPD patients.

In addition, postoperative complications require special attention for the LCPD patients. In the current study, seven hips sustained a total of 8 complications. For the femoral fracture, 2 (2%) cases occurred, which was a low rate compared with the fracture rate that has been reported to vary between 0 and 34.1% for cementless THA in LCPD [6, 8, 10]. Lee et al. demonstrated that a wedge-shaped stem with bulky proximal design seemed unsuitable for femurs with anatomical deformity

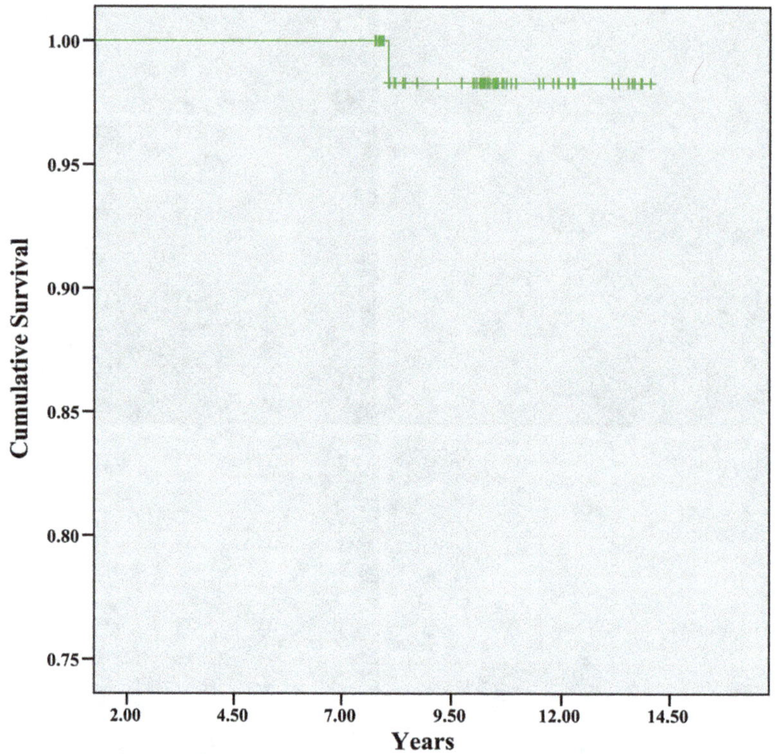

Fig. 3 A Kaplan-Meier survivorship curve with any revision for any component as the end points

due to the risk of intraoperative femoral fracture [6]. Seufert et al. recommended a modular prosthesis which could make appropriate contact of the metaphysis and the diaphysis. In the current study, a monobloc stem could be available for LCPD with 2 cases of fracture. Use of a monobloc stem for LCPD should be recommended and carefully planned during preoperative planning according to preoperative templating and the degree of anatomical deformity. Careful templating aids in selecting the type of implant that would restore the center of rotation of the hip, provide the best femoral fit and decrease the femoral fracture.

Nerve injury is another complication we need to carefully monitor. An analysis of the literature by Goetz et al. determined the risk of nerve palsy after primary total hip arthroplasty to be 0.5% for arthritis, 2.3% for hip dysplasia, and 3.5% for revision surgery [30]. In the current study, two patients (2%) sustained a sciatic nerve paralysis with a leg lengthening of 3.1 cm and 3.6 cm and all the two cases were resolved at the final follow-up. Baghdadi et al. detected three cases (3%) of sciatic nerve paralysis that were lengthened by 2, 1.3, and 3.2 cm (mean, 2.2 cm) at the time of THA compared with a mean of 1.4 ± 1 cm in the patients who did not sustain a neurologic injury (P = 0.3) [11]. In the prior study, the association between limb lengthening and sciatic nerve palsy has been studied with varying conclusions. Edwards et al. correlated the amount of lengthening with the development of sciatic palsy and complete sciatic palsy occurred with a lengthening of 4.0 to 5.1 cm [31]. In contrast, Eggli S et al. found nerve palsy had no correlation with the amount of lengthening, which was most commonly caused by direct or indirect mechanical trauma [32]. The cause of sciatic palsy is still not clear, and we believe the excessive lengthening and mechanical trauma can both be potential causes. For patients with LCPD with severe leg-length discrepancy, shortening osteotomies may be considered to avoid nerve injury. In addition, careful exposing, mobilizing, and protecting the nerve and avoiding a stretch injury or direct contusion of the nerve are needed.

Finally, one patient conducted a revision and the Kaplan-Meier survival estimate at 10 years was 98.3% (95% confidence interval [CI], 94.9%–99.9%). Traina et al. reported the THA survivorship in patients with a history of LCPD at a 96% survivorship at 15 years [12]. Seufert et al. reported one revision (3%) at 3 years with a modular stem in patients with a history of LCPD [8]. Lee et al. reported no revision was required during a 9–15 years of follow-up with a monobloc stem of LCPD [5]. From the results of the present and prior studies, the survivorship of the monobloc stem was shown to be satisfactory.

There are several limitations to our study. First, it was a retrospective review at a single center. Second, the

Table 4 Overview of Relevant Literature in the Treatment of Legg–Calve–Perthes Disease with Total Hip Arthroplasty

Study	Year	Patient (Hips)	Mean Age(y)	Mean FollowUp (yrs)	Implantation Type	Preoperative LLD(mm)	Postoperative LLD(mm)	Preoperative Function	Postoperative Function	Revision	Complication	Survival
Lee et al.	2017	68 (68)	48(16–73)	8.5(5.2–10)	Monobloc Cementless[Corail, DePuy]	NA	2.2(−2–14)	NA	HHS: 91 (73–100) UCLA activity: 5.5 (3–8)	None	Sciatic nerve palsy: 1 Ectopic ossification: 9	100%
Huang et al.	2016	33(33)	46.8 (24–72)	4.5 (2.2–11.3)	Various: Monobloc cementless: 22 Modular Femoral Component[SROM, DePuy]: 11	NA	NA	HHS: 37.6 (15–56)	HHS: 92.8(70–100) Diminished or no limping: 45% (15/33) dissatisfied: 9.1%(3/33)	None	Ectopic ossification: 2 Sciatic nerve palsy: 1 Intraoperative fracture: 4	NA
Lee et al.	2016	37(41)	43.8 ± 12.7 (18.9–66.3)	10.4 ± 3.3 (5.2–16.0)	Aluminae-alumina Cementless	20 ± 12	2 ± 9	HHS:66.7 ± 17.4	HHS: 96.8 ± 6.8 Lengthening: 17 ± 9 Diminished or no limping: 97% (36/37)	None	Intraoperative fracture: 14 Peroneal nerve palsy: 1 Deep vein thrombosis: 1	NA
Seufert et al.	2015	28(35)	51.6 (22–74)	8.2 (2–14)	Modular Femoral Component[SROM, DePuy]	18.6	7	HHS: 49.8 ± 9.2	HHS: 93.9 ± 8.5 Diminished or no limping: 94.3% (33/35)	Deep Infection: 1	Ectopic ossification: 2 Dislocation: 1	NA
Lim et al.	2014	23(23)	49.2 (25–69)	3.5 (2–7)	Monobloc Cementless: Bencox II 22,Accolade 1	15 (7–25)	3 (1–7)	HHS: 48.3 (42–67)	HHS: 92.4 (79–97)	Sciatic nerve palsy: 1	Sciatic nerve palsy: 1 Intraoperative fracture: 3	96%
Al-Khateeb et al.	2014	14(15)	32.8 (23–55)	10.1 (5–15)	Custom-made Cementless	NA	NA	HHS: 41(27–57) Trendelenburg sign(+): 11(78%) Walking aids: 8	HHS: 80(51–94) Trendelenburg sign(+): 3(21%) Walking aids: 1	Aseptic loosening: 3 Deep infection: 1	Ectopic ossification: 1 Dislocation: 1	Femoral stem: 100% Acetabular components: 79%
Baghdadi et al.	2013	95(99)	48 ± 15	8 ± 5	Cementless implants: 76 Hybrid implants21	NA	NA	HHS: 56 (25–85)	HHS: 88 (50–100)	Aseptic loose stem component: 5 Liner wear: 3 Aseptic loose cup component: 1 Deep infection: 1	Intraoperative fracture: 8 (femoral), 1 (acetabular) Sciatic nerve palsy: 3 Thromboembolic: 1 Infection: 1 Dislocation: 1 Adductor tenotomy: 1	Cementless implants: 90% (76%–96%) Hybrid implants:86% (57%–96%)
Traina et al.	2011	27(32)	37.8(19–65)	12.3(5–21)	Cement-less: 31 Cemented:1	NA	9(0–26)	HHS: 50.1(25–75)	HHS: 87.5 (73–96) Average Lengthening: 12 (6–27)	Failure for cemented component: 1	Sciatic nerve palsy: 2 Intraoperative fracture: 1 Hematoma: 1	96.9%(90.8% -100.0%)
Pietrzak et al.	2011	9(9)	56(41–69)	15(11–21)	Cement-less: 6 Cemented:3	NA	NA	HHS: 34 WOMAC: 77	HHS: 93 WOMAC: 6	None	NA	100%
Current study	2017	71(88)	49.94 ± 11.40 (36–73)	10.09 ± 1.84 (7.7–14)	Monobloc cementless: 88	24.3 ± 7.8 (8–36)	2.4 ± 2.8 (−2–10)	HHS: 46.42 ± 6.11, Sym: 11.37 ± 2.40, Pain:19.39 ± 5.90, DL: 34.80 ± 3.78, SARA: 8.07 ± 1.77, QOF: 6.62 ± 1.21, PCS: 15.80 ± 2.69, MCS: 16.63 ± 2.80	HHS: 89.70 ± 5.46, Sym: 17.19 ± 1.45, Pain:37.32 ± 2.05, DL: 65.77 ± 1.17, SARA: 14.55 ± 1.96, QOF: 13.42 ± 1.31, PCS: 23.11 ± 2.78, MCS: 24.55 ± 3.13	Fracture: 1	Intraoperativel fracture: 2 Sciatic nerve palsy:2 Heterotopic ossification: 2 Dislocation: 1 Thigh pain: 1	98.3%(94.9%–99.9%)

LLD Limb length discrepancy, *HHS* Harris Hip Score, *UCLA* University of California activity, Los Angeles activity scales, *WOMAC* The Western Ontario and McMaster Universities Osteoarthritis Index, *Sym* Symptoms, *DL* Daily living, *SARA* Sports and recreational activities, *QOF* Quality of life, *PCS* physical component summary, *MCS* mental component summary, *NA* not applicable

number of patients was relatively small. However, our study group is the largest series of patients with such an uncommon diagnosis. Third, two kinds of monobloc stems and three combinations of bearing were used. Fourth, all the patients' functional outcomes were based on conventional questionnaire-based outcome measures. It would be more objective and reliable if a quantitative gait analysis was conducted for the patient. Finally, all operations were performed by five senior surgeons, which may affect the validity of our findings. However, in this series, all of the chosen implants and the surgical techniques were decided by the five senior surgeons together for all THAs.

Conclusion

These data suggest that the monobloc stem can lead to satisfactory outcomes of the clinical function, radiological evaluation, restoration of normal limb lengths, complications, and survivorship among LCPD patients undergoing total hip arthroplasty.

Abbreviations

DL: Daily living; HHS: Harris Hip Score; HOOS: Hip dysfunction and osteoarthritis outcome score; LCPD: Legg-Calve-Perthes disease; LLD: Limb length discrepancy; MCS: Mental component summary; NA: Not applicable; PCS: Physical component summary; QOF: Quality of life; ROM: Range of motion; SARA: Sports and recreational activities; SF-12: 12-item short-form health survey questionnaire; Sym: Symptoms; THA: Total hip arthroplasty; UCLA: University of California activity, Los Angeles activity scales; VAS: Visual Analogue Scale; WOMAC: The Western Ontario and McMaster Universities Osteoarthritis Index

Acknowledgements

We are thankful for the support of the nursing staffs from the Department of Orthopedic Surgery, West China Hospital and the patients enrolled in this study. We are thankful for the language assistant from "American Journal Experts".

Funding

This research was funded by the China Health Ministry Program (201302007).

Authors' contributions

ZYL performed the data collection and analysis and participated in manuscript writing. HYW and HP performed the database setup and statistical analysis. ZYL, HYW, WD, FXP and ZKZ performed the operations. ZYL and HYW participated in the study design and coordination and helped to draft the manuscript. All the authors have read and approved the final manuscript.

Consent for publication

Not applicable.

Competing interests

The authors declare that they have no competing interests.

Author details

[1]Department of Orthopedics, West China Hospital/West China School of Medicine, Sichuan University, 37# Wuhou Guoxue Road, Chengdu 610041, People's Republic of China. [2]Department of Hematology, The First Affiliated Hospital of Chongqing Medical University, No. 1 Youyi Road, Yuzhong District, Chongqing 400016, People's Republic of China.

References

1. Gower WE, Johnston RC. Legg-Perthes disease. Long-term follow-up of thirty-six patients. J Bone Joint Surg Am. 1971;53(4):759–68.
2. Kelly FB Jr, Canale ST, Jones RR. Legg-calve-Perthes disease. Long-term evaluation of non-containment treatment. J Bone Joint Surg Am. 1980;62(3):400–7.
3. Kim J, Cho YJ, Kim HJ. Role of total hip arthroplasty and resurfacing in Legg-calve-Perthes disease. J Pediatr Orthop. 2011;31(2 Suppl):S241–4.
4. National Clinical Guideline C: National Institute for health and clinical excellence: guidance. In: Osteoarthritis: care and Management in Adults. edn. London: National Institute for Health and Care Excellence (UK) Copyright (c) National Clinical Guideline Centre, 2014.; 2014.
5. Lee KH, Jo WL, Ha YC, Lee YK, Goodman SB, Koo KH. Total hip arthroplasty using a monobloc cementless femoral stem for patients with childhood Perthes' disease. Bone Joint J. 2017;99-b(4):440–4.
6. Lee SJ, Yoo JJ, Kim HJ. Alumina-alumina total hip arthroplasty for the sequelae of Legg-calve-Perthes disease: a comparative study with adult-onset osteonecrosis. J Orthop Sci. 2016;21(6):836–40.
7. Deyong H, Dewei H, Liang Z, Yong H, Yixin Z. Total hip arthroplasty for treatment of sequelae of Legg-Cavé-Perthes disease: a mid-term follow-up results. Orthopedic J China. 2016;24(13):1189-93.
8. Seufert CR, McGrory BJ. Treatment of arthritis associated with Legg-calve-Perthes disease with modular Total hip Arthroplasty. J Arthroplast. 2015;30(10):1743–6.
9. Lim YW, Kim MJ, Lee YS, Kim YS. Total hip Arthroplasty in patient with the Sequelae of Legg-calve-Perthes disease. Hip Pelvis. 2014;26(4):214–9.
10. Al-Khateeb H, Kwok IH, Hanna SA, Sewell MD, Hashemi-Nejad A. Custom cementless THA in patients with Legg-calve-Perthes disease. J Arthroplast. 2014;29(4):792–6.
11. Baghdadi YM, Larson AN, Stans AA, Mabry TM. Total hip arthroplasty for the sequelae of Legg-calve-Perthes disease. Clin Orthop Relat Res. 2013;471(9): 2980–6.
12. Traina F, De Fine M, Sudanese A, Calderoni PP, Tassinari E, Toni A. Long-term results of total hip replacement in patients with Legg-calve-Perthes disease. J Bone Joint Surg Am. 2011;93(7):e25.
13. Pietrzak K, Strzyzewski W, Pucher A, Kaczmarek W. Total hip replacement after Legg-calve-Perthes disease. Chir Narzadow Ruchu Ortop Pol. 2011;76(3):129–33.
14. Greidanus NV, Mitchell PA, Masri BA, Garbuz DS, Duncan CP. Principles of management and results of treating the fractured femur during and after total hip arthroplasty. Instr Course Lect. 2003;52:309–22.
15. Stulberg SD, Cooperman DR, Wallensten R. The natural history of Legg-calve-Perthes disease. J Bone Joint Surg Am. 1981;63(7):1095–108.
16. Wan Z, Malik A, Jaramaz B, Chao L, Dorr LD. Imaging and navigation measurement of acetabular component position in THA. Clin Orthop Relat Res. 2009;467(1):32–42.
17. Engh CA Jr, Culpepper WJ 2nd, Engh CA. Long-term results of use of the anatomic medullary locking prosthesis in total hip arthroplasty. J Bone Joint Surg Am. 1997;79(2):177–84.
18. Gruen TA, McNeice GM, Amstutz HC. "Modes of failure" of cemented stem-type femoral components: a radiographic analysis of loosening. Clin Orthop Relat Res. 1979;141:17–27.
19. Weber M, Lechler P, von Kunow F, Vollner F, Keshmiri A, Hapfelmeier A, Grifka J, Renkawitz T. The validity of a novel radiological method for measuring femoral stem version on anteroposterior radiographs of the hip after total hip arthroplasty. Bone Joint J. 2015;97-b(3):306–11.
20. Biant LC, Bruce WJ, Assini JB, Walker PM, Walsh WR. The anatomically difficult primary total hip replacement: medium- to long-term results using a cementless odular stem. J Bone Joint Surg Br. 2008;90(4):430–5.
21. Engh CA, Massin P, Suthers KE. Roentgenographic assessment of the biologic fixation of porous-surfaced femoral components. Clin Orthop Relat Res. 1990;257:107–28.

22. Engh CA, Bobyn JD, Glassman AH. Porous-coated hip replacement. The factors governing bone ingrowth, stress shielding, and clinical results. J Bone Joint Surg Br. 1987;69(1):45–55.
23. Loudon JR, Charnley J. Subsidence of the femoral prosthesis in total hip replacement in relation to the design of the stem. J Bone Joint Surg Br. 1980;62-b(4):450–3.
24. Brooker AF, Bowerman JW, Robinson RA, Riley LH Jr. Ectopic ossification following total hip replacement. Incidence and a method of classification. J Bone Joint Surg Am. 1973;55(8):1629–32.
25. Lloyd-Roberts GC. Osteoarthritis of the hip; a study of the clinical pathology. J Bone Joint Surg Br. 1955;37-b(1):8–47.
26. Boyd HS, Ulrich SD, Seyler TM, Marulanda GA, Mont MA. Resurfacing for Perthes disease: an alternative to standard hip arthroplasty. Clin Orthop Relat Res. 2007;465:80–5.
27. Amstutz HC, Su EP, Le Duff MJ. Surface arthroplasty in young patients with hip arthritis secondary to childhood disorders. Orthop Clin North Am. 2005;36(2):223–30. x
28. Upadhyay SS, Burwell RG, Moulton A. Femoral anteversion in Perthes' disease with observations on irritable hips. Application of a new method using ultrasound. Clin Orthop Relat Res. 1986;209:70–6.
29. Costa CR, Johnson AJ, Naziri Q, Mont MA. Review of total hip resurfacing and total hip arthroplasty in young patients who had Legg-calve-Perthes disease. Orthop Clin North Am. 2011;42(3):419–22. viii
30. Goetz MB, Seybold D, Gosse F, Muhr G, Roetman B. The risk of nerve lesions in hip alloarthroplasty. Z Orthop Unfall. 2010;148(2):163–7.
31. Edwards BN, Tullos HS, Noble PC. Contributory factors and etiology of sciatic nerve palsy in total hip arthroplasty. Clin Orthop Relat Res. 1987;218: 136–41.
32. Eggli S, Hankemayer S, Muller ME. Nerve palsy after leg lengthening in total replacement arthroplasty for developmental dysplasia of the hip. J Bone Joint Surg Br. 1999;81(5):843–5.

19

Bone turnover and periprosthetic bone loss after cementless total hip arthroplasty can be restored by zoledronic acid

Tsan-Wen Huang[1,2,7], Chao-Jan Wang[2,4,6], Hsin-Nung Shih[2,3,6], Yuhan Chang[2,3,6], Kuo-Chin Huang[2,5,8], Kuo-Ti Peng[1,2,7] and Mel S. Lee[2,5*]

Abstract

Background: Although the loss of bone mineral density (BMD) after total hip arthroplasty (THA) is a known problem, it remains unresolved. This study prospectively examined the effect of zoledronic acid (ZA) on bone turnover and BMD after cementless THA.

Methods: Between January 2010 and August 2011, 60 patients who underwent cementless THA were randomly assigned to receive either ZA infusion or placebo (0.9% normal saline only) postoperatively. ZA was administered at 2 day and 1 year postoperatively. Periprosthetic BMD in seven Gruen zones was assessed preoperatively and at given time points for 2 years. Serum markers of bone turnover, functional scales, and adverse events were recorded.

Results: Each group contained 27 patients for the final analysis. The loss of BMD across all Gruen zones (significantly in zones 1 and 7) up to 2 years postoperatively was noted in the placebo group. BMD was significantly higher in the ZA group than in the placebo group in Gruen zones 1, 2, 6, and 7 at 1 year and in Gruen zones 1, 6, and 7 at 2 years ($p < 0.05$). Compared with baseline measures of BMD, the ZA group had increased BMD in zones 1, 2, 4, 5, 6, and 7 at 1 year and in zones 1, 4, 6, and 7 at 2 years ($p < 0.05$). Serum bone-specific alkaline phosphatase and N-telopeptide of procollagen I levels were significantly increased at 6 weeks in the placebo group and decreased after 3 months in the ZA group. A transient decrease in osteocalcin level was found at 6 months in the ZA group. Functional scales and adverse events were not different between the two groups.

Conclusions: The loss of periprosthetic BMD, especially in the proximal femur (zones 1 and 7), after cementless THA could be effectively reverted using ZA. In addition, bone turnover markers were suppressed until 2 years postoperatively following ZA administration.

Keywords: Cementless total hip arthroplasty, Bone mineral density, Bisphosphonate, Stress shielding, Zoledronic acid, Bone turnover markers

* Correspondence: bone@doctor.com
[2]Chang Gung University, Taoyuan, Taiwan
[5]Department of Orthopaedic Surgery, Kaohsiung Chang Gung Memorial Hospital, No. 123, Dapi Rd., Niaosong District, Kaohsiung City 83301, Taiwan
Full list of author information is available at the end of the article

Background

Cementless total hip arthroplasty (THA) has become popular in recent decades [1, 2], but its long-term stability may be limited by progressive bone loss around the prosthetic implant [3, 4]. Periprosthetic bone loss is associated with reduced bone mineral density (BMD) in the periprosthetic Gruen zones [5–7] and may increase the risk of migration, implant loosening, and periprosthetic fractures [8].

A reduction in BMD, especially in the calcar region, is a common sequela of THA [6, 9–11]. Thus, preserving bone mineral content is important. Bisphosphonates are anti-resorptive agents that promote bone mineralization and inhibit farnesyl pyrophosphate synthase [12]. Their protective effects after joint arthroplasty have been shown in recent meta-analysis studies [13–15] wherein the periprosthetic BMD continued to increase by 9.40% at 18–70 months after discontinuation of bisphosphonate therapy.

Zoledronic acid (ZA), a third-generation bisphosphonate, is several times more potent than the first- or second-generation bisphosphonates. It is well tolerated and can rapidly lower bone turnover rates in children and adults at high risk of fractures [16–19]. In the pivotal Health Outcomes and Reduced Incidence with ZA Once-Yearly Trial (HORIZON-PFT), a once-yearly infusion of 5-mg intravenous ZA for a 3-year period significantly reduced the risk of vertebral fractures by 70%, hip fractures by 41%, and non-vertebral fractures by 25% in post-menopausal women with osteoporosis [20]. ZA protects against osteoporotic fractures [21]. Recently, two studies demonstrated the efficacy of ZA in patients who underwent cementless THA [22, 23], but ZA was administered on different schedules, leaving questions about the optimal dose timing of ZA unanswered.

In the present study, we administered ZA during the early postoperative period after cementless THA, and as a booster dose at 1 year postoperatively. The effects of ZA on periprosthetic BMD and functional outcome measures were assessed prospectively. Additionally, we examined safety concerns surrounding the dosing of ZA.

Methods

Study design

This prospective, randomized, open-label clinical trial was registered in ClinicalTrials.gov (NCT02838121). The Institutional Review Board of the study institution approved the study protocol (Reference number 98-1150A3), which adhered to the Declaration of Helsinki. All of the study participants provided written informed consent.

Based on Arabmotlagh et al. [10], the assumption of mean BMD change was −8% in the placebo group and 6% in the ZA group, with a standard deviation (SD) of 15%. Power analysis indicated that 25 patients were required, per group, to achieve a power of 0.9 with a 5% significance level. To avoid drop off and loss to follow-up, we recruited 30 patients in each group, for a total study sample of 60 patients. The assumptions were proven to be adequate because a similar sample size was reported by another prospective randomized trial [22]. Eligible patients were randomly assigned to either the ZA or placebo groups by an envelope drawing.

On the day following cementless THA, and at 1-year post-THA, the ZA group received 5 mg ZA (Aclasta®; Novartis Pharmaceuticals Corporation) via intravenous infusion with 0.9% normal saline (500 mL). The control group received only an intravenous saline infusion. All patients received oral calcium (600 mg) and vitamin D3 supplements (800 IU) daily throughout the course of the study [24]. Follow-up for radiographic and functional assessments was conducted at 2, 6, and 12 weeks, 6 months, and 1 and 2 years postoperatively.

Patients

Patients aged 35–85 years undergoing THA, who received dual-energy x-ray absorptiometry (DXA) scanning within the 3 months preceding surgery, were considered for enrollment. Exclusion criteria included use of bisphosphonates during the preceding 2 years; uncontrolled seizure disorders; invasive malignancy within the preceding 5 years; osteogenesis imperfect; multiple myeloma; Paget's disease; iritis; uveitis; diabetic neuropathy/retinopathy; active primary hyperthyroidism; Aspartate aminotransferase (AST), alanine aminotransferase (ALT), or bone-specific alkaline phosphatase levels more than twice the normal limit; serum calcium level >11 mg/dL; hypocalcemia; renal insufficiency (creatinine clearance ≤35 mL/min); use of investigational drugs; and the use of hip protectors or implants on the contralateral hip joint.

The patients' demographic data, body mass index, pre-operative diagnoses, and baseline characteristics were recorded.

Total hip arthroplasty

All of the patients underwent standardized THA via direct lateral approach [25, 26] using a Zimmer Trilogy Cup, VerSys Fiber Metal Taper Stem, and highly cross-linked polyethylene, coupled with a 32 mm metal head. An experienced surgeon performed all of the procedures. Based on our standard of care following cementless THA, the patients were encouraged to ambulate as soon as possible after surgery and advised to protect against weight bearing for 6 weeks.

Assessments

An experienced clinician, blinded to group assignment and patients' demographic data, performed all radiographic and clinical assessments.

On each follow-up visit, radiographic evaluation of the total hip prosthesis was performed on each standard antero-posterior views of the pelvis and lateral views of the operated hip according to methods described by Engh et al. [27] and Johnston et al. [28]. The vertical distance between the lateral shoulder of the prosthesis and the superior tip of the greater trochanter on the radiograph was measured. This served as the reference distance for monitoring implant migration. At each study visit, this distance was measured and recorded.

The patients underwent DXA scanning of the operated hip using a densitometer (Hologic Inc., Waltham, MA) for quantifying bone mass and density changes [7]. To estimate the precision of the densitometer, double measurements involving repositioning of the patient and the scanner between the first and second scans were made in 10 patients [29]. The DXA method had a measurement error of 1%–3% in Gruen zones. BMD was measured in the frontal plane, throughout seven Gruen zones, and changes in BMD ratios from baseline were estimated for each zone.

Functional assessments included the Hip Harris Score (HHS), UCLA activity score, Short-Form (SF)-12 Physical Component Summary (PCS), and SF-12 Mental Component Summary (MCS). Renal function (glomerular filtration rate [GFR] and creatinine level), hepatic function (AST and ALT), serum calcium, and levels of bone turnover biomarkers (osteocalcin, bone-specific alkaline phosphatase, and N-telopeptide of procollagen I) were also assessed [30, 31].

Complications, including reported need for analgesics, were recorded. Any medical or surgical event that compromised clinical recovery was defined and recorded as an adverse event. A relatively poorer and slower functional recovery beyond 3 months and an HHS score <80 were considered adverse events.

The primary endpoint was the change in periprosthetic BMD, between baseline and all other time points. Secondary endpoints included radiologic analyses, implant migration, levels of serum markers for bone metabolism, functional outcomes, and safety and tolerability of the experimental drug.

Statistical analysis

Values are presented as mean (±SD). Group differences were analyzed using independent-samples *t*-test. Time-based differences were analyzed by repeated measures analysis of variance (ANOVA) using a general linear model with Greenhouse-Geisser correction. Significance was set at $p < 0.05$. Post hoc comparisons were performed using Bonferroni corrections for multiple comparisons. SPSS software version 13.0 (SPSS Inc., Chicago, IL) was used for all analyses.

Results

Patient demographics

Between January 2010 and August 2011, 60 patients were enrolled. Following randomization into either the ZA or placebo control groups, four patients (one in the ZA group and three in the control group) were excluded due to periprosthetic fractures and an additional two (both from the ZA group) were excluded due to missing BMD data at 1 year (Fig. 1). Each group had 27 patients for the final analysis and no significant differences in baseline characteristics were found between the two groups (Table 1).

Radiographic analysis

All implants showed stable osteo-integration without evidence of early or late migration. There were no radiolucent lines at the prosthesis-bone interface of the cups and stems, and no pedestal formation in any stem, in either group.

Bone mineral density

At baseline, both groups had similar BMD. The delta BMD at each time point revealed that at 12 weeks, the ZA group had significantly higher BMD than the control group in Gruen zones 2, 6, and 7. Increases in BMD persisted at 6 months in zones 6 and 7, at 1 year in zones 1, 2, 6, and 7, and at 2 years in zones 1, 6, and 7 (Table 2). The BMD changes from baseline (BMD ratio) were significantly higher for the ZA group in Gruen zones 2, 4, 6, and 7 at 12 weeks; in zones 1, 6, and 7 at 6 months; in zones 1, 2, 4, 5, 6 and 7 at 1 year, and in zones 1, 4, 6, and 7 at 2 years (Table 3).

Time-based BMD differences in each Gruen zones were analyzed by repeated measure ANOVA (Fig. 2). In zone 1, the mean BMD change was 111% in the ZA group and 88% in the control group (95% CI, 10%–36%; $p = 0.001$). In zone 2, the mean BMD change was 114% (ZA) and 103% (control) (95% CI, 2%–20%; $p = 0.018$). In zone 4, the mean BMD change was 105% (ZA) and 95% (control) (95% CI, 5%–15%; $p = 0.001$). In zone 5, the mean BMD change was 108% (ZA) and 99% (control) (95% CI, 1%–18%; $p = 0.024$). In zone 6, the mean BMD change was 114% (ZA) and 98% (control) (95% CI, 7%–25%; $p = 0.001$). In zone 7, the mean BMD change was 110% (ZA) and 84% (control) (95% CI, 14%–37%; $p < 0.001$).

Functional outcomes

There were no significant differences in HHS, SF-12 (PCS), SF-12 (MCS), and UCLA scores between the

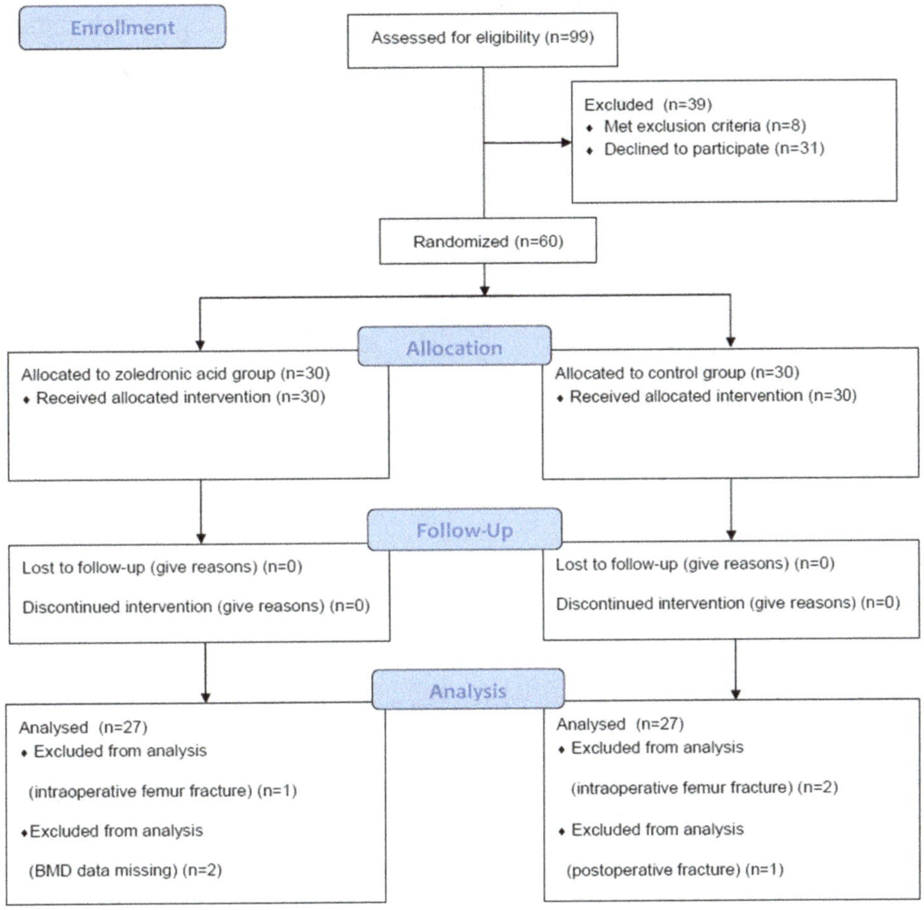

Fig. 1 Patient disposition

groups at any point in the study. However, the within-group functional scores changed significantly throughout the study period ($p < 0.001$) (Table 4). HHS increased significantly from baseline to 6 weeks, and thereafter up to 2 years, in both groups ($p < 0.001$). SF-12 (PCS) scores were lower at 2 weeks compared to baseline ($p < 0.001$), but increased significantly from baseline to 12 weeks, and thereafter up to 2 years, in both groups ($p < 0.001$).

Table 1 Patient demographics and surgical results

	ZA group ($n = 27$)	Control group ($n = 27$)
Age (years), mean (SD)	60.1 (11.7)	59.4 (13.3)
Sex, female:male	15:12	14:13
BMI (kg/m^2), mean (SD)	26 (4)	25 (5)
Operation time (minutes), mean (SD)[a]	118 (27)	103 (17)
Blood loss (mL), mean (SD)	502 (312)	387 (162)
Diagnosis (OA/AVN)	16/11	17/10

BMI body mass index, *SD* standard deviation, *ZA* zoledronic acid, *OA* osteoarthritis, *AVN* avascular necrosis
[a]statistically significant difference between the ZA and control groups ($P < 0.05$)

The SF-12 (MCS) scores of both groups were significantly lower at 1 year compared to 6 weeks ($p < 0.05$). Compared to baseline, the UCLA scores of both groups were significantly lower at 2 and 6 weeks ($p < 0.01$), but significantly increased by 1 year ($p < 0.001$).

Renal and hepatic function and serum calcium levels

There were no significant differences in creatinine levels between the two groups at baseline or at any time point throughout the study. GFR increased within both groups between baseline and 6 months ($p < 0.01$) and baseline and 1 year ($p < 0.001$) (Table 5). The AST and ALT values at baseline and at 6 and 12 weeks were within normal limits and had no group differences were realized at any time point. Serum calcium levels were similar in both groups at all time points.

Biomarkers of bone turnover

There was a significant reduction, from baseline, in levels of bone-specific alkaline phosphatase for the ZA group at 12 weeks, 6 months, 1 year, and 2 years postoperatively ($p < 0.01$). In the control group, bone-specific

Table 2 Mean (SD) BMD (g/cm^2) for both groups in all gruen zones

Gruen zones	1	2	3	4	5	6	7	Delta
Baseline								
ZA group	0.64(0.14)	1.26(0.21)	1.52(0.24)	1.63(0.19)	1.57(0.19)	1.24(0.21)	0.96(0.19)	1.15(0.16)
Control	0.64(0.16)	1.24(0.22)	1.53(0.21)	1.66(0.21)	1.61(0.23)	1.25(0.22)	0.97(0.24)	1.15(0.17)
p-value	0.863	0.778	0.779	0.522	0.446	0.951	0.830	0.968
12 weeks								
ZA group	0.74(0.38)	1.46(0.28)	1.69(0.88)	1.73(0.35)	1.75(0.58)	1.40(0.21)	1.09(0.22)	1.38(0.60)
Control	0.59(0.14)	1.28(0.21)	1.50(0.21)	1.61(0.21)	1.61(0.22)	1.23(0.23)	0.88(0.20)	1.16(0.14)
p-value	0.060	0.010[a]	0.276	0.142	0.238	0.009[a]	0.001[a]	0.077
6 months								
ZA group	0.65(0.14)	1.40(0.17)	1.55(0.17)	1.68(0.19)	1.62(0.27)	1.40(0.19)	1.04(0.25)	1.26(0.12)
Control	0.59(0.15)	1.31(0.26)	1.51(0.22)	1.62(0.23)	1.63(0.23)	1.26(0.23)	0.84(0.30)	1.17(0.16)
p-value	0.109	0.144	0.529	0.301	0.922	0.021[a]	0.008[a]	0.021[a]
1 year								
ZA group	0.66(0.15)	1.38(0.19)	1.50(0.24)	1.68(0.19)	1.66(0.16)	1.40(0.22)	1.01(0.27)	1.25(0.13)
Control	0.54(0.20)	1.19(0.38)	1.44(0.38)	1.54(0.38)	1.51(0.39)	1.20(0.36)	0.80(0.30)	1.11(0.28)
p-value	0.021[a]	0.035[a]	0.434	0.096	0.057	0.014[a]	0.011[a]	0.021[a]
2 years								
ZA group	0.67(0.15)	1.38(0.20)	1.49(0.25)	1.68(0.19)	1.65(0.20)	1.44(0.21)	1.01(0.27)	1.26(0.13)
Control	0.55(0.15)	1.35(0.77)	1.51(0.23)	1.59(0.23)	1.62(0.21)	1.21(0.24)	0.78(0.22)	1.14(0.15)
p-value	0.013[a]	0.870	0.786	0.167	0.612	0.001[a]	0.003[a]	0.011[a]

[a]statistically significant difference between ZA and control groups
BMD bone mineral density, *SD* standard deviation, *ZA* zoledronic acid

alkaline phosphatase was significantly increased at 6 and 12 weeks postoperatively ($p < 0.05$) (Table 5). In the ZA group, osteocalcin was significantly reduced between baseline and 6 months, 1 year, and 2 years ($p < 0.05$). The control group demonstrated significant increases in osteocalcin between baseline and 1 year ($p < 0.05$).

In the ZA group, levels of N-telopeptide of procollagen I were significantly reduced from baseline at 12 weeks, 6 months, 1 year, and 2 years postoperatively

Table 3 Mean (SD) bone mineral density ratio (the BMD changes from baseline) for each group by gruen zone at different time points

Gruen zones	1	2	3	4	5	6	7
12 weeks							
ZA group	1.20(0.74)	1.18(0.28)[a]	1.13(0.62)	1.07(0.23)[a]	1.13(0.41)	1.13(0.13)[a]	1.15(0.21)[a]
Control	0.93(0.14)	1.04(0.12)	0.98(0.08)	0.97(0.04)	1.00(0.07)	1.00(0.15)	0.93(0.22)
6 months							
ZA group	1.05(0.19)[a]	1.13(0.12)	1.05(0.21)	1.04(0.07)	1.04(0.18)	1.14(0.12)[a]	1.09(0.20)[a]
Control	0.92(0.18)	1.07(0.19)	0.99(0.08)	0.97(0.06)	1.01(0.07)	1.02(0.18)	0.88(0.29)
1 year							
ZA group	1.05(0.19)[a]	1.10(0.10)[a]	1.00(0.09)	1.03(0.08)[a]	1.07(0.12)[a]	1.13(0.13)[a]	1.07(0.22)[a]
Control	0.86(0.24)	0.98(0.25)	0.95(0.22)	0.93(0.20)	0.95(0.24)	0.97(0.28)	0.84(0.29)
2 years							
ZA group	1.08(0.21)[a]	1.12(0.11)	1.00(0.11)	1.04(0.09)[a]	1.08(0.15)	1.16(0.13)[a]	1.06(0.22)[a]
Control	0.89(0.14)	1.10(0.46)	1.00(0.08)	0.96(0.07)	1.02(0.10)	1.00(0.19)	0.83(0.20)

[a]statistically significant difference between the ZA and control groups ($P < 0.05$)
BMD bone mineral density, *SD* standard deviation, *ZA* zoledronic acid

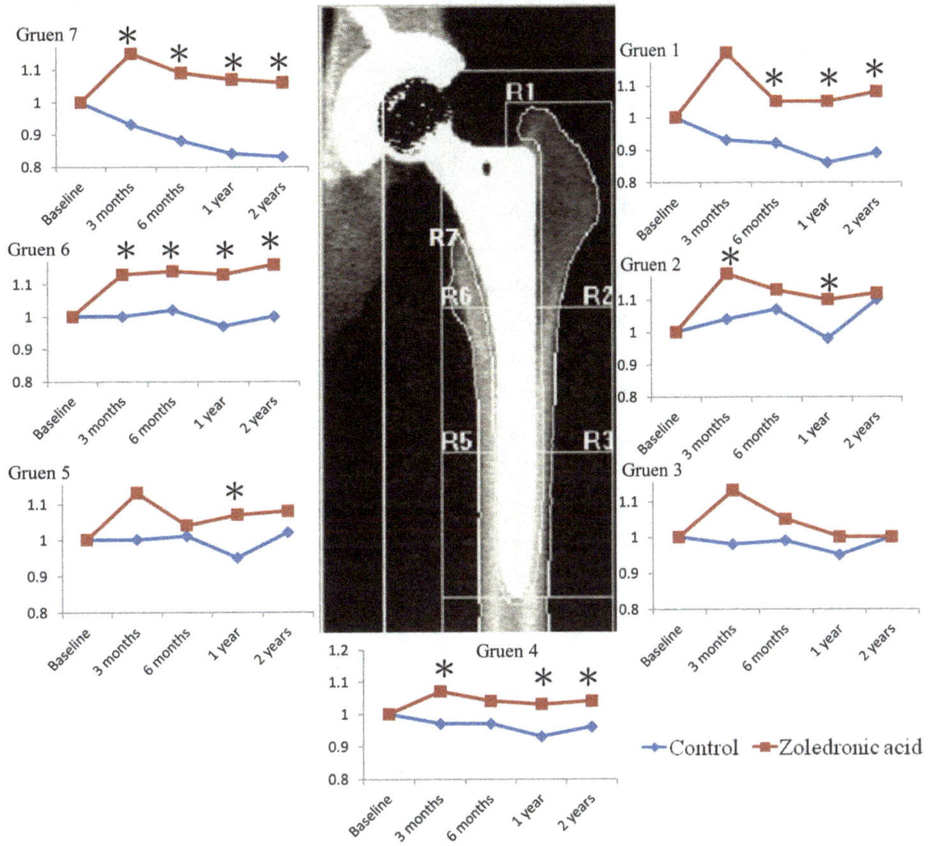

Fig. 2 Bone mineral density changes in the zoledronic acid and control groups in Gruen zones

Table 4 Clinical assessments in each group at different time intervals ($n = 54$)

	Preop		2 week		6 week		3 months		6 months		1 year		2 years	
	N	mean ± SD	N	mean ± SD	N	mean ± SD	N	mean ± SD	N	mean ± SD	N	mean ± SD	N	mean ± SD
Harris hip score														
Group ZA	27	60.31 ± 10.49	27	56.23 ± 14.06	27	70.96 ± 13.03[a]	27	77.93 ± 10.63[a]	27	83.60 ± 7.52[a]	27	86.34 ± 7.08[a]	27	90.18 ± 2.11[a]
Group N/S	27	60.88 ± 11.63	27	58.80 ± 10.13	27	71.08 ± 12.26[a]	27	79.89 ± 9.42[a]	27	81.50 ± 9.87[a]	27	85.16 ± 7.28[a]	27	87.67 ± 5.44[a]
SF-12(PCS)														
Group ZA	27	27.53 ± 10.13	27	18.96 ± 7.48[a]	27	28.23 ± 11.35	27	40.01 ± 13.54[a]	27	48.09 ± 6.95[a]	27	51.29 ± 4.45[a]	27	53.69 ± 3.79[a]
Group N/S	27	29.16 ± 11.31	27	21.37 ± 8.34[a]	27	27.79 ± 11.99	27	42.12 ± 10.61[a]	27	48.96 ± 7.90[a]	27	50.53 ± 6.95[a]	27	52.50 ± 4.16[a]
SF-12(MCS)														
Group ZA	27	57.65 ± 12.57	27	60.87 ± 9.51	27	59.23 ± 10.59	27	60.3 ± 6.86	27	58.85 ± 4.95	27	58.49 ± 4.07	27	58.61 ± 5.98
Group N/S	27	59.17 ± 11.99	27	60.08 ± 7.29	27	63.72 ± 3.84	27	59.9 ± 4.77	27	55.97 ± 8.34	27	56.96 ± 7.20	27	59.01 ± 4.05
UCLA activity score														
Group ZA	27	3.96 ± 1.16	27	2.56 ± 0.80[a]	27	3.41 ± 0.97[a]	27	4.22 ± 0.93	27	4.63 ± 1.15	27	5.74 ± 1.06[a]	27	7.00 ± 0.90[a]
Group N/S	27	4.33 ± 1.59	27	2.56 ± 0.70[a]	27	3.44 ± 0.97[a]	27	4.52 ± 0.94	27	4.70 ± 0.95	27	5.52 ± 1.19[a]	27	6.50 ± 0.74[a]

Statistically significant difference between ZA and control groups
[a]significant difference between each time point and baseline
SD Standard deviation, *ZA* zoledronic acid, *SF* short form, *PCS* physical component summary, *MCS* mental component summary, *N/S* normal saline

Table 5 Mean serum creatinine (Cr) level, glomerular filtration rate (GFR), and bone turnover biomarkers in the ZA (zoledronic acid) and control groups as a function of time

	Baseline	6 weeks	12 weeks	6 months	1 year	2 years
Renal function						
Cr (mg/dL)						
ZA group	0.79 (0.23)	0.76 (0.27)	0.81 (0.28)	0.85 (0.59)	0.78 (0.24)	0.76 (0.26)
Control	0.83 (0.2)	0.81 (0.22)	0.79 (0.18)	0.79 (0.19)	0.76 (0.23)	0.79 (0.22)
GFR (mL/min)						
ZA group	59.39 (2.21)	60.08 (5)	61.84 (10.78)	77.56 (27.24)	83.8 (28.48)	93.9 (23.3)
Control	59.63 (1.28)	59.78 (1.15)	63.16 (12.83)	73.82 (23.6)	79.45 (25.96)	87.3 (19.5)
Ca *(mg/dL)*						
ZA group	9.53 (0.49)	9.34 (0.57)	9.52 (0.44)	9.46 (0.46)	9.43 (0.49)	9.37 (0.39)
Control	9.57 (0.43)	9.2 (1.77)	9.54 (0.36)	9.47 (0.52)	9.13 (1.89)	9.24 (0.29)
Bone turnover biomarkers						
Bone-specific alkaline phosphatase (μg/L)						
ZA group	78.6 (17.7)	77.3 (19.2)[a]	65.6 (11.7)[b]	67.5 (26.6)	68.7 (24.5)	66.5 (18.1)
Control	76 (17.6)	89.4 (21.7)	83.3 (22.8)	74.5 (19.9)	73.2 (22.9)	74 (15.9)
Osteocalcin (ng/mL)						
ZA group	21.1 (8.7)	18.1 (7.9)	17.2 (10.2)	14.7 (5)	16.8 (7.2)	14.9 (7.2)
Control	18.5 (10.3)	20.9 (13.2)	20.8 (11.5)	17.7 (6.4)	20.5 (10.4)	18.8 (8.6)
N-telopeptide of procollagen I (ng/mL)						
ZA group	53.9 (23.1)	57.1 (24.6)[a]	38.8 (16.9)[b]	30.5 (11.9)[b]	34.6 (19.5)	28.3 (11.3)[a]
Control	43.2 (21.8)	80.7 (44)	69.7 (38)	57.5 (24.9)	50.4 (35.4)	44.3 (19.3)

[a]significant difference between groups ($P < 0.05$)
[b]significant difference between groups ($P < 0.001$)

($p < 0.05$). In the control group, these levels significantly increased from baseline at 6 weeks, 12 weeks, and at 6 months postoperatively ($p < 0.05$). There were significant differences in bone turnover biomarkers between the ZA and control groups (Table 5).

Adverse events

Complications included fever ($n = 3$) and hypocalcemia ($n = 1$) but were mild-to-moderate in severity, and believed to be related to the investigational drug. No patient sustained osteonecrosis of the jaw or atypical femoral fracture. Three patients (one in the ZA group and two in the control group) had intra-operative periprosthetic fractures, and one (control) subject had postoperative periprosthetic fracture. These individuals were excluded from the final analysis.

Discussion

The present study shows that ZA infusions on the day after cementless THA, and as a booster at 1 year postoperatively, significantly reduced periprosthetic femoral BMD loss. In the control group, BMD decreased significantly in Gruen zones 1 and 7 up to 2 years postoperatively. In contrast, for the ZA group, BMD significantly increased in all Gruen zones (except for zone 3) between baseline and 1 year postoperatively. At 2 years postoperatively it remained significantly increased in zones 1, 6, and 7. The greatest effect of ZA was observed in the proximal femur at 2 years, with BMD changes of +6% (control: −17%) in zone 7 and +8% (control: −11%) in zone 1. However, this improvement does not necessarily reflect better functional outcomes.

Only two reports have previously studied ZA in patients after cementless THA. Scott et al. [23] reported that ZA significantly prevented BMD loss in Gruen zones 1, 4, and 6 at 1 year, and in zones 1 and 6 at 2 years. However a decrease in BMD was still evident in zone 7 (calcar region) at 1 and 2 years. Our results were different. We found increased BMD after ZA across all Gruen zones at 1 year (though this difference did not rise to the level of statistical significance for zone 3), including Gruen zone 7. We thought the difference may be related to differences in Scott et al.'s timing of ZA administration (2 weeks postoperatively), or differences among the various types of prosthesis (two types of modular stems). The present study always administered ZA at 2 days postoperatively and used only one type of prosthesis. Periprosthetic BMD varies as a function of stem type. Patients with large and stiff femoral stems experience greater stress shielding, which results in more resorption of the proximal femur [15]. The modular femoral prosthesis has a larger proximal implant segment (for the neck-body taper junction) and is stiffer proximally. Proximal stiffness mismatches may increase proximal femoral stress shielding and subsequent bone loss. Moreover, more proximal bone loss occurs in femur preparation for larger femoral prosthesis. A femur with less bone mass is less stiff, relative to the implanted stem, and this will increase stress-related bone resorption [32]. In this study, we used a flat and double-tapered non-modular femoral stems. This design decreases the cross-sectional area moment of inertia and achieves initial stability by wedging into the proximal femur. It is considerably less stiff than the modular design and prevents periprosthetic bone loss.

In the second study, ZA (4 mg) was administered on the first postoperative day to 25 patients after cementless THA. Periprosthetic BMD was not analyzed but ZA improved the initial fixation of the cementless implant and prevented early implant migration, compared to 24 control patients [22]. The current study also used ZA in the acute postoperative period and did not find severe adverse events related to the drug. ZA infusion was deemed safe during the acute phase after THA. Taken together, early timing for postoperative ZA treatment may be a safe and effective means of preventing BMD loss after cementless THA.

Since periprosthetic bone loss is most pronounced in the early postoperative period [9], administering bisphosphonates soon after surgery is logical [22]. Ericksen and colleagues reported that the timing of the first ZA infusion changes BMD for patients who recently underwent hip surgery [33]. At 1 year postoperatively, all patients treated with ZA had increased BMD except for the group that received an early dose (≤2 weeks postoperatively). This group also demonstrated worse anti-fracture outcomes. While the current findings seem to contradict those of Ericksen et al., the patients in their study who received ZA ≤2 weeks after surgery had a higher risk of mortality due to older age and a greater number of comorbidities. Moreover, their study had a smaller sample size and therefore group heterogeneity may have affected their findings. The current study provides a consolidated examination of BMD and revealed biochemical data supporting the use of ZA in the early postoperative period (2 days postoperatively). Since THA or bipolar hemiarthroplasty are common surgeries for patients with hip fractures, early initiation of ZA or other bisphosphonates is practical and may lead to superior outcomes.

In their meta-analysis, Bhandari et al. [13] suggested that bisphosphonates had a beneficial effect in maintaining periprosthetic BMD after THA or total knee arthroplasty. Arabmotlagh et al. [10] reported long-standing beneficial effects of alendronate in the prevention of periprosthetic bone loss 6 years after cementless THA. A single-dose of ZA can restore BMD beyond 1 year, with an effect comparable to that obtained with three annual ZA infusions [34]. In addition, ZA can prevent bone loss for long time periods. The HORIZON-PFT study reports a 6.02% increase in total hip BMD in patients, at risk of hip fractures, following 3 years of annual ZA treatment [19, 35]. Improvements in BMD continued for 6 years in these patients, suggesting a lasting effect of ZA.

Measuring serum calcium levels during ZA treatment is recommended [23]. In this study, both groups were administered oral calcium supplements. Serum calcium levels were within normal range throughout the study period (Table 5). Since ZA can lead to reduced serum calcium levels 6 weeks after its administration, providing calcium supplements is imperative.

Previous studies report short-term increases in creatinine after treatment, which typically resolve quickly, and without long-term impact on renal function [35]. In this study, there were no significant differences in renal function between the ZA and control groups, supportive of improved GFR over time.

This study found that bone turnover markers were significantly altered by the administration of ZA. Decreased bone turnover markers may contribute to the development of complications such as bisphosphonate-induced osteonecrosis of the jaw (ONJ) [23, 36] or atypical femoral fractures [37, 38]. ZA was administered over two doses in this study. This dosing was different from past studies of fracture prevention or studies that reported on complications such as ONJ and atypical femoral fractures related to prolonged use of bisphosphonates. Extending the current study period will be beneficial since our data revealed changes in bone turnover markers toward the conclusion of the study. By following patients for more than 2 years, we may learn more about these changes, as well as the risks of bisphosphonate-related complications.

The main limitation of this study was the sample size. Nonetheless, the findings are compelling and consistent with those of previous reports [12, 18, 20]. Although this study was powered to show changes in BMD throughout various Gruen zones, at various time points postoperatively, some zones exhibited borderline significances. It is possible that the study was underpowered and a larger sample size may be needed to demonstrate significant changes in BMD following administration of ZA. Bone mineral homeostasis correlates with the calcium and vitamin D metabolism. Another limitation of the current study was our failure to measure vitamin D levels at baseline. Although all study subjects had normal BMDs, labs, and no osteoporosis, we cannot rule out the possibility of an underlying vitamin D deficiency in study subjects. A future studies should clarify the effects of vitamin D levels.

Conclusions

In conclusion, initiation of ZA treatment in the acute postoperative period preserves periprosthetic BMD in the proximal femur (zones 1 and 7). ZA may be effective prophylaxis against periprosthetic bone loss and implant migration. Future large-scale, longitudinal studies are necessary to demonstrate clinical effectiveness and investigate the risk of treatment-related complications.

Abbreviations

ALT: Alanine aminotransferase; ANOVA: Analysis of variance; AST: Aspartate aminotransferase; BMD: Bone mineral density; DXA: Dual-energy x-ray absorptiometry; GFR: Glomerular filtration rate; HHS: Hip Harris Score; MCS: Mental Component Summary; PCS: Physical Component Summary; SD: Standard deviation; SF-12: Short-Form-12; THA: Total hip arthroplasty; ZA: Zoledronic acid

Acknowledgments

We thank Ms. Yu-Shuan Lin for recording radiographic and functional data and for assisting with the statistical analyses.

Funding

This study (CZOL446HTW07T study) was sponsored by Novartis. No additional grant support was provided.

Authors' contributions

MSL and H-NS contributed substantially to the conception and design of the study. C-JW, YC, K-CH, and K-TP analyzed and interpreted the data. T-WH drafted the article and revised it critically for important intellectual content. All authors reviewed and edited the manuscript and approved the final version of the manuscript.

Competing interests

All authors declare that they have no competing interests.

Consent for publication

Consents regarding individual details, images, and videos have been obtained from all patients.

Author details

[1]Department of Orthopaedic Surgery, Chang Gung Memorial Hospital, Chiayi, Taiwan. [2]Chang Gung University, Taoyuan, Taiwan. [3]Department of Orthopaedic Surgery, Chang Gung Memorial Hospital, Linkou, Taiwan. [4]Department of Diagnostic and Interventional Radiology, Chang Gung Memorial Hospital, Linkou, Taiwan. [5]Department of Orthopaedic Surgery, Kaohsiung Chang Gung Memorial Hospital, No. 123, Dapi Rd., Niaosong District, Kaohsiung City 83301, Taiwan. [6]5 Fu-Hsin Street, Kweishan, Taoyuan, Taiwan. [7]No. 6, West Section, Chia-Pu Road, Pu-Tzi City, Chia-Yi Hsien 613, Taiwan. [8]No. 123, Dapi Rd., Niaosong District, Kaohsiung City 83301, Taiwan.

References

1. Stephen R, Burnett J. Total hip arthroplasty: techniques and results. BCMJ. 2010;52:455–64.
2. Markel DC, Hoard DB, Porretta CA. Cemented total hip arthroplasty with Boneloc bone cement. J South Orthop Assoc. 2001;10:202–8.
3. Chen G, Shukeir N, Potti A, et al. Up-regulation of Wnt-1 and beta-catenin production in patients with advanced metastatic prostate carcinoma: potential pathogenetic and prognostic implications. Cancer. 2004;101:1345–56.
4. Yamada H, Yoshihara Y, Henmi O, et al. Cementless total hip replacement: past, present, and future. J Orthop Sci. 2009;14:228–41.
5. Oh I, Harris WH. Proximal strain distribution in the loaded femur. An in vitro comparison of the distributions in the intact femur and after insertion of different hip-replacement femoral components. J Bone Joint Surg Am. 1978;60:75–85.
6. Alm JJ, Makinen TJ, Lankinen P, et al. Female patients with low systemic BMD are prone to bone loss in Gruen zone 7 after cementless total hip arthroplasty. Acta Orthop. 2009;80:531–7.
7. Iolascon G, Di Pietro G, Capaldo A, et al. Peri-prosthetic bone density as outcome of therapeutic response. Clin Cases Miner Bone Metab. 2010;7:27–31.
8. Aro HT, Alm JJ, Moritz N, et al. Low BMD affects initial stability and delays stem osseointegration in cementless total hip arthroplasty in women: a 2-year RSA study of 39 patients. Acta Orthop. 2012;83:107–14.
9. Venesmaa PK, Kröger HP, Miettinen HJ, et al. Monitoring of peri-prosthetic BMD after uncemented total hip arthroplasty with dural-energy X-ray absorptiometry – a 3-year follow-up study. J Bone Miner Res. 2001;16:1056–61.
10. Arabmotlagh M, Pilz M, Warzecha J, et al. Changes of femoral periprosthetic bone mineral density 6 years after treatment with alendronate following total hip arthroplasty. J Orthop Res. 2009;27:183–8.
11. Smolders JM, Hol A, Rijnders T, et al. Changes in bone mineral density in the proximal femur after hip resurfacing and uncemented total hip replacement: A prospective randomised controlled study. J Bone Joint Surg (Br). 2010;92:1509–14.
12. Ott SM. What is the optimal duration of bisphosphonate therapy? Cleve Clin J Med. 2011;78:619–30.
13. Bhandari M, Bajammal S, Guyatt GH, et al. Effect of bisphosphonates on periprosthetic bone mineral density after total joint arthroplasty. A meta-analysis. J Bone Joint Surg Am. 2005;87:293–301.
14. Lin T, Yan SG, Cai XZ, et al. Bisphosphonates for peri-prosthetic bone loss after joint arthroplasty: a meta-analysis of 14 randomized controlled trials. Osteoporos Int. 2012;23:1823–34.
15. Knusten AR, Ebramzadeh E, Longjohn DB, et al. Systematic analysis of bisphosphonate intervention on periprosthetic BMD as a function of stem design. J Arthroplasty. 2014;29:1292–7.
16. Yoshimura M, Kohno N, Yamada K, et al. (89)Sr imaging with bremsstrahlung in patients with metastatic breast cancer. Clin Nucl Med. 2012;37:1035–40.
17. Rakel A, Boucher A, Ste-Marie LG. Role of zoledronic acid in the prevention and treatment of osteoporosis. Clin Interv Aging. 2011;6:89–99.
18. Simm PJ, Johannesen J, Briody J, et al. Zoledronic acid improves bone mineral density, reduces bone turnover and improves skeletal architecture over 2 years of treatment in children with secondary osteoporosis. Bone. 2011;49:939–43.
19. Orwoll ES, Miller PD, Adachi JD, et al. Efficacy and safety of a once-yearly i.v. Infusion of zoledronic acid 5 mg versus a once-weekly 70-mg oral alendronate in the treatment of male osteoporosis: a randomized, multi-center, double-blind, active-controlled study. J Bone Miner Res. 2010;25:2239–50.
20. Black DM, Delmas PD, Eastell R, et al. HORIZON Pivotal Fracture Trial, Once-yearly zoledronic acid for treatment of post-menopausal osteoporosis. N Engl J Med. 2007;356:1809–22.
21. Jansen JP, Bergman GJ, Huels J, et al. The efficacy of bisphosphonates in the prevention of vertebral, hip, and non-vertebral-nonhip fractures in osteoporosis: a network meta-analysis. Semin Arthritis Rheum. 2011;40:275–84. e1-2.
22. Friedl G, Radl R, Stihsen C, et al. The effect of a single infusion of zoledronic acid on early implant migration in total hip arthroplasty. A randomized, double-blind, controlled trial. J Bone Joint Surg Am. 2009;91:274–81.

23. Scott DF, Woltz JN, Smith RR. Effect of Zoledronic acid on reducing femoral bone mineral density loss following total hip arthroplasty: preliminary results of a prospective randomized trial. J Arthroplasty. 2013;28:671–5.
24. Lambrinoudaki I, Vlachou S, Galapi F, et al. Once-yearly zoledronic acid in the prevention of osteoporotic bone fractures in post-menopausal women. Clin Interv Aging. 2008;3:445–51.
25. Lee MS. Minimally invasive total hip arthroplasty. Formosan J Musculoskeletal Dis. 2011;2:41–4.
26. Chen D, Hu C, Chang Y, et al. Comparison of clinical outcome in primary total hip arthroplasty by conventional antero-lateral trans-gluteal or 2-incision approach. J Arthroplasty. 2009;24:528–32.
27. Engh CA, Massin P, Suthers KE. Roentgenographic assessment of the biologic fixation of porous-surfaced femoral components. Clin Orthop Relat Res. 1990;257:107–28.
28. Johnston RC, Fitzgerald Jr RH, Harris WH, et al. Clinical and radiographic evaluation of total hip replacement. A standard system of terminology for reporting results. J Bone Joint Surg Am. 1990;72:161–8.
29. Bodén H, Adolphson P. No adverse effects of early weight bearing after uncemented total hip arthroplasty: a randomized study of 20 patients. Acta Orthop Scand. 2004;75:21–9.
30. Kamiya N, Suzuki H, Endo T, et al. Clinical usefulness of bone markers in prostate cancer with bone metastasis. Int J Urol. 2012;19:968–79.
31. Savarino L, Granchi D, Cenni E, et al. Systemic cross-linked N-terminal telopeptide and procollagen I C-terminal extension peptide as markers of bone turnover after total hip arthroplasty. J Bone Joint Surg (Br). 2005;87:571–6.
32. Glassman AH, Bobyn JD, Tanzer M. New femoral designs: do they influence stress shielding? Clin Orthop Relat Res. 2006;453:64–74.
33. Eriksen EF, Lyles KW, Colon-Emeric CS, et al. Anti-fracture efficacy and reduction of mortality in relation to timing of the first dose of zoledronic acid after hip fracture. J Bone Miner Res. 2009;24:1308–13.
34. Reid IR, Black DM, Eastell R, et al. HORIZON Pivotal Fracture Trial and HORIZON Recurrent Fracture Trial Steering Committees, Reduction in the risk of clinical fractures after a single dose of zoledronic Acid 5 milligrams. J Clin Endocrinol Metab. 2013;98:557–63.
35. Black DM, Reid IR, Boonen S, et al. The effect of 3 versus 6 years of zoledronic acid treatment of osteoporosis: a randomized extension to the HORIZON-Pivotal Fracture Trial (PFT). J Bone Miner Res. 2012;27:243–54.
36. Mehrotra B, Ruggiero S. Bisphosphonate complications including osteonecrosis of the Jaw. Hematol Am Soc Hematol Educ Program. 2006;515:356–60.
37. Shane E, Burr D, Abrahamsen B, et al. Atypical subtrochanteric and diaphyseal femoral fractures: second report of a task force of the American Society for Bone and Mineral Research. J Bone Miner Res. 2014;29:1–23.
38. Unnanuntana A, Saleh A, Mensah KA, et al. Atypical femoral fractures: what do we know about them? AAOS Exhibit Selection. J Bone Joint Surg Am. 2013;95:1–13. e8.

Finite Element Analysis of porously punched prosthetic short stem virtually designed for simulative uncemented hip arthroplasty

Matthew Jian-Qiao Peng[1], Hai-Yan Chen[1], Yong Hu[2], XiangYang Ju[3] and Bo Bai[1*]

Abstract

Background: There is no universal hip implant suitably fills all femoral types, whether prostheses of porous short-stem suitable for Hip Arthroplasty is to be measured scientifically.

Methods: Ten specimens of femurs scanned by CT were input onto Mimics to rebuild 3D models; their *stl format dataset were imported into Geomagic-Studio for simulative osteotomy; the generated *.igs dataset were interacted by UG to fit solid models; the prosthesis were obtained by the same way from patients, and bored by punching bears designed by Pro-E virtually; cements between femora and prosthesis were extracted by deleting prosthesis; in HyperMesh, all compartments were assembled onto four artificial joint style as: (a) cemented long-stem prosthesis; (b) porous long-stem prosthesis; (c) cemented short-stem prosthesis; (d) porous short-stem prosthesis. Then, these numerical models of Finite Element Analysis were exported to AnSys for numerical solution.

Results: Observed whatever from femur or prosthesis or combinational femora-prostheses, "Kruskal-Wallis" value $p > 0.05$ demonstrates that displacement of (d) ≈ (a) ≈ (b) ≈ (c) shows nothing different significantly by comparison with 600 N load. If stresses are tested upon prosthesis, (d) ≈ (a) ≈ (b) ≈ (c) is also displayed; if upon femora, (d) ≈ (a) ≈ (b) < (c) is suggested; if upon integral joint, (d) ≈ (a) < (b) < (c) is presented.

Conclusions: Mechanically, these four sorts of artificial joint replacement are stabilized in quantity. Cemented short-stem prostheses present the biggest stress, while porous short-stem & cemented long-stem designs are equivalently better than porous long-stem prostheses and alternatives for femoral-head replacement. The preferred design of those two depends on clinical conditions. The cemented long-stem is favorable for inactive elders with osteoporosis, and porously punched cementless short-stem design is suitable for patients with osteoporosis, while the porously punched cementless short-stem is favorable for those with a cement allergy. Clinically, the strength of this study is to enable preoperative strategy to provide acute correction and decrease procedure time.

Keywords: Uncemented short stem, Porously punched prosthesis, Artificial joint replacement, Contact stress, Finite Element Analysis

* Correspondence: 18922346634@163.com
[1]Guangdong Orthopedics Implantation key Lab, Orthopedics Department of 1st Affiliated Hospital, Guangzhou Medical University, 151 YanJiangXi Rd, Guangzhou 510120, China
Full list of author information is available at the end of the article

Background

A meticulous preoperative strategy is of paramount importance before performing a complex operation that could employ multiple available reconstructive techniques. Additionally, proper modular implants of artificial prostheses in terms of type and length must be selected prior to hip surgery. There are various procedures for treating femoral neck fractures. For fresh fracture without dislocation, internal fixation is preferable. For elderly patients with osteoarthritis or rheumatoid arthritis, Hip Arthroplasty (HA) is a prevalent approach to achieve function restoration of degenerative joint diseases in the twentieth century. However, there is no universal hip implant to suitably treat all femoral types, and appropriate design is demanded that could prevent complications from the implant's geometric mismatch. The previous literature indicates that joint fracture is quite likely to occur if there are high stresses in the fixation areas [1, 2], and conventional stems have showed disadvantages, such as proximal stress shielding, loss of bone stock, and a risk of fracture [3]. Dennis et al. suggests that cement carries a risk of fatigue failure than bone since more cracks were formed in cement than in bone in this study [4]. Fawzi et al. posited that bone cement material, stem material and shape significantly affect the Total Hip Joint performance, as well as that the stem length has significant effects on resultant Von Mises stresses for bone, stem and cement [5]. Short-stem prostheses were reported primarily to preserve femoral bone stock, reduce the amount of osteotomy during femoral preparation and facilitate future revision surgery possibly [6], but there has been doubt that they can maintain stability, osseointegration and survival of the femoral stem [5]. Walker et al. suggests that the femoral moment of the compressive strain of an uncemented prosthesis is only 30% of that for cemented prostheses [7]. Whiteside et al. declared that cementless short-stem prostheses preserve femoral neck with greater torsional stability while reducing distal migration of the stem [8]. Because uncemented straight stems have demonstrated excellent long-term results into the third decade, we hypothesize that the stem type or size may affect the value and distribution of mechanical stress, but newly designed short-stem designs need to be critically evaluated. The issues of "Long or short stem?" & "Cementlss or cement stem?" will therefore be investigated in this study. To realize this aim, first of all, a three-dimensional (3D) femoral model for pre-operative planning is achieved by Reverse Engineering Software that mimicked operative protocol virtually; then, four sorts of simulative stems (Cemented stem of long and short without pore, Cementless stem of long and short with pore) were designed and compared by Finite Element (FE) method mechanically. Finally, clinical contention concerning the bio-mechanism is discussed in the conclusion.

Methods

Experimental material

The facilities needed are listed as: 10 sets of specimens (female patients aged 20 ~ 40 yrs) of femora with prostheses from our hospital (in accordance with standards of Guangzhou Medical University Committee (#2014A0 20215035) and with the 1964 Helsinki declaration) scanned by Computed Tomography (CT, Toshiba, Japan), medical Image Processor Mimics (Materialise, Leuvan, Belgium), Reverse Engineering software Geomagic-Studio-12 (3D Systems, Rock Hill, USA), interactive Computer Aided Design (CAD) / Computer Aided Manufacturing (CAM) package UG-8.0 (Siemens, Germany), 3D drawing processor ProE/Engineer-5 (Parametric Tech Corp, USA), and Finite Element Analysis (FEA) package AnSys-14 (ANSYS, Inc. Pennsylvania, USA), pre-FEA processor Hypermesh-13 (Altair Engineering, USA), and Universal Testing Machine (UTM, Zwick Roell, Germany).

Experimental procedure

Reconstruction of the femoral model

Ten femora scanned by CT in Dicom format were exported to Mimics. The default bony gray value range of 226 ~ 2311 was set to the threshold so that the femur was separated from the proximal femur extracted by "Region Growing". The "Edit mask" function on the "Mask" module was then executed to erasure / protract / calculate the 3D model [9], and a proximal femur model of the *.stl format was developed for accurate measurement.

Distal femur developed

The aforementioned 3D model was imported to Reverse Engineering software Geomagic Studio and then faired-up by the function of "Grid doctor". The osteotomy along the base line of femoral neck was processed by "Plane section" module so that 1.5 cm medial femoral cortex is remained (Fig. 1a), which was performed through a series of procedures called "Probe curvature" (Fig. 1b) → "Degraded contour" (Fig. 1c) → "Construct surface patches" (Fig. 1d) → "Construct grid" (Fig. 1e) → "Fitting surface" (Fig. 1f) etc. A curve contour graph, called Non-uniform rational Basis spline (NURBS) cyrtography, was then fitted (Fig. 1).

Solid model fit

The above acquired cyrtograph models of the femoral shaft were exported to commercially available "Interactive CAD/CAM software", UG-8.0, for further refinement. An entity model of solid was conversed by its functions of "Insert → Combine → Fit", and clicking the "Checking Geometric Solid" module with the Surface Sweeping Method to check model until complete.

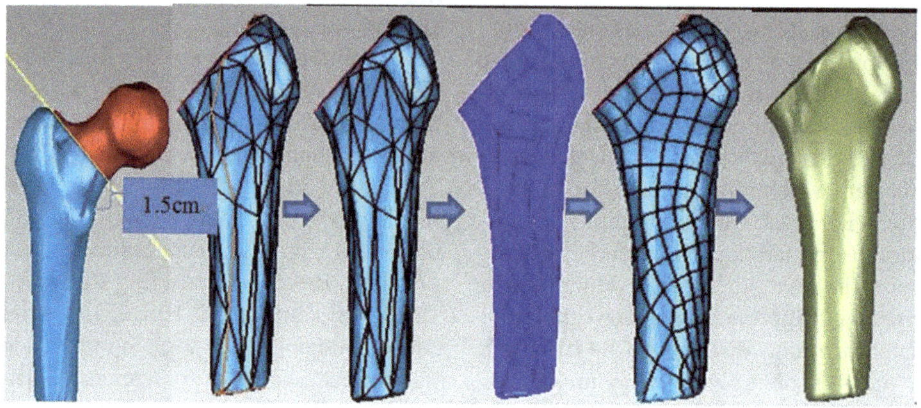

Fig. 1 NURBS kyrtograph fitted for femoral shafts. **a** Simulative osteotomy. **b** Curvature detected. **c** Outline downgraded. **d** Patch constructed. **e** Grating constructed. **f** Kyrtograph fitting

Femoral prostheses preparation

(1) A "Long-stem femoral prosthesis" of 135 mm was obtained (Fig. 2b) when patients with femoral head replacement underwent CT and were similarly processed as the aforementioned "***Distal femur developed***" session.

(2) A "Long-stem femoral porous prosthesis": a punching-bear with 27 cylinders of 4 mm diameter was created by Pro-E (Fig. 2a), and was then imported onto Hypermesh together with the (1) "Long-stem femoral prosthesis" so that this long-stem is punched to be "porous prosthesis" (Fig. 2c) through "Boolean calculation".

(3) A "Short-stem femoral prosthesis" of 100 mm (Fig. 2d) was developed after simulatively osteotomized by 35 mm from the (1) "Long-stem femoral prosthesis".

(4) A "Short-stem femoral porous prosthesis" with 23 cylinders that had diameters of 4 mm (Fig. 2e) was acquired after (3) "Short-stem femoral prosthesis" was punched with a "Boolean calculation", similarly to procedure of item (2).

Osseous cement preparation

The total hip prostheses were amplified by 2 pixels during the Mimics execution and then extracted by *.stl format. Simulative osteotomy occurred on Geomagic-studio along the break-angle of prosthesis by same direction. The remaining prosthetic stem, which was amplified by 2 voxels, was imported onto UG to fit 3D-solid model. The models were then exported to Hypermesh to remove the original prosthetic stem from the amplified prosthetic stem by Boolean calculation. The virtual model of the bony cement layer with 3 mm-thickness [10] and a cavity are shown in Fig. 2f & 2g.

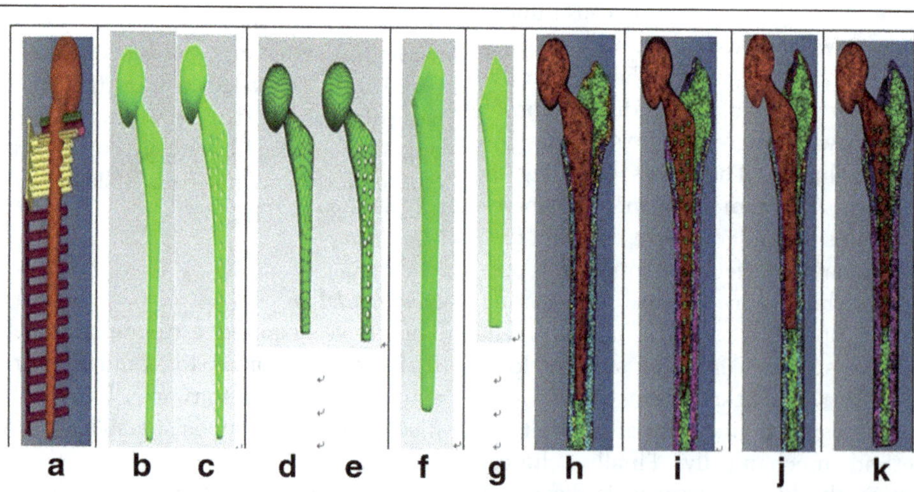

Fig. 2 Prosthesis model & Punching-bear model. Cemented model & Sectional views of Grid model

Assemblies of the replacement model
The above models of the femora, prostheses and cement were synthetized in Hypermesh to assemble the following four replacement types: (a) long-stem cemented prosthesis (Fig. 2h), (b) long-stem porous prosthesis (Fig. 2i), (c) short-stem cemented prosthesis (Fig. 2j), and (d) short-stem porous prosthesis (Fig. 2k).

Joint material assignment
A distal femur can be obtained after removing the space occupied by the prosthetic cemented stem or porous stem by Boolean calculation. The femora and other compartments were volume-meshed with cell-attribute assignment. All models of femora, prostheses and cement were exported back into Mimics for materials assignment. Then, the elastic modulus was automatically calculated. Based on CT gray-scale for bone, the elastic modulus was divided into five uniform scale so that five types of bony materials were assigned (with the minimum for inner and maximum for outer) according to a known formula [such as: Density p = 1017 × Grayvaluscale - 13.4 (g/cm^3), Modulus = 5925 × Density-388.8 (MPa)]. Poisson's ratio was assumed to be 0.3. The properties of the remaining materials are based on prior studies [11, 12]. In this way, the geometrical 3D FE models of classic stems were obtained.

Loads configuration & boundary constraint
The above grid models are to be imported back to Hypermesh so that a compressive preload of 600 N was applied vertically and applied on the bone structures symmetrically. The degree of freedom on a node basis of x-y-z direction of Cartesian coordinate was constrained to 0, and translational displacements at the distal nodes of the femur were inhibited (Fig. 3a, 3b & 3c) [13, 14].

Model validation test
There are two ways to validate FE Models, which include the following: (1), Numerous model testing — To compare the present method with previous studies of

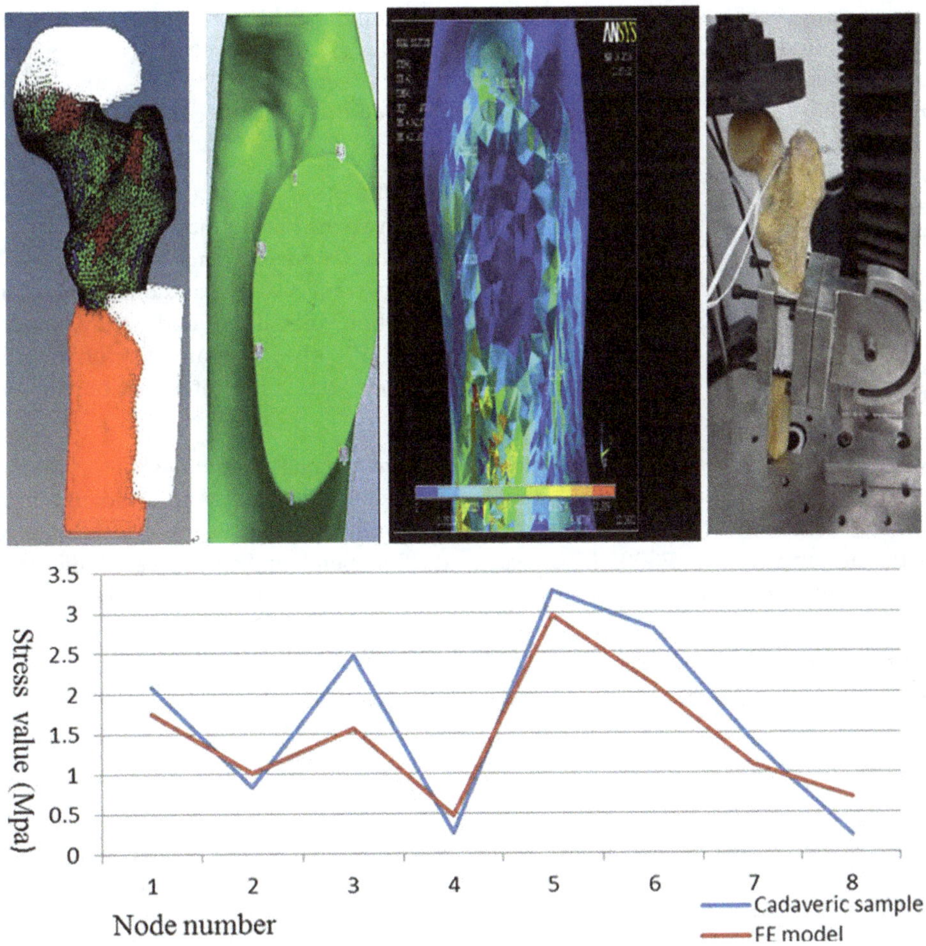

Fig. 3 Verification of model validity. **a** Constrain. **b** Node plane. **c** Model validity. **d** Cadaveric validity. **e** Line chart for stress comparison between FE model and cadaveric femur

Table 1 Stress values for each 8-node of 12 FE samples

Position # Sample #	1	2	3	4	5	6	7	8
1	0.95962	1.08178	0.722216	0.222289	2.21429	1.231093	0.725866	0.600427
2	2.365501	0.522318	2.214457	0.290111	4.60191	2.907203	1.0395	0.713425
3	1.89497	1.204012	1.012684	0.467758	2.768523	2.102543	1.328077	0.819144
4	0.620409	0.399854	1.045387	0.371484	2.942854	2.261493	0.730747	0.462416
5	3.186124	1.094655	2.260299	0.609772	2.836237	2.868277	1.982035	0.202032
6	1.23152	2.22689	2.58363	0.754154	4.946323	2.627293	1.195486	0.950645
7	1.54106	1.06443	1.885397	0.354257	2.39623	1.369875	0.971287	0.798693
8	1.703297	0.650252	1.278543	0.205116	1.87754	1.337363	1.518337	1.046773
9	2.173445	1.507025	1.764093	0.862081	3.858323	3.472113	1.147653	0.367901
10	2.38251	0.916799	1.276729	0.970677	3.069833	2.331347	0.668171	0.883533
11	1.507317	0.710776	1.338166	0.412746	2.74588	1.366152	0.683243	0.581944
12	1.417896	0.720122	1.34875	0.19126	1.19263	1.19263	1.249671	0.896941
Average (MPa)	1.748639	1.008243	1.560863	0.475975	2.954214	2.088949	1.103339	0.693656

similar stress / displacement, and (2), Cadaveric model testing — To develop a cadaveric model that resembles FEM in vitro. Its validity will be verified by comparing the similarity of outcomes for each experiment based on equal status.

It is assumed that FE model of the femoral neck is resected by a plane horizontally, and the circumference is intercrossed by four lines at 45° angles, forming 8 nodes (8 × 45° = 360°). When 600 N is vertically pressed on each of the corresponding 8 nodes of 12 samples [15] (these 12 samples are for model validation which are different from those 10 sets of spacemen for virtual surgery), the average values of stresses were acquired, as presented in Table 1. On the other hand, strain-foils were attached at relative positions of an intact cadaveric femur corresponding to FE model and mounted to UTM [12] (Fig. 3d). The load-strain curve was observed by recording the strain value when the maximal pressure of 600 N was reached. Force values were calculated to form Table 2 with these formulas: Actual-force = 10 × Measured-force - 6 (Mpa), Stress = Actual-force × Elastic-modulus (here, 7300 Mpa was chosen according to a reference [16]).

Finite element solution

This generated FE model was exported onto AnSys package for computation and analysis, and the peak and distribution yield were measured. The observation index includes (1) Von Mises stress / displacement contours of femur / cement / prosthesis, and (2) Stress / displacement contours of the general model.

Results

Observations during model testing

Numerous model validations

The current testing outcome was consistent with the validation technique and study conducted by Zhang et al. [17], the comparability of the current result and previous results indicates that our FE model is valid.

Cadaveric model validations

Tables 1 and 2 can be consolidated into Table 3 and are interpreted in Fig. 3e. A significance of $p > 0.05$ from the Independent Sample Test indicates that in vitro cadaveric testing and the FE models are not significantly

Table 2 Stress values for each 8-node of cadaveric femur

Node #	Strain #1	Strain #2	Strain #3	Strain average	Absolute value	Stress (MPa)
1	250	290	315	285	285	2.0805
2	−110	−120		−115	115	0.8395
3	−325	−350		−337.5	337.5	2.46375
4	−35	−35	−35	−35	35	0.2555
5	425	455	460	446.6667	446.7	3.26091
6	380	385		382.5	382.5	2.79225
7	190	185		187.5	187.5	1.36875
8	−30	−30	−30	−30	30	0.219

Table 3 Stress comparison on correspond positions of FE model to cadaveric femur

Node # Sample #	1	2	3	4	5	6	7	8
FE model	1.7486	1.0082	1.5609	0.4760	2.9542	2.0889	1.1033	0.6937
Cadaver	2.0805	0.8395	2.4638	0.2555	3.2609	2.7923	1.3688	0.2190

different (they are agreeable to each other), which validates our approach for further simulation and analysis.

Observation of stress distribution

Stress of prostheses

As depicted by Fig. 4, generally, the contact stresses of all femoral-head prostheses are concentrated around prosthetic stems equably. For model (a), the pressure crest value is across the edge of femoral-head intersecting the prosthetic stem. For style (b), the summit value is along the middle of prosthetic stem. For style (c), the stress peak appears at the intersection of prosthetic terminus and bony cement. For style (d), the stress apex is located at prosthetic head crossing neck as well as the middle stem. The prostheses are easier to damage from these locations [18].

As depicted by Table 4, the mean stress value of each model is as follows: (a) = 46.7682, (b) = 57.5332, (c) = 57.2927, and (d) = 48.8891 (MPa). The variance homogeneity test and analysis demonstrates that these

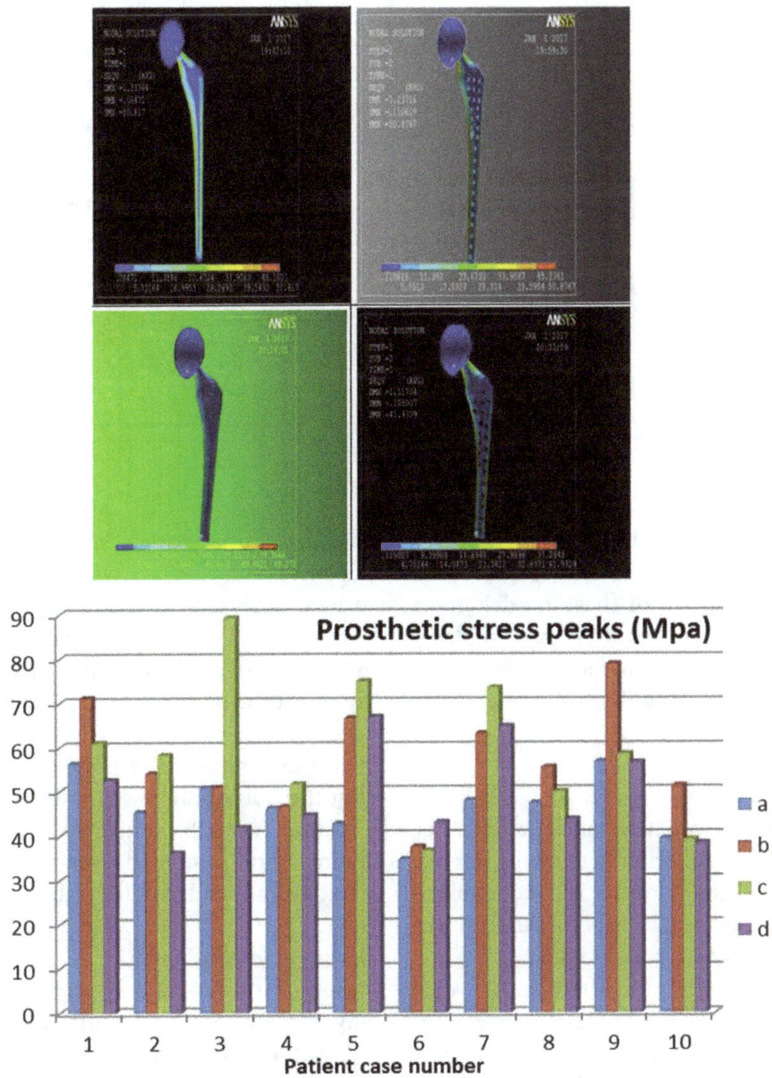

Fig. 4 Stress distribution of femoral prostheses & Histogram of femoral prosthetic stresses

Table 4 Statistics of prosthetic stresses peak (variance homogeneity test & analysis)

ANOVA

	Sum of Squares	df	Mean Square	F	Sig.
Between Groups	1158.257	3	386.086	2.643	.064
Within Groups	5259.760	36	146.104		
Total	6418.017	39			

Test of Homogeneity of Variances force

Levene Statistic	df1	df2	Sig.
1.929	3	36	.142

	N	Mean
a	10	46.7682
b	10	57.5332
c	10	59.2927
d	10	48.8891
Total	40	53.1208

	(I) model	(J)model	Mean Difference (I-J)	Std. Error	Sig.	95% Confidence Interval Lower Bound	95% Confidence Interval Upper Bound
LSD	a	b	-10.76509	5.40563	.054	-21.7282	.1980
		c	-12.52459(*)	5.40563	.026	-23.4877	-1.5615
		d	-2.12098	5.40563	.697	-13.0841	.8422
	b	a	10.76509	5.40563	.054	-.1980	21.7282
		c	-1.75950	5.40563	.747	-12.7226	9.2036
		d	8.64411	5.40563	.119	-2.3190	19.6072
	c	a	12.52459(*)	5.40563	.026	1.5615	23.4877
		b	1.75950	5.40563	.747	-9.2036	12.7226
		d	10.40361	5.40563	.062	-.5595	21.3667
	d	a	2.12098	5.40563	.697	-8.8422	13.0841
		b	-8.64411	5.40563	.119	-19.6072	2.3190
		c	-10.40361	5.40563	.062	-21.3667	.5595
	a	b	-10.76509	5.40563	.054	-21.7282	.1980

four types are indifferent significantly ($p = 0.064 > 0.05$) according to SPSS-13, which could be simplified as (a) ≈ (b) ≈ (c) ≈ (d). However, all of these models meet the mechanical prerequisite of femoral-head replacement because the maximum stress of each model is less than the Yield Strength of the titanium alloy, which is 600 ~ 900 MPa.

Stress on femora

By reviewing the Von Mises variation of FEA data, the reaction stresses of femora are distributing equally inferior to femoral trochanter and superior to the constrained position. Additionally, stress peaks disperse around the interface of the prostheses terminus and femur.

When observed within Table 5, the stress mean-value of each model is as follows: (a) = 10.6316, (b) = 9.5798, (c) = 17.4404, and (d) = 9.5140 (MPa), which are less than the Yield Strength of femur (104 ~ 120 MPa) according to previously published studies [19]. Based on the factor of variance, all were $p < 0.001 < 0.05$, which suggests the four styles were significantly different. When analyzed by pairwise comparison between the other three models to determine the biggest stress (c), $p < 0.05$ indicated that the cemented short-stem (c) was the most unsuitable type for hip joint implantation [shortened by (d) < (b) < (a) < (c)]. When further analyzed by pairwise comparison among (a) (b) & (d), $p > 0.05$ implies that the porous short-stem design (d) was not significantly different from the long-stem (b), and (d) was also indifferent from cemented long-stem (a) significantly, which can be simplified as d (d) ≈ (b) ≈ (a) < (c).

Stress on integral joints

Based on the Von Mises outcome, the contact stresses of any type of integral joint distributed similarly as the prostheses, the stresses peaked on the prostheses and decreased from the maximum value at the femoral fixation point to the minimum values at the proximal end. By

Table 5 Statistics of femoral stresses peak (pairwise comparison among 4 models)

Test of Homogeneity of Variances force

Levene Statistic	df1	df2	Sig.
.520	3	36	.672

ANOVA

	Sum of Squares	df	Mean Square	F	Sig.
Between Groups	433.343	3	144.448	8.698	.000
Within Groups	597.819	36	16.606		
Total	1031.162	39			

	(I) model	(J)model	Mean Difference (I-J)	Std. Error	Sig.	95% Confidence Interval Lower Bound	95% Confidence Interval Upper Bound
LSD	a	b	1.05184	1.82242	.567	-2.6442	4.7479
		c	-6.80879(*)	1.82242	.001	-10.5048	-3.1128
		d	1.11765	1.82242	.544	-2.5784	4.8137
	b	a	-1.05184	1.82242	.567	-4.7479	2.6442
		c	-7.86063(*)	1.82242	.000	-11.5567	-4.1646
		d	.06582	1.82242	.971	-3.6302	3.7619
	c	a	6.80879(*)	1.82242	.001	3.1128	10.5048
		b	7.86063(*)	1.82242	.000	4.1646	11.5567
		d	7.92644(*)	1.82242	.000	4.2304	11.6225
	d	a	-1.11765	1.82242	.544	-4.8137	2.5784
		b	-.06582	1.82242	.971	-3.7619	3.6302
		c	-7.92644(*)	1.82242	.000	-11.6225	-4.2304

reviewing Table 6, the stress mean-value of each model is as follows: (a) = 47.4895, (b) = 58.5053, (c) = 60.4703, and (d) = 45.8822 (MPa). These values were analyzed by a factor of variance: all $p = 0.031 < 0.05$, suggesting a significant discrepancy [simply described by (d) < (a) < (b) < (c)]. When analyzed by pairwise comparison, $p < 0.05$ indicates they are significantly different, but $p > 0.05$ suggests the difference between (a) v.s. (d) was not significant statistically, which is (d) ≈ (a) < (b) < (c). Mechanically, the (a) cemented long-stem and (d) porous short-stem are the least stressed.

Observation of displacement distribution

Displacement of femora

Femur displacement implies its magnitude of stability relative to femoral joint. Through observation of Fig. 5, we found that peak displacement of all models was concentrated near the greater-trochanter adjacent region, which decreases distally in concentric circles. The direction of migration was vertical downward. The displacement mean-value of each model is as follows: (a) = 0.8484, (b) = 0.8269, (c) = 0.8179, and (d) = 0.7658 (mm); a significance of $p > 0.05$ when analyzed by pairwise comparison suggests the difference is not significant.

Displacement of integral joint

The displacement of integral joint implies its magnitude of fastness relative to the entire femoral joint. By observation of finite element data, we found that the direction of displacement was vertically downwards, the all peak displacements were concentrated on the head of prostheses and decrease distally in concentric circles. The displacement mean-value of each model was as follows: (a) = 1.0257, (b) = 0.9984, (c) = 0.9915, and (d) = 0.9849 (mm), a significance of $p > 0.05$ when analyzed by pairwise comparison suggested the risk of coxa adducta among all joint types was significantly indifferent.

Displacement of prostheses

The distribution of prosthetic displacement behaves similarly to that of the integral joint.

Table 6 Statistics of integral joint stresses peak (pairwise comparison among 4 models)

Test of Homogeneity of Variances

force

Levene Statistic	df1	df2	Sig.
2.172	3	36	.108

ANOVA

	Sum of Squares	df	Mean Square	F	Sig.
Between Groups	1671.117	3	557.039	3.305	.031
Within Groups	6068.176	36	168.560		
Total	7739.293	39			

Multiple Comparisons

Dependent Variable: force

	(I) model	(J)model	Mean Difference (I-J)	Std. Error	Sig.	95% Confidence Interval	
						Lower Bound	Upper Bound
LSD	a	b	-11.01579	5.80621	.066	-22.7913	.7598
		c	-12.98078(*)	5.80621	.032	-24.7563	-1.2052
		d	1.60729	5.80621	.783	-10.1683	13.3828
	b	a	11.01579	5.80621	.066	-.7598	22.7913
		c	-1.96499	5.80621	.737	-13.7405	9.8106
		d	12.62308(*)	5.80621	.036	.8475	24.3986
	c	a	12.98078(*)	5.80621	.032	1.2052	24.7563
		b	1.96499	5.80621	.737	-9.8106	13.7405
		d	14.58807(*)	5.80621	.017	2.8125	26.3636
	d	a	-1.60729	5.80621	.783	-13.3828	10.1683
		b	-12.62308(*)	5.80621	.036	-24.3986	-.8475
		c	-14.58807(*)	5.80621	.017	-26.3636	-2.8125

Discussion

Artificial short stems for uncemented total HA have been alternatively practiced to conventional stem designs. However, there is little biomechanical examination for effects of stem length and stem character on surgical complications [20]. To isolate clinical variables, the theoretic test performed by FEA is essential to Mimic ultimate prosthetic geometry prior to actual fabrication because it is rectified to fail practically if a stem fails at this stage. Computational FEM has been extensively employed in predicting optimized implants prescribed by surgeons [21]. The strength of FEA carried out by computer aided simulation enables preoperative strategy and decreases procedure time. This experiment of "outside bone and outside body" is also harmless for humans or animals. Our models were not only consistent with predecessors, and they were also similar to cadaveric data. These punched prostheses were designed virtually with mechanic compatibility and bio-compatibility for clinical application. These structures may induce bony ingrowth at the porous interface, which is beneficial to bioactivity. Additionally, all the four femoral stems were anatomically tailored to individualize the femoral structure towards stress and displacement.

Displacement is an indicator for determining the stability of newly designed stems. Several factors such as implant shape, stem size, bone-implant gap are accounted for micromotion [22]. Regarding cemented stems, fastness between bone and cement relies on penetration of the cement upon cortex. The mechanical interlocking between these two constituents is correlated with bony stress surrounding the cement. A Load-transfer mechanism takes place at this interface, and cementing mechanization is driven by friction rather

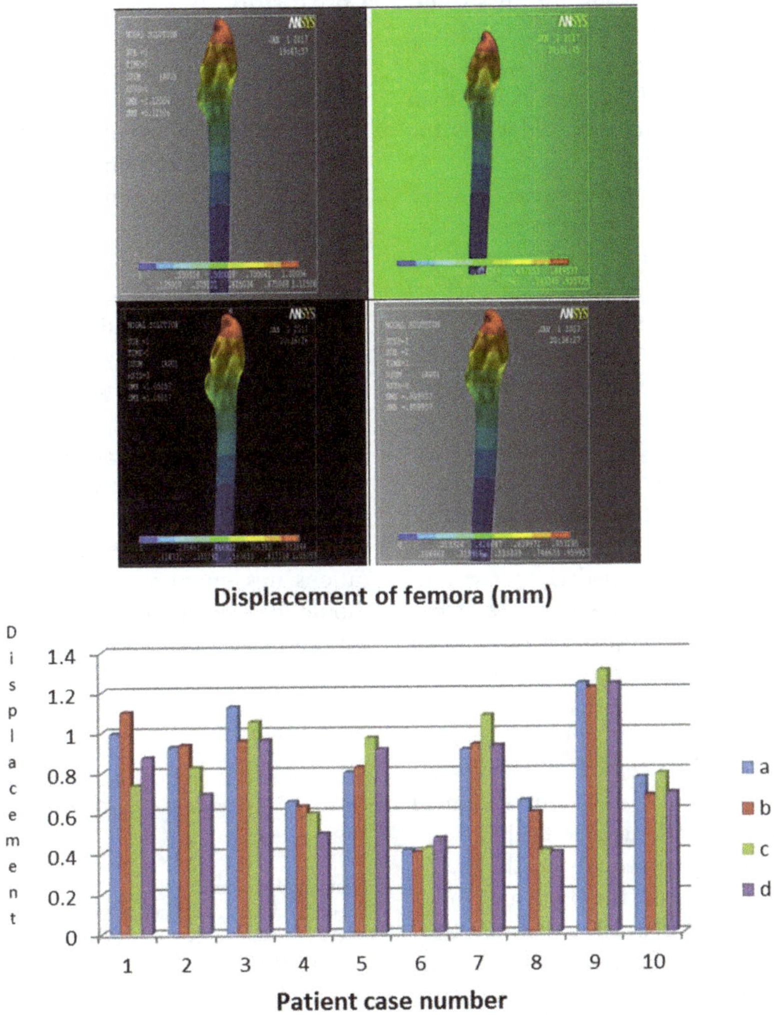

Fig. 5 Von Mises of displacement for femurs & Femoral displacement Histogram

than adhesive properties [23]. Cemented prostheses (a) / (c) achieve primary stability mechanically through locks between cement surrounding the bone and implant, which inhibits distal migration by osseointegration. Cementless prostheses (b) / (d) induce bony ingrowth onto the implant surface, which is biologically referred to as secondary stability. Previous studies indicate that the amount of ongrowth is inversely proportional to the amount of micromotion [24]. With respect to porous stems, Manley et al. reported that uncemented porous prostheses allow for bone ingrowth to achieve rigid fixations, but the shortcoming of osteolysis influences their long-term stability [25]. These results conflict with Ellison's view that the "porous stem encourages stable fixation and securely seals joint space by preventing migration" [26]. At this time, we numerically demonstrated the degree of stabilization using the analytical FE approach. When double tested statistically by SPSS, $p > 0.05$ for displacements of (a) / (b) / (c) / (d) implied that these four sorts of stems attain fastened equally after installation.

Pre-stress to bones can be created in femoral canal by internal fixation, which is probably susceptible to failure based on the stresses distribution onto the modular junctions of the implants. Suppose the joint with implant is loaded in equivalency. In terms of contact stresses upon femoral-head prostheses, the statistical dataset [(d) ≈ (a) ≈ (b) ≈ (c) in simplification] demonstrates these four types behave similarly in quantitation; In terms of the stresses upon femurs, the statistical data in order of (d) ≈ (a) ≈ (b) < (c) demonstrates that type (c), the "Cemented short-stem", performs the worst; In terms of the stresses on the whole joints, the statistical data supporting (d) ≈ (a) < (b) < (c) demonstrates that type (b), "Porous long-stem", is also not a good option. In sequence, the least stress (d) ≈ (a) supports that type (a) "Cemented long-stem" and (d) "Porous short-stem" distribute optimal loads and can be used in practice. There are several possible mechanical reasons for these outcomes: (1), If designed with cemented, when considering the stem, because quota-stress is shared by wider area when length is extended, stress on long-stem is less than short-stem. When considering the cement, which is the weakest material and has a higher risk of fatigue failure at the cement-bone interface, maximum stress on the cement increases when the length increases, a longer distance between the loading-point and fixation-point induces larger bending-stress at the distal end. (2), If designed with uncemented, long-stem appears to be superior to short-stem by the reasoning in (1), but this statement is actually controversial as follows: short-stems enable sufficient space for complete osseous ingrowth, preserving greater stability, this design also confers higher resistance from torsional forces and has a lower risk of peri-prosthetic fracture than long-stems. With respect to the survival rate (99 ~ 100% for 10 years) reported by McLaughlin et al. [23, 27], short stem designs are suggested as alternative to longer stem designs. (3), If designed with "punched", porous stems provide meaningful structural support. The porous nature enables bony ingrowth, and the new bones can handle load and enlarge surface area [28]. As a result, stress on cementless-stem with pore is sequentially less than cemented-stem without porous coating [4, 29]. Therefore, short-stemmed punched-prostheses are generally thought to facilitate surgery compared to long-stemmed cemented-prostheses.

However, "the least" doesn't mean "the best" and "minimal" isn't equal to "optimal", because minimal stress doesn't guarantee the best choice for a clinical trial. The prostheses inserted into the femoral cavity might change the normal stresses distributions. Stress can be spread to the distal femur via intramedullary prosthesis despite its support by the proximal femur, which leads to stress-shielding, affecting the osseous integrity and resistance [30]. Longer stems are believed to give higher stresses at the femur and then be capable of reducing stress shielding problems, whereas shorter stems decrease the load-transfer to the cortical bone and encourages stress shielding and bone resorption, which results in failure of the prosthesis sometimes [31]. Chen WP et al. revealed that less stress shielding occurs in those femurs with fully cemented fixation [32]. For an uncemented short stem, even if Maier reported it is curved stems but not straight stems that cause cortical hypertrophy, there is no significant effect on the clinical outcome at early follow-up [33]. Regarding porous prostheses, Ellison et al. provides evidence that these prostheses do not cause stress shielding in 14-year follow-up [26]. As another result, the module that achieves the minimum stress-shielding is the cementless prosthesis, due to poor results of cemented components after revision surgery, short-stem of porously punched uncemented prosthesis has become more popular.

Conclusion

In summary, this study proposes long v.s. short stems of cementless v.s. cement in 3D models providing statistical analysis in comparison with conventional methods. The data support the hypothesis that stresses and distributions of prosthetic stems are various from types or sizes: Mechanically, displacement outcome has equal fastness for these four types of femoral stems, and the mechanic result is positive for both cemented long-stem and uncemented short-stem designs. Clinically, the cemented long-stem design is suitable for patients with osteoporosis, while the porously punched cementless short-stem is preferable for those with easy osseo-ingrowth or with cement allergy. Functionally, the advantage of the punched-prosthesis designed by virtual computation without a cement matrix is that it could be immobilized by the flesh bone structure growing inside the prosthesis orifices. Not only is the contract stress reduced, complications in cement are also avoidable, and this approach should be recommended as reasonable alternative for femoral-head replacement.

Abbreviations

3D: Three Dimensional; CAD: Computer Aided Design; CAM: Computer Aided Manufacturing; CT: Computed Tomography; FE: Finite Element; FEA: Finite Element Analysis; HA: Hip Arthroplasty; THA: Total Hip Arthroplasty

Acknowledgements

Thanks for detailed comments from Dr. Nagano & Dr. Rahmatullah. Thanks for Dr. Liu Yueju's direction for correction requested. Thanks a lot for additional chance given by Dr. James Mockridge!

Funding

This work is supported by: 1. "Guangdong Dept. of Science Technology" granted project (#2014A020215035); 2. Guangzhou Dept. of Education granted project: "High Educational 12-5 Plan" project (#1201420813); 3. Innovation and Technology Fund of Hong Kong / Guangdong Collaborative Plan (#20170506).

Authors' contributions

Informed consent was obtained from all participants included in the study. All authors have read and approved the final submitted manuscript. MJ-QP: Conception Designer, applied for research project, created the idea of "Finite Element Analysis of porously punched prosthetic short stem virtually designed for simulative uncemented Hip Arthroplasty" based on reference, design experimental software, materials, method and procedure, edited manuscript in English. H-YC: Searched experimental literature, carried out specimen preparation, CT scanning / image processing, numerous model validations, and cadaveric model validations, prepare the images and histology work. YH: Performed clinical testing & data interpretation primarily, monitored stability of fixations in clinical cases, feedback information to experiment procedure, interpreted the result data into tables, provided opinion based on surgical experience and direct further operation. XJ: Performed mechanical analysis, examination and observations of Stress distribution, examination and observations of Displacement distribution, and assisted in drafting manuscript. BB: General instruction & coordination, distributed research teamwork to group, helped any member's difficulties in need, compared and drew conclusion from testing data, control funding support financially, managed the process of experiment, approval of submission and publication.

Consent for publication
Not applicable.

Competing interests
No author associated with this paper has disclosed any potential or pertinent conflicts which may be perceived to have impending conflict with this work.

Author details
[1]Guangdong Orthopedics Implantation key Lab, Orthopedics Department of 1st Affiliated Hospital, Guangzhou Medical University, 151 YanJiangXi Rd, Guangzhou 510120, China. [2]Neural Electrophysiology Lab, University of Hong Kong, Room 501, Haking Wong Building, Pokfulam Road, Pok Fu Lam, Hong Kong. [3]Clinical Physics & Bioengineering Department, University of Glasgow, 378 Sauchiehall St., Glasgow G2 3JZ, UK.

References
1. Gillies RM, Morberg PH, Bruce WJ, Turnbull A, Walsh WR. The influence of design parameters on cortical strain distribution of a cement less titanium femoral stem. Med Eng Phys. 2002;24:109–14.
2. Kim SC, Lim YW, Jo WL, et al. Surgical accuracy, function, and quality of life of simultaneous versus staged bilateral Total hip Arthroplasty in patients with Osteonecrosis of the femoral head. BMC Musculoskeletal Disorders 2017;18:266.
3. Yerasimides JG. Use of the Fitmore (R) hip stem bone-preserving system for the minimally invasive anterior-supine approach in hip replacement. Am J Orthop (Belle Mead NJ). 2010;39:13–6.
4. Janssen D, Mann KA, Verdonschot N. Finite element simulation of cement-bone interface micromechanics; a comparison to experimental results. J Orthop Res. 2009;27(10):1312–8.
5. Fawzi F, Jassir A, Fouad H, Alothman OY. In vitro assessment of Function Graded (FG) artificial Hip joint stem in terms of bone/cement stresses: 3D Finite Element (FE) study. Biomed Eng Online. 2013;12:5. 1–17
6. Kim YH, Park JW, Kim JS. Is diaphyseal stem fixation necessary for primary total hip arthroplasty in patients with osteoporotic bone (Class C bone)? J Arthroplast. 2013;28(1):139–46.
7. Walker PS, Schneeweis D, Murphy S. Strains and micro motions of press-fit femoral stem prostheses. J Biomech. 1987;20:693–702.
8. Whiteside LA, White SE, McCarthy DS. Effect of neck resection on torsional stability of cementless total hip replacement. Am J Orthop (Belle Mead NJ). 1995;24:766–70.
9. Peng MJ, Hu Y, Ju X, Cai DZ. Clinical Significance Of Creative 3D-Image Fusion Across [CT+MR] Modalities Based On Approach Of Characteristic Co-Registration. J Med Imaging Health Inf. 2016;6(6):e71–7.
10. Joshi RP, Efekhar NS, McMahon DJ, Nercessian OA. Osteolysis afer Charnley primary low-friction arthroplasty. A comparison of two matched paired groups. J Bone Joint Surg. 1998;80(4):585–90.
11. Senalp AZ, Kayabasi O, Kurtaran H. Static, dynamic and fatigue behavior of newly designed stem shapes for hip prosthesis using finite element analysis. Mater Des. 2007;28(5):1577–83.
12. Joshi MG, Advani SG, Miller F, Santare MH. Analysis of a femoral hip prosthesis designed to reduce stress shielding. J Biomech. 2000;33(12):1655–62.
13. Kayabasi O, Ekici B. Te effects of static, dynamic and fatigue behavior on three-dimensional shape optimization of hip prosthesis by fnite element method. Mater Des. 2007;28(8):2269–77.
14. Viceconti M, Muccini R, Bernakiewicz M, Baleani M, Cristofolini L. Large-sliding contact elements accurately predict levels of bone-implant micromotion relevant to osseointegration. J Biomech. 2000;33(12):1611_8.
15. Ramos A, Simoes J. Tetrahedral versus hexahedral fnite elements in numerical modelling of the proximal femur. Med Eng Phys. 2006;28(9):916–24.
16. Reggiani B, Cristofolini L, Varini E, Viceconti M. Predicting the subject-specifc primary stability of cementless implants during pre-operative planning: preliminary validation of subject-specifc fnite-element models. J Biomech. 2007;40(11):2552–8.
17. Zhang GD, Liao WJ, Tao SX. Exploration for Material Assignment and Effectiveness Validation of femoral neck FEA. J Tissue Eng Reach. 2009; 52(3):10263–8.
18. Pitto RP, Hayward A, Walker C, et al. Femoral bone density changes after total hip arthroplasty with uncemented taper-design stem: a five year follow-up study. Int Orthop. 2010;34:783–7.
19. Balasubramaniam U, Dowsey M, Ma F, et al. Functional and clinical outcomes following anterior hip replacement: a 5-year comparative study versus posterior approach. ANZ J Surg. 2016;86:589–93.
20. Kang KT, Koh YG, Son J, et al. Measuring the effect of femoral malrotation on knee joint biomechanics for total knee arthroplasty using computational simulation. Bone Joint Res. 2016;5:552–9.
21. Moussa ME, Esposito CI, Elpers ME, et al. Hip Dislocation Increases Roughness of Oxidized Zirconium Femoral Heads in Total Hip Arthroplasty: An Analysis of 59 Retrievals. J Arthroplast. 2015;30(4):713–7.
22. Viceconti M, Brusi G, Pancanti A, Cristofolini L. Primary stability of an anatomical cementless hip stem: a statistical analysis. J Biomech. 2006;39(7):1169–79.
23. McLaughlin JR, Lee KR. Cementless total hip replacement using second-generation components: a 12- to 16-year follow-up. J Bone Joint Surg Br. 2010;92:1636–41.
24. Janssen D, Mann KA, Verdonschot N. Micromechanical modeling of the cement-bone interface: the effect of friction, morphology and material properties on the micromechanical response. J Biomech. 2008;41(15):3158–63.
25. Manley MT, D'Antonio JA, Capello WN, Edidin AA. Osteolysis: a disease of access to fixation interfaces. Clin Orthop Relat Res. 2002;405:129–37.
26. Ellison B, Cheney NA, Berend KR, Lombardi AV, Mallory TH. Minimal stress shielding with a Mallory-Head titanium femoral stem with proximal porous coating in total hip arthroplasty. J Orthop Surg Res. 2009;4:42.
27. Sariali E, Mouttet A, Mordasini P, Catonne Y. High 10-year survival rate with an anatomic cementless stem (SPS). Clin Orthop Relat Res. 2012;470:1941–9.
28. Chen YL, Lin T, Liu A, et al. Does hydroxyapatite coating have no advantage over porous coating in primary total hip arthroplasty? A meta-analysis. Clin Orthop Relat Res. 2015;10:21.
29. Varitimidis SE, Dimitroulias AP, Karachalios TS, Dailiana ZH. Konstantinos N Malizos Outcome after tantalum rod implantation for treatment of femoral head osteonecrosis 26 hips followed for an average of 3 years. Acta Orthop. 2009;80(1):20–5.
30. Oba M, Inaba Y, Kobayashi N, et al. Effect of femoral canal shape on mechanical stress distribution and adaptive bone remodelling around a cementless tapered-wedge stem. Bone Joint Res. 2016;5:362–9.
31. Huiskes R, Weinans H, Dalstra M. Adaptive bone remodelling and biomechanical design considerations for noncemented total hip arthroplasty. Orthopedics. 1989;12:1255–67.
32. Chen WP, Tai CL, Lee MS, Lee PC, Liu CP, Chun-Hsiung Shih H. Comparison of stress shielding among different cement fixation modes of femoral stem in total Hip arthroplasty–a three-dimensional finite element analysis. J Med Biol Eng. 2004;24:183–7.
33. Maier MW, Streit MR, Innmann MM, Krüger M, Nadorf J, Kretzer P, Ewerbeck V, Gotterbarm T. Cortical hypertrophy with a short, curved uncemented hip stem does not have any clinical impact during early follow-up. BMC Musculoskelet Disord. 2015;16:371.

Risk factors for failure of revision total hip arthroplasty using a Kerboull-type acetabular reinforcement device

Shinya Hayashi[1*], Takayuki Nishiyama[2], Shingo Hashimoto[1], Tomoyuki Matsumoto[1], Koji Takayama[1], Kazunari Ishida[3], Kotaro Nishida[1] and Ryosuke Kuroda[1]

Abstract

Background: The present study aimed to identify the risk factors associated with revision total hip arthroplasty (THA) failure using a Kerboull-type (KT) plate.

Methods: We analyzed 77 revision THAs using cemented acetabular components with a KT plate for aseptic loosening between May 2000 and March 2012. We examined the association of bone graft type, acetabular bone defects, age at the time of surgery, preoperative Japanese Orthopaedic Association (JOA) score, postoperative JOA hip score, and body mass index, with radiographic failure as the outcome.

Results: The 7.4-year radiographic failure survival rate was 81.6%. The survival rate was significantly different between the beta-tricalcium phosphate (β-TCP) group and the bulk allograft group ($p = 0.019$). The survival curves were also significantly different between the β-TCP group and bulk allograft group ($p = 0.036$). American Academy of Orthopaedic Surgeons type IV was significantly associated with radiographic failure (odds ratio [OR]: 15.5, 95% confidence interval [CI]: 1.4–175.4; $p = 0.032$).

Conclusions: The midterm outcomes of revision THA indicate that type of bone graft and bone defect size may affect radiographic survival rate when using a KT plate.

Keywords: Revision total hip arthroplasty, KT plate, Allograft, Beta-tricalcium phosphate, Hydroxyapatite

Background

Outcomes following THA have improved owing to advancements in prostheses and surgical procedures [1–3]. However, failure of acetabular components can lead to large bone defects with residual bone loss. It is well documented that bone defects determine outcome and management after revision hip surgery [4].

To compensate for large bone loss, prosthetic augmentation with bone grafting was developed, and several types of reinforcement devices are currently in use for revision THA, including the Burch-Schneider anti-protrusion cage [5], Mueller support ring [6], Ganz reinforcement ring [7], Kerboull device [8, 9], and Kerboull-type (KT) device [10, 11] (Table 1).

* Correspondence: s11793290@yahoo.co.jp
[1]Department of Orthopaedic Surgery, Kobe University Graduate School of Medicine, 7-5-1 Kusunoki-cho, Chuo-ku, Kobe 650-0017, Japan
Full list of author information is available at the end of the article

The use of a Kerboull reinforcement device can reduce excessive bone graft loading during incorporation and remodeling processes [12, 13]. The KT plate, a modified Kerboull plate made of titanium with a similar shape, has various offsets and vertical lengths (Fig. 1). Therefore, it is particularly useful for treating severe dysplasia or large bone defects of the acetabulum. Since 2000, we have used the KT plate with artificial bone materials or bulk grafts fashioned from a femoral head allograft.

Bone graft substitutes in combination with or without human bone are widely used for reconstruction of massive acetabular bone defects in revision surgery [13–16]. Good results have been associated with bone graft substitutes for acetabular bone defects [13–16] (Table 2).

Factors such as bone defect size, bone graft, age, and postoperative activity level may affect implant survival

Table 1 Results of previous studies

Authors	Device type	Cases	Bone defect classification	Mean f/u years	Survival rate (loosening endpoint)
Ilyas et al. [5]	Burch-Schneider cage	33	AAOS III, IV	6.2y	85%
Schlegel et al. [6]	Mueller reinforcement ring	164	AAOS I-IV	8y	95%
Kerboull et al. [8]	Kerboull reinforcement device	53	AAOS III-IV	13y	92.1%
Kawanabe et al. [9]	Kerboull reinforcement device	42	AAOS II-IV	8.7y	67%
Baba et al. [10]	KT-plate	18	AAOS II, III	5y	87.5%
Hori et al. [11]	KT-plate	32	AAOS III, IV	10y	82.1%

following revision THA, but no study has identified the critical risk factors for failure of revision THA using a KT plate. We hypothesized that factors specific to patient status or bone grafting may be predictive of poorer radiographic outcomes after revision THA. Therefore, the aim of this study was to evaluate the association between survival rates for radiological loosening and results according to bone defect or type of graft. Factors such as age and postoperative activity level were also considered.

Clinical relevance

- Unlike prior reports, our study analyzed predictive factors for radiographic failure after revision THA.

Methods

Patients and surgery

A total of 95 consecutive revision THAs (86 patients) for aseptic loosening using cemented acetabular components with a KT acetabular reinforcement device (KT plate; KYOCERA Medical Corporation, Kyoto, Japan) were performed between May 2000 and March 2012. Exclusion criteria were recurrent dislocations and revision due to infection (8 cases); 10 cases were excluded because of loss to follow-up. Therefore, the data from 77 hips (6 men and 71 women) were included in the analysis. Initial diagnoses comprised osteoarthritis (59 hips), idiopathic osteonecrosis of the femoral head (4 hips), and rheumatoid arthritis (14 hips) (Fig. 1). Thirty-one patients underwent both acetabular- and femur-side revision surgery (cemented stem: 11 patients; cementless-stem: 20 patients), and 46 patients underwent only acetabular-side surgery (Fig. 3). The KT plate is available with an inside dome diameter of 44 mm, 48 mm, or 52 mm, and a vertical offset of +0 mm, +10 mm, or +15 mm. We used the 44-mm model in 20 patients, the 48-mm model in 35 patients, and the 52-mm model in 22 patients; we used the +0-mm vertical offset in 37 patients, the +10-mm vertical offset in 31 patients, and the +15-mm vertical offset in 9 patients. The inner head size diameter was 28 mm or 32 mm. We used an inner head size of 28 mm in 43 patients and 32 mm in 34 patients (Fig. 3).

Surgeries were performed using a direct lateral approach. All surgeries were performed by three experienced senior surgeons. The degree of acetabular bone defect was assessed after removal of the loosened implant, and the acetabular bone defect was augmented with a bone graft. The KT plate was fixed firmly by an inferior hook to the teardrop and a superior flange with at least two screws to the ilium. The polyethylene component was then cemented into the dome of the plate. When fixation of the inferior hook to the teardrop was not possible due to loss of host bone, the inferior hook of the KT plate was fixed to the ischium, inferior acetabular dome, or allograft. Between May 2000 and February 2003, bone defects were filled with β-TCP granules (OSferion; Olympus, Tokyo, Japan). Between February 2003 and March 2009, the bone defect was filled with HA block (Osteograft, Apaceram; KYOCERA Medical Corporation, Kyoto, Japan). Since 2009, we have used femoral head allografts that were harvested under sterile conditions and stored at −80 °C. After removing the remaining cartilage and soft tissue, the femoral head was cut using an oscillating saw into an appropriate shape and size to be used as a bulk allograft. A representative case with preoperative and postoperative X-rays is shown in Fig. 2. Postoperatively, full weight-bearing

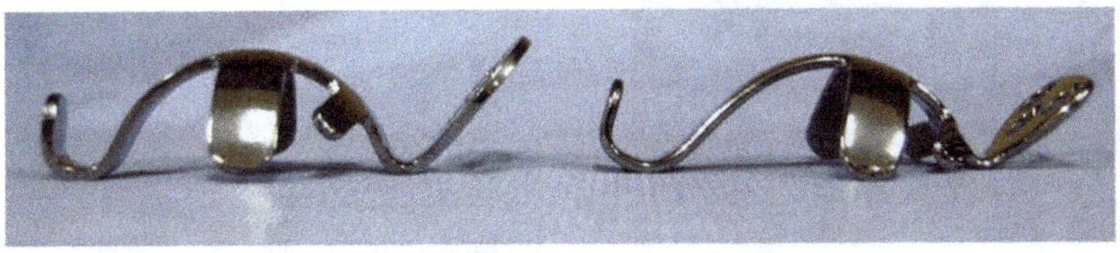

Fig. 1 Photographs of the KT plate in the original position (*left*) and high placement position (*right*)

Table 2 Results of previous studies

Authors	Type of graft	Cases	Bone defect classification	Mean f/u duration	Survival rate (loosening endpoint)
McNamara et al. [13]	allograft and hydroxyapatite	37	AAOS I-III	56.9m	95%
Oonishi et al. [14]	hydroxyapatite	40	AAOS I-II	4-10y	93%
Schwartz et al. [15]	biphasic calcium phosphate ceramics	29	Data not specified	more than 6m	100%
Blom et al. [16]	allograft and tricalcium phosphate-hydroxyapatite	43	Data not specified	24m	98%

was tolerated by all patients within 3 days of surgery and patients were discharged from the hospital with a T-cane gait at 3 weeks postoperatively. The weight-bearing protocol was not changed over the course of the study period. All data were obtained in accordance with the World Medical Association Declaration of Helsinki Ethical Principles for Medical Research Involving Human Subjects.

Postoperative evaluation

Hip function was evaluated using the Japanese Orthopaedic Association (JOA) score, which allocates 40 points for pain, 20 points for range of motion, 20 points for walking ability, and 20 points for activities of daily living, with a maximum total score of 100 points [17]. The JOA score was evaluated preoperatively and at the final follow-up assessment. Body mass index (BMI) and University of California, Los Angeles (UCLA) activity scores were also evaluated at the final follow-up assessment. Acetabular defects were classified by one senior experienced surgeon according to the American Academy of Orthopedic Surgeons (AAOS) grading system [11]. Type II defects (cavitary bone loss) were found in 6 hips (7.8%), type III defects (cavitary and segmental bone loss) in 66 hips (85.7%), and type IV defects (pelvic discontinuity) in 5 hips (6.5%) (Fig. 3).

Radiological failure was defined by any of the following three criteria, according to Kawanabe [9]: 1. substantial migration defined as a change in the inclination angle of greater than 3° or migration greater than 2 to 3 mm; 2. progressive radiolucent line greater than 2 mm wide in all three zones as defined by DeLee and Charnley [18]; or 3. breakage of screws or device without migration or change in inclination. The postoperative and final follow-up radiographs were compared to assess radiological failure of the implant. The failure rate may be affected by the follow-up duration. Therefore, we performed survivorship analysis using radiographic failure as the endpoint.

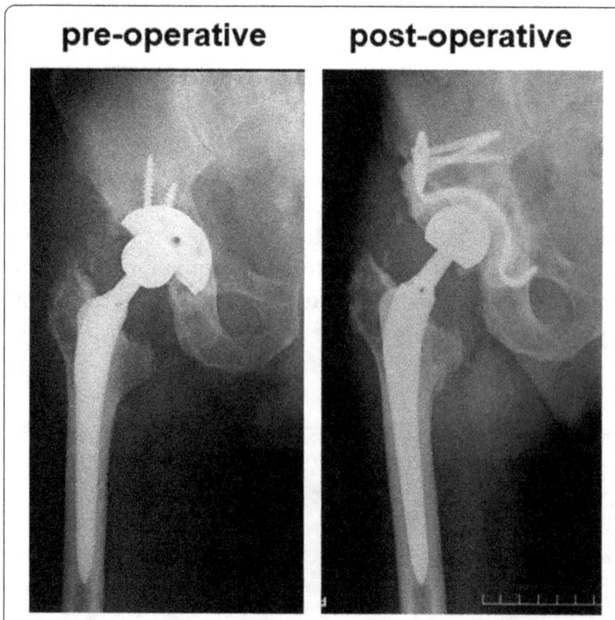

Fig. 2 Representative case of preoperative and postoperative X-rays

revision sides	number of cases
both acetabular side and femur side	31
acetabular side	46
Fixation type (femur side)	
cementless	20
cemented	11
Size variation of KT-plate	
44mm	20
48mm	35
52mm	22
+0mm offset	37
+10mm offset	31
+15mm offset	9
Size of inner head	
28mm	43
32mm	34

AAOS classification	number of cases
Type II	6
Type III	66
Type IV	5

Fig. 3 Summary of revision THA and number of patients according to AAOS classification. AAOS: American Academy of Orthopaedic Surgeons

Statistical analysis

Demographic data were recorded as the mean ± standard deviation (SD) unless otherwise indicated. All data were normally distributed. Statistical analysis was performed using one-way analysis of variance with the Tukey post hoc test for multiple comparisons of paired samples. Cumulative probabilities of radiographic failure rate were estimated by using the Kaplan-Meier method. The survivorship curves for various subgroups were compared using the log-rank test. Logistic regression was performed to examine the association of age at the time of the operation, preoperative JOA score, postoperative JOA score, BMI, UCLA activity score, and AAOS classification with radiographic failure. Odds ratios (ORs) and 95% confidence interval (CIs) were calculated. Multivariate analysis was performed to adjust for potential confounders of age at the time of operation, preoperative JOA score, postoperative JOA score, BMI, UCLA activity score, and AAOS classification. The database was analyzed using SPSS software (IBM Corp., Armonk, NY, USA). Values of $p < 0.05$ were considered significant.

Results

Patient background

This study is a retrospective review of patient records. The patient background is shown in Fig. 4. The JOA score at the final follow-up examination increased significantly ($p < 0.001$). The patient background including pre- and postoperative JOA score, BMI, and UCLA score at final follow-up were not significantly changed according to the bone defect type or type of bone graft.

number of cases	77
sex	male 6, female 71
age	66.6±10.4 y.o.
preoperative JOA score	53.5±16.0 points
postoperative JOA score	69.2±13.6 points
BMI	22.4±4.0 kg/mm^2
UCLA score at final follow-up	4.2±1.5 points
Follow-up duration	7.4±4.1 yrs

Fig. 4 Patient demographic data. JOA: Japanese Orthopaedic Association, THA: total hip arthroplasty, BMI: body mass index, UCLA; University of California, Los Angeles

Radiographic survival rate

Radiographic failure was evaluated for revision THA with β-TCP, hydroxyapatite (HA), and bulk allografts using cemented sockets with a KT plate. The total survival rate was 81.6%. The survival rate was 74.2% in the β-TCP group, 81.5% in the HA group, and 94.7% in the bulk allograft group (Fig. 5). However, the survival rate in the β-TCP group was significantly lower than in the HA ($p = 0.048$) or bulk allograft groups ($p = 0.019$). We also evaluated the stability of the acetabular component using the AAOS classification. The survival rate was 100% in the AAOS type II group, 83.3% in the type III group, and 40% in the type IV group (Fig. 5). The survival rate in the AAOS type IV group was significantly lower than in the type III group ($p = 0.033$).

We further performed survivorship analysis using radiographic failure as the endpoint. The survival curves were significantly different between the β-TCP group and bulk allograft group ($p = 0.036$), but were not significantly different between the HA group and bulk allograft group (Fig. 6).

Risk factors for radiographic failure

To identify risk factors for radiographic failure, we performed multivariate analysis to test the association of AAOS classification, clinical factors including age, pre- and postoperative JOA scores, BMI, UCLA activity score, and follow-up duration with radiographic failure and revision. AAOS type IV defect was found to be a risk factor for radiographic failure (OR: 15.5, 95% CI: 1.4–175.4, $p = 0.032$).

Discussion

The core evaluation in this study focuses on the relationship between survival rates for radiological loosening and results according to bone defect or type of graft. We demonstrated that the 7.4-year survival rate was 81.6% when radiographic failure was the endpoint. These results are similar to those reported by previous studies [9–11].

Various types of graft have been used for reconstruction of acetabular bone defects. Blom et al. reported a 2-year survival rate of 100% in revision THA with impaction bone grafting of the acetabulum using a mix of bone chips and 80% TCP/20% HA [16]. In an in vitro study, Bolder reported that impaction bone grafting using TCP/HA and human bone chips significantly decreased socket migration in comparison with the use of human bone chips alone [19]. Aulakh et al. reported that the 13-year survival rate in revision THA with impaction bone grafting using a

AAOS classification	β-TCP		HA		Bulk allograft		total	survival rate
	stable	failure	stable	failure	stable	failure		
II	3	0	2	0	1	0	6	100%
III	20	8	19	2	16	1	66	83.3%
IV	0	0	1	3	1	0	5	40%
total	23	8	22	5	18	1	77	81.6%
survival rate (mean follow-up duration)	74.2% (8.9 ± 5.0)		81.5% (8.3 ± 2.3)		94.7% (5.1 ± 2.5)			

Fig. 5 Number of radiographic failure cases according to type of bone graft and AAOS classification. AAOS: American Academy of Orthopaedic Surgeons, β-TCP: beta-tricalcium phosphate, HA: hydroxyapatite

mix of 50% HA and 50% bone chips was 82%, and 84% with impaction bone grafting using only bone chips [20]. There was no significant difference between the two groups [20]. Tanaka et al. reported a 5-year survival rate of 100% in THA using a KT plate with HA granules [19].

Many good outcomes accompanied acetabular reconstructions of revision THA using artificial bone grafts [16, 19–21]. Kawanabe et al. compared the outcomes of morselized allografts and bulk allografts, and found the 10-year survival rate was 53% for morselized allografts and 82% for bulk grafts [9]. The authors also found the failure rate in the morselized allograft group was significantly higher than in the bulk allograft group when the acetabular defect was large (i.e., AAOS type III/IV) [9]. Based on our observations, the survival curves were significantly different between the β-TCP group and bulk allograft group. These results indicate the type of bone graft may affect radiographic survival rate when using a KT plate.

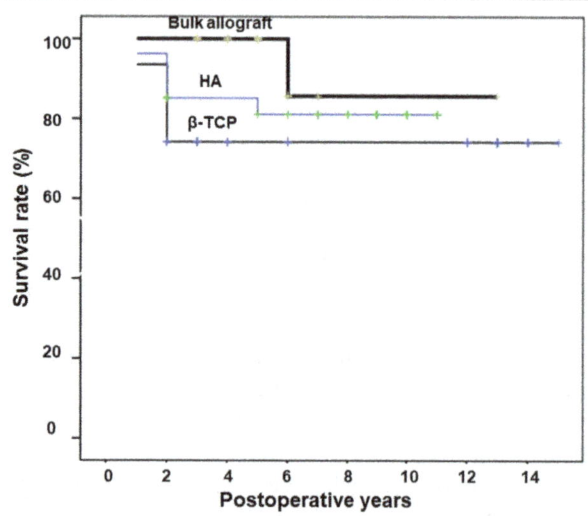

Fig. 6 A Kaplan-Meier survival curve with radiographic failure as the endpoint. β-TCP: beta-tricalcium phosphate, HA: hydroxyapatite

We further evaluated risk factors for failure of revision THA in association with clinical factors (age at the time of the operation, preoperative JOA score, postoperative JOA score, BMI at final follow-up assessment, follow-up duration, and UCLA activity score at final follow-up assessment), type of bone graft (β-TCP, HA, bulk allograft), and AAOS bone defect classifications. Only AAOS type IV was found to be a significant risk factor for failure of revision THA. Based on this finding, bone defect size is the critical risk factor for failure of revision THA using a KT plate.

Other reconstruction devices can fix the posterior wall in the case of massive host bone defect [20, 21]. Rogers et al. reported that an ilioischial cage or cup cage was able to fix the device to both the superior and inferior host bone with screws [20]. Friedrich et al. reported reconstruction for pelvic discontinuity using a patient-specific custom-made implant [21]. We are not aware of any reports of posterior plating combined with the use of a KT plate for pelvic discontinuity. Nonetheless, posterior plating might improve the survival rate of revision surgery with a KT plate in pelvic discontinuity.

A major limitation of this study is its small cohort size for statistical analysis. However, the number of hips evaluated in the study was quite high in comparison with other clinical studies of acetabular revision surgery [9–11, 19]. Another limitation is that three types of bone grafts were used at different times. Further, the mean follow-up duration was longer in the β-TCP group (mean: 8.9 ± 5.0 y) and HA group (mean: 8.3 ± 2.3 y) compared to the bulk allograft group (mean: 5.1 ± 2.5 y). These limitations may affect the survival result.

Conclusion

The midterm outcomes of revision THA indicate that type of bone graft and bone defect size may affect radiographic survival rate when using a KT plate. New devices and techniques for KT plates are needed to improve the treatment of pelvic discontinuity.

Abbreviations

β-TCP: beta-tricalcium phosphate; AAOS: American Academy of Orthopaedic Surgeons; BMI: Body mass index; HA: Hydroxyapatite; JOA: Japanese Orthopaedic Association; OR: Odds ratio; THA: Total hip arthroplasty; UCLA: University of California, Los Angeles

Acknowledgements

Not applicable.

Funding

The authors have no funding

Authors' contributions

SHay participated in the study design, drafting of the manuscript, and data collection. TN participated in the data collection and drafting of the manuscript. SHas carried out data collection and drafting of the manuscript. TM participated in the data collection and drafting of the manuscript. KT participated in the study design and helped to revise the manuscript. KI participated in the data collection and drafting of the manuscript. KN carried out data collection and drafting of the manuscript. RK participated in the study design and helped to revise the manuscript. All authors read and approved the final manuscript.

Consent for publication

Not applicable.

Competing interests

The authors declare that they have no competing interests.

Author details

[1]Department of Orthopaedic Surgery, Kobe University Graduate School of Medicine, 7-5-1 Kusunoki-cho, Chuo-ku, Kobe 650-0017, Japan. [2]Department of Orthopaedic Surgery, Kakogawa City Hospital, Kakogawa, Japan. [3]Department of Orthopaedic Surgery, Kobe Kaisei Hospital, Kobe, Japan.

References

1. Caton J, Prudhon JL. Over 25 years survival after Charnley's total hip arthroplasty. Int Orthop. 2011;35(2):185–8.
2. Aldinger PR, Jung AW, Breusch SJ, Ewerbeck V, Parsch D. Survival of the cementless Spotorno stem in the second decade. Clin Orthop Relat Res. 2009;467(9):2297–304.
3. Suckel A, Geiger F, Kinzl L, Wulker N, Garbrecht M. Long-term results for the uncemented Zweymuller/Alloclassic hip endoprosthesis. A 15-year minimum follow-up of 320 hip operations. J Arthroplast. 2009;24(6):846–53.
4. Boscainos PJ, Kellett CF, Maury AC, Backstein D, Gross AE. Management of periacetabular bone loss in revision hip arthroplasty. Clin Orthop Relat Res. 2007;465:159–65.
5. Ilyas I, Alrumaih HA, Kashif S, Rabbani SA, Faqihi AH. Revision of Type III and Type IVB Acetabular defects with Burch-Schneider Anti-Protrusio Cages. J Arthroplast. 2015;30(2):259–64.
6. Schlegel UJ, Bitsch RG, Pritsch M, Clauss M, Mau H, Breusch SJ. Mueller reinforcement rings in acetabular revision: outcome in 164 hips followed for 2-17 years. Acta Orthop. 2006;77(2):234–41.
7. Gerber A, Pisan M, Zurakowski D, Isler B. Ganz reinforcement ring for reconstruction of acetabular defects in revision total hip arthroplasty. J Bone Joint Surg Am. 2003;85-A(12):2358–64.
8. Kerboull M, Hamadouche M, Kerboull L. The Kerboull acetabular reinforcement device in major acetabular reconstructions. Clin Orthop Relat Res. 2000;378(9):155–68.
9. Kawanabe K, Akiyama H, Onishi E, Nakamura T. Revision total hip replacement using the Kerboull acetabular reinforcement device with morsellised or bulk graft: results at a mean follow-up of 8.7 years. J Bone Joint Surg Br Vol. 2007;89(1):26–31.
10. Baba T, Shitoto K. Revision of total hip arthroplasty using the Kerboull and KT plates. Int Orthop. 2010;34(3):341–7.
11. Hori J, Yasunaga Y, Yamasaki T, Yoshida T, Oshima S, Yamasaki K, Matsuo T, Ochi M. Mid-term results of acetabular reconstruction using a Kerboull-type acetabular reinforcement device. Int Orthop. 2012;36(1):23–6.
12. Kawanabe K, Akiyama H, Goto K, Maeno S, Nakamura T. Load dispersion effects of acetabular reinforcement devices used in revision total hip arthroplasty: a simulation study using finite element analysis. J Arthroplast. 2011;26(7):1061–6.
13. McNamara I, Deshpande S, Porteous M. Impaction grafting of the acetabulum with a mixture of frozen, ground irradiated bone graft and porous synthetic bone substitute (Apapore 60). J Bone Joint Surg Br Vol. 2010;92(5):617–23.
14. Oonishi H, Iwaki Y, Kin N, Kushitani S, Murata N, Wakitani S, Imoto K. Hydroxyapatite in revision of total hip replacements with massive acetabular defects: 4- to 10-year clinical results. J Bone Joint Surg Br Vol. 1997;79(1):87–92.
15. Schwartz C, Liss P, Jacquemaire B, Lecestre P, Frayssinet P. Biphasic synthetic bone substitute use in orthopaedic and trauma surgery: clinical, radiological and histological results. J Mater Sci Mater Med. 1999;10(12):821–5.
16. Blom AW, Wylde V, Livesey C, Whitehouse MR, Eastaugh-Waring S, Bannister GC, Learmonth ID. Impaction bone grafting of the acetabulum at hip revision using a mix of bone chips and a biphasic porous ceramic bone graft substitute. Acta Orthop. 2009;80(2):150–4.
17. Hasegawa Y, Iwata H, Mizuno M, Genda E, Sato S, Miura T. The natural course of osteoarthritis of the hip due to subluxation or acetabular dysplasia. Arch Orthop Trauma Surg. 1992;111(4):187–91.
18. DeLee JG, Charnley J. Radiological demarcation of cemented sockets in total hip replacement. Clin Orthop Relat Res. 1976;121(11):20–32.
19. Tanaka C, Shikata J, Ikenaga M, Takahashi M. Acetabular reconstruction using a Kerboull-type acetabular reinforcement device and hydroxyapatite granules: a 3- to 8-year follow-up study. J Arthroplast. 2003;18(6):719–25.
20. Rogers BA, Whittingham-Jones PM, Mitchell PA, Safir OA, Bircher MD, Gross AE. The reconstruction of periprosthetic pelvic discontinuity. J Arthroplast. 2012;27(8):1499–506. e1491
21. Friedrich MJ, Schmolders J, Michel RD, Randau TM, Wimmer MD, Kohlhof H, Wirtz DC, Gravius S. Management of severe periacetabular bone loss combined with pelvic discontinuity in revision hip arthroplasty. Int Orthop. 2014;38(12):2455–61.

Conversion to total hip arthroplasty after failed proximal femoral nail antirotations or dynamic hip screw fixations for stable intertrochanteric femur fractures

Xianshang Zeng[1†], Ke Zhan[1†], Lili Zhang[2†], Dan Zeng[3†], Weiguang Yu[1†], Xinchao Zhang[4*] and Mingdong Zhao[4†]

Abstract

Background: Conversion to total hip arthroplasty (CTHA) is a relatively common procedure after a failed dynamic hip screw (DHS) or proximal femoral nail anti-rotation (PFNA) fixation of intertrochanteric fractures, but there have been far fewer reports specifically describing the long-term results of CTHA after failed treatments of stable intertrochanteric fractures with DHS or PFNA. The aim of the present study was to compare the clinical and radiological outcomes of CTHA after failed PFNA or DHS fixations of stable intertrochanteric fractures after a minimum follow-up of 3 years.

Methods: Between January 2005 and April 2014, we retrospectively reviewed 142 active elderly patients treated at our institution (a single institution study). A total of 72 patients (72 hips; 41 women, 31 men; mean age 76.9 years old; range 60–92 years old) who underwent conversion of a failed PFNA to a THA were compared with 70 patients (70 hips; 36 women, 34 men; mean age 75.0 years old; range 60–90 years old) who underwent CTHA after a failed DHS fixation. The mean follow-up periods were 48 (range 43–52) and 48 (range 44–52) months for the DHS and PFNA groups, respectively. Clinical and radiologic evaluations were performed on all patients. The primary outcome was the Harris Hip Score (HHS). The secondary outcomes were the complication rates.

Results: The Harris Hip Score (HHS) improved from 50.61 ± 3.23 preoperatively to 85.28 ± 4.45 at the last follow-up in the PFNA group and from 51.46 ± 3.90 to 84.50 ± 4.34 in the DHS group, with no significant differences noted between the groups at each follow-up ($P > 0.05$). However, the complication rate in the converted DHS patients was significantly higher (42.9%) than that in the converted PFNA patients (20.8%; $P = 0.003$). Thirty-seven PFFs (2.4%) occurred during a mean follow-up of 44.4 months. The incidence of periprosthetic fractures was found to be significantly higher ($P = 0.021$) for the DHS group (15.7%) than for the PFNA group (4.2%).

(Continued on next page)

* Correspondence: zhangxc401@aliyun.com
†Equal contributors
[4]Department of Orthopaedics, Jinshan Hospital, Fudan University, Longhang Road No. 1508, Jinshan District, Shanghai City 201508, China
Full list of author information is available at the end of the article

(Continued from previous page)

Conclusions: CTHA after failed DHS fixations of stable intertrochanteric fractures might be associated with a significantly higher complication rate than CTHA after failed PFNA fixations. Therefore, PFNA patients with stable intertrochanteric fractures may be more suitable for CTHA.

Keywords: Intertrochanteric fracture, Total hip arthroplasty, Complication, Proximal femoral nail antirotation, Dynamic hip screw

Background

Intertrochanteric fractures are among the most important health care issues facing orthopaedic surgeons today [1, 2]. These fractures are well known to cause significant physical and functional impairment for patients and require substantial financial resources for both perioperative and rehabilitative care [3]. Proximal femoral nail anti-rotation (PFNA) and dynamic hip screw (DHS) fixation are accepted treatment options that are currently widely used as the primary treatment for stable intertrochanteric fractures (AO/OTA Type 3.1A1) [4, 5]. There is generally agreement that failed PFNA or DHS fixations of intertrochanteric fractures should be treated with a conversion to total hip arthroplasty (CTHA) whenever possible [3]. In China, an increasing incidence of intertrochanteric fractures has led to higher rates of CTHA [5].

Prior studies have reported that CTHA was a successful procedure that could be used to treat failed DHS or PFNA fixations of intertrochanteric fractures [3–5]. However, it has been unclear whether there are differences in the success rates for converting PFNA or DHS to a THA [3]. On the other hand, numerous studies have been published regarding comparisons of PFNA and DHS for the fixation of intertrochanteric fractures in active elderly patients [4–6]. Thus far, there has been no clear conclusion regarding the superiority of one of the approaches over the other. Some researchers hold that, for the management of stable intertrochanteric fractures, DHS should usually be recommended as the first choice and, in contrast, PFNA should be recommended for the treatment of unstable intertrochanteric fractures [4–8]. However, for stable intertrochanteric fractures, PFNA has also been shown to be an acceptable approach in extensive studies [4, 6]. In spite of some reports of good results, not all researchers have reported success with either DHS or PFNA [5, 7]. Thus, many active elderly patients with a failed DHS or PFNA are converted to a THA as a last option to salvage hip function. However, the failure rate for CTHA in active elderly patients remains high despite continuous improvements in the design and technique [6, 7]. With reported rates of dislocation greater than 22.5% and rates of periprosthetic fracture greater than 30% [9], it is very important to continue to monitor the clinical and radiological outcomes and to improve the treatment strategies for failed DHS or PFNA-II fixations of stable IFFs to reduce the complications in these patients [4–6]. In addition, the results of CTHA after failed DHS or PFNA are still controversial, although some studies have reported no differences [9–11]. To date, none of the previous reports have directly compared the clinical and radiological outcomes of CTHA after failed DHS or PFNA fixations of stable intertrochanteric fractures.

The aim of the present study was to compare the clinical and radiological outcomes of CTHA after failed PFNA or DHS fixations of stable intertrochanteric fractures after a minimum follow-up of 3 years.

Methods

Between January 2005 and April 2014, 192 patients (192 hips) underwent CTHA following failed treatment of stable intertrochanteric fractures with DHS or PFNA devices at our institution (a single centre). The average time interval from the initial fracture fixation (PFNA or DHS) to CTHA fixation was 11 (range 3–16) months. The inclusion criteria were: active elderly patients aged 60–92 years old; a prior intertrochanteric fracture (type AO/OTA 31. A1); failed fixation due to screw cut-out, nonunion, avascular necrosis or insufficient initial fixation; normal cognitive function; ability to walk independently without aids before fracture; and eligibility to receive a standard CTHA device (Standard-device, Stryker, Mahwah, New Jersey). The exclusion criteria were: pathological fractures, metastatic disease, infection, neoplasia, arthritis, ASA score V, ipsilateral lower-limb surgery, contralateral hip fracture or other revision procedures. Based on these criteria, 29 patients were excluded. Another 16 refused to participate, leaving 147 patients eligible for the study. The patient characteristics are expressed as the means with SDs or as frequencies and percentages. The primary outcome was the clinical outcome, as defined by the Harris Hip Score (HHS), which was collected at 1 h preoperatively and post-operatively at 2, 6, 12, 24, 36 months and at the last follow-up. The secondary outcomes were the incidence and distribution of complications.

Surgical methods

All of the patients were treated with CTHA by the surgeons (WY, XCZ, XZ and KZ) after failed fixation (PFNA or DHS) for stable intertrochanteric fractures. All of the operations were carried out under general anaesthesia. Two surgical approaches for conversion to a THA were performed according to standard protocols for CTHA, which were recommended by the manufacturers and have been previously described in the literature [11, 12]. All of the CTHAs were carried out through a posterolateral approach with the patient in a lateral decubitus position. The previous DHS or PFNA was removed. With the hip joint dislocated, osteotomy of the femoral neck was performed with an oscillating saw. After removal of the femoral head, the acetabulum was reamed [13]. The details of each surgical approach are almost identical. Immediate postoperative radiographs and ultrasonic examination were used to evaluate the quality of operation. All of the patients underwent a clinical evaluation to determine the HHS. Intra- and post-operative complications were recorded.

Fisher's exact test and the chi-square test were utilized for categorical variables and numerical variables, respectively. All of the reported P values were two-sided, and a P value < 0.05 was considered to be significant for all of the statistical tests. All hips were assumed to be independent in the statistical analysis. All statistical analyses were performed using the SPSS software program (version 22.0, IBM Inc. Chicago, Illinois).

Results

During the follow-up period, 3 patients in the PFNA group died in car accidents, and 2 patients from the DHS group died of heart attacks. Therefore, 142 patients (142 secondary operations, all were CTHAs) were included in the final analysis and their records were retrospectively reviewed (2 groups: DHS [$n = 70$] and PFNA [$n = 72$]) (Fig. 1). The patient demographics are shown in Table 1. None of 142 patients were lost to follow-up, and all 142 patients were available for review (zero mortality). Sixty-eight male patients and 74 female patients were evaluated in the current study. The PFNA group

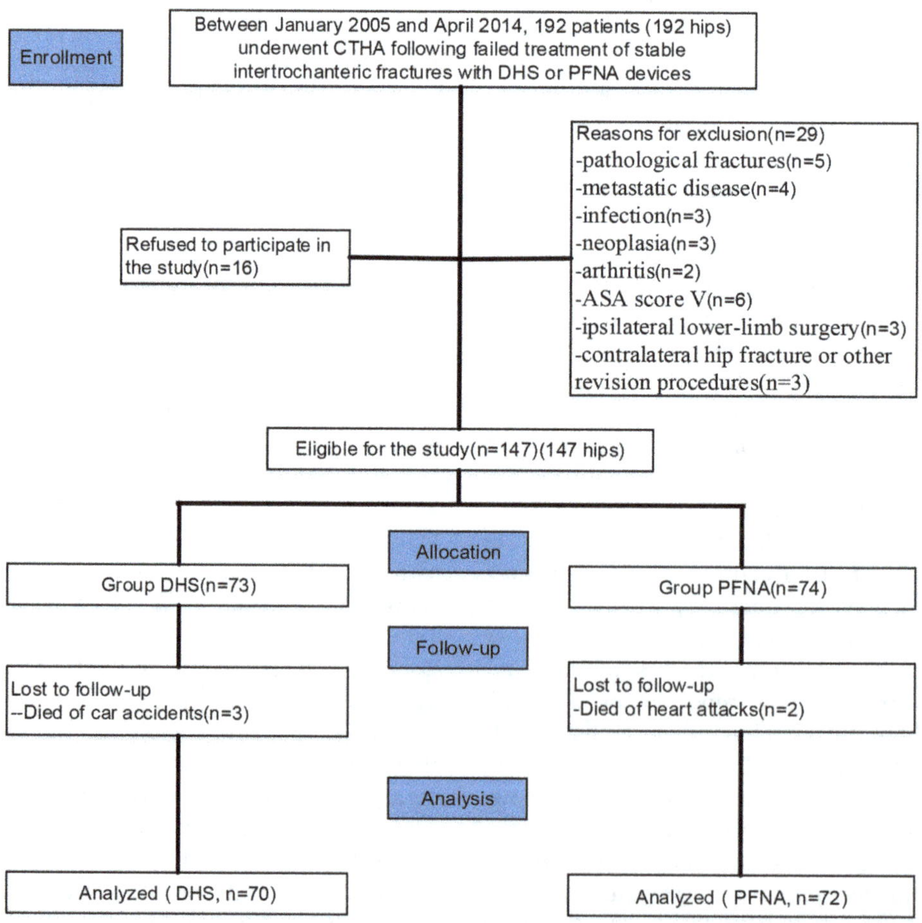

Fig. 1 Flow diagram demonstrating methods for identification of studies to assess the treatment of CTHA after failed PFNA or DHS fixations of stable intertrochanteric fractures in the elderly

Table 1 Patient demographics in the groups with different implant types

Variable	PFNA (*n* = 72)	DHS (*n* = 70)	*P* value
Age (years)	76.93 ± 9.25	74.96 ± 8.59	0.19
Sex (M:F)	31:41	34:36	0.51
Modes of prior failure fixation			0.94
Screw cut-out	24	23	0.95
Nonunion	21	18	0.65
Avascular necrosis	16	16	0.93
Insufficient initial fixation	11	13	0.60
ASA score, No.			0.82
1	10	12	0.59
2	18	17	0.92
3	22	24	0.64
4	22	17	0.40
Femoral fixation (NO.)			0.41
Cemented	30 (41.7%)	34 (48.6%)	
Uncemented	42 (58.3%)	36 (51.4%)	
Length of follow-up (months)	47.92 ± 4.31	48.10 ± 4.12	0.80
Body Mass Index (BMI, kg/m2)	29.50 ± 2.70	28.90 ± 1.50	0.10
AO/OTA classification (NO.)			0.88
3.1A1.1	12	13	0.77
3.1A1.2	37	33	0.61
3.1A1.3	23	24	0.77

had 31 (43.1%) men and 41 (56.9%) women. The DHS group had 34 (48.6%) men and 36 (51.4%) women. There were no significant differences between the groups regarding sex, the modes of prior failed fixation, ASA score, AO/OTA classification, BMI, initial complication rates before the CTHA procedure, length of stay in the hospital, intraoperative blood loss, length of the operation or preoperative HHS. The average age at the CTHA procedure was 76.93 years old (range, 60–92 years; SD, 9.25) in the PFNA group and 74.96 years old (range, 60–90 years; SD, 8.59) in the DHS group (P = 0.19). There were no significant differences in the medical complications between groups (P = 0.442) with 3 of 72 (4.2%) patients affected in the PFNA group and 5 of 70 (7.1%) patients affected in the DHS group (Table 3).

Clinical outcomes

There was an improvement in the HHS between the preoperative evaluation and the last follow-up in both groups (Table 2). The mean lengths of follow-up were 47.92 months (interquartile range [IQR] 43 to 52) and 48.10 months (IQR 44 to 52) for the PFNA and DHS groups, respectively.

The HHS in the PFNA group improved significantly from 50.61 ± 3.23 to 85.28 ± 4.45, and that in the DHS group improved significantly from 51.46 ± 3.90 to 84.50 ± 4.34. There were no significant differences between groups in terms of the HHS at the last follow-up (P = 0.29).

Table 2 Comparison of the Harris Hip Scores at 1 h preoperatively; 2, 6, 12, 24 and 36 months postoperatively; and at the last follow-up

	PFNA	DHS	*p*
1 h Pre-operatively	50.61 ± 3.23	51.46 ± 3.90	0.16
2 Months Postoperatively	78.33 ± 1.65	77.90 ± 1.77	0.13
6 Months Postoperatively	79.31 ± 2.09	78.53 ± 2.98	0.08
12 Months Postoperatively	82.54 ± 2.49	81.91 ± 4.36	0.30
24 Months Postoperatively	86.35 ± 4.38	85.03 ± 4.47	0.78
36 Months Postoperatively	86.14 ± 3.22	85.30 ± 3.72	0.15
Last follow-up	85.28 ± 4.45	84.50 ± 4.34	0.29

Radiological outcomes

Postoperative radiographs were available for all patients, with a mean follow-up of 48 months (43–52 months). No intra-operative fractures were observed in either group. There were no significant differences in the rate of periprosthetic fracture between cemented and uncemented implants.

The complication rate in the PFNA group was 16.7% (12/72) compared with 37.1% (26/70) in the DHS group. Three (4.2%) periprosthetic fractures occurred. There was a statistically significant difference regarding the rate of periprosthetic fractures between the groups. Ten complications in 10 patients were observed in the PFNA group, including postoperative periprosthetic fractures, prosthetic instability, dislocation, limb length discrepancy (>2.5 cm), abductor tendon deficiency, Brooker class 6 heterotopic ossification, and aseptic loosening (Table 3).

In the DHS group, orthopaedic complications were significantly more common, at a rate of 37.1%. Twenty-four complications were identified in 24 patients, including postoperative periprosthetic fractures, prosthetic instability, dislocation, limb length discrepancy (>2.5 cm), Brooker class 6 heterotopic ossification, aseptic loosening and late deep infection requiring removal of hardware. Eleven (15.7%) periprosthetic fractures occurred. More than one-third (37.1%; 26/70) of the patients had experienced an orthopaedic complication by the last follow-up in the DHS group compared with a 16.7% (12/72) orthopaedic complication rate in the PFNA group (P = 0.003) (Table 3).

Discussion

Most retrospective studies have investigated intertrochanteric fractures in a comprehensive manner. However, most follow-up period is commonly reduced to 2-years postoperation, and the implants are often compared in terms

Table 3 Complications of conversion to total hip arthroplasty

Variable	PFNA ($n = 72$)	DHS ($n = 70$)	P value
Total complications	15	31	0.003
Patients affected	15 (20.8%)	31 (42.9%)	0.003
Medical complications	3	5	0.442
Patients affected	3 (4.2%)	5 (7.1%)	0.442
Urinary tract infection	1	1	1.000
Pulmonary embolism	0	2	0.241
Atrial fibrillation	2	0	0.497
Acute renal failure	0	2	0.241
Orthopaedic complications	12	26	0.011
Patients affected	12 (16.7%)	26 (37.1%)	0.011
Periprosthetic fracture	3 (4.2%)	11 (15.7%)	0.021
Prosthetic instability	1	2	0.617
Dislocation	1	3	0.363
Limb length discrepancy (>2.5 cm)	1	2	0.617
Abductor tendon deficiency	2	2	1.000
Heterotopic ossification	1	1	1.000
Intraoperative nerve injury	1	1	1.000
Aseptic loosening	0	1	0.241
Periprosthetic infection	2	2	1.000

of their use [8, 11, 12]. Consequently, these studies had substantial differences compared with our study in terms of the inclusion criteria and the parameters investigated.

The evidence in the literature regarding the optimal method that should be used for the initial internal fixation of stable intertrochanteric fractures is inconclusive [8, 11, 12, 14]. Prior evidence has suggested that DHS may be superior to PFNA, but these findings were based on studies with small sample sizes and low event numbers [15]. Moreover, in China, 70% of surgeons prefer PFNA over DHS for treating a stable intertrochanteric fracture in active elderly patients [10]. Other studies have previously reported that DHS was the best choice for the initial treatment of stable intertrochanteric fractures [6, 7, 9, 16, 17]. Although the complication rates of DHS devices ranged from 12 to 34% [10], DHS was still regarded as a preferred device for stable intertrochanteric fractures in active elderly patients. However, another problem that must be considered is that the results of CTHA after a failed DHS fixation compared to a failed PFNA fixation are relatively controversial [7, 8, 16–18]. There is currently no consensus about which type of implant to use or what technique to perform in patients with stable intertrochanteric fractures previously treated with DHS fixation or PFNA. Some studies reported no difference in the clinical and radiological outcomes [7–12, 19, 20], while others reported higher complication rates and revision rates for one approach after CTHA [17, 21]. To address this controversy, we compared the clinical and radiological outcomes of CTHA after a failed PFNA or DHS fixation for stable intertrochanteric fractures.

There have only been a few previous reports that have focused on CTHA after a failed PFNA or DHS fixation for stable intertrochanteric fractures. Furthermore, the majority of these studies had low numbers of patients and short follow-up periods, and therefore, drawing conclusions about the relative superiority of one implant over the other is inappropriate. Unnanuntana et al. [22] retrospectively reviewed 78 patients who underwent CTHA after failed DHS fixations of stable intertrochanteric fractures and found that orthopaedic complications were more frequent. Diwanji et al. [9] performed 163 CTHAs after failed DHS fixations of a prior stable intertrochanteric fracture and noted a 14.1% (23/163) orthopaedic complication rate, including 11 dislocations (6.7%) and 12 femur fractures (7.4%). In the current study, a 37.1% orthopaedic complication rate (42.9% total complication rate) was identified in the DHS group compared with a 16.7% orthopaedic complication rate (20.8% total complication rate) in the PFNA group. The present complication rate in the DHS group was comparable to those of other series using similar osteosynthesis techniques.

In the previous study [3, 8, 19, 23], the incidence of periprosthetic fractures after CTHA ranged from 11.9% to 28%. The incidence of periprosthetic fractures in these studies was higher in comparison with the results of our study (14 out of 142, 9.9%). A recent study has reported the incidence of periprosthetic fractures after CTHA was used to treat failed PFNA or DHS fixations of intertrochanteric fractures in a large cohort [12]. Fifty-two of the 594 patients (8.8%) sustained a periprosthetic fracture during a mean follow-up of 4 years, and 71% of the fractures occurred within 1 year. The incidence of periprosthetic fractures in that study was consistent with the results of our study. In this study, prior DHS-treated patients receiving CTHA tended to have less resistance to periprosthetic fractures. One of the major reasons for this finding might be that the patients sustaining stable intertrochanteric fractures treated with a DHS tended to have poorer bone quality caused by stress shielding, which was in line with the prior consensus that a high incidence of mechanical complications (periprosthetic fractures) was recorded in patients who had received prior DHS treatment [7, 9, 16, 24]. As demonstrated by recent biomechanical testing [19], patients undergoing DHS may have poorer bone quality caused by stress-shielding than patients undergoing PFNA, which might partly explain the destruction of the bone and the disuse and atrophy of the proximal femur.

Both cemented and uncemented CTHA designs are being successfully used for the treatment of failed DHS fixations of stable intertrochanteric fractures, despite the fact that uncemented CTHAs are commonly offered to youthful patients [16]. Moreover, previous studies had evaluated the outcome of the cemented and uncemented CTHA, and reported no difference between cemented and uncemented CTHA was observed with respect to stem performance [2, 22, 24]. That was consistent with our conclusion.

A growing but still very limited body of literature has shown that conversion from prior PFNA fixation is better compared with conversion from prior DHS fixation with regard to the postoperative HHS after 0.5–1.5 years of follow-up [8, 15, 17, 25]. However, similar to a multicentre, randomized study [26], we found no obvious differences in the postoperative HHS between the groups treated with the two types of conversions after a median of 3 years of follow-up. An obvious explanation for this may be the differences in the follow-up period compared to other studies. In addition, our results were also in line with other previous studies based on data acquired from the Healthcare Cost and Utilization Project's Nationwide Inpatient Sample [13, 21, 23, 27].

This study should be interpreted in light of important limitations. First, this study is observational and it is possible that we failed to address every potential confounding variable in our analyses. Second, it is a retrospective study with all the problems inherent with this methodology. Third, because the conversion often occurred several years after the initial treatment with PFNA or DHS, the initial fracture pattern of stable intertrochanteric fractures may not have been recorded. It is possible that the fractures treated with DHS may have been more complex than those treated with PFNA, which might have eventually led to more malunions and fractures in the DHS group, thus making intra- and post-operative complications more common than in randomized, controlled cohorts.

Conclusions

We found significant complication rates associated with the conversion of both DHS and PFNA to THA. Moreover, CTHA after a failed DHS was associated with a higher complication rate. Thus, prior PFNA-treated patients with stable intertrochanteric fractures appear to be more suitable for treatment with CTHA. Further follow-up is needed to confirm whether these results persist over a longer term.

Abbreviations

CTHA: Conversion total hip arthroplasty; DHS: Dynamic hip screw; HHS: Harris hip score; IQR: Interquartile range; PFNA: Proximal femoral nail anti-rotation; SD: Standard deviation

Acknowledgements

The authors would like to thank Jun Hu for help with retrieval of patients' notes and radiographs.

Funding

No funding was received for this study or for the writing of this manuscript.

Authors' contributions

WY performed the data collection and analysis and participated in manuscript writing. DZ and LZ performed the database setup and statistical analysis. WY, XCZ, XZ and KZ performed the operations. XCZ and MZ participated in the study design and coordination and helped to draft the manuscript. All of the authors have read and approved the final manuscript.

Competing interests

The authors declare that they have no competing interests.

Consent for publication

Not applicable as no identifying personal information is being published in this manuscript.

Author details

[1]Department of Orthopedics, The First Affiliated Hospital of Sun Yat-sen University, Huangpu East Road No. 183, Huangpu District, Guangzhou City, Guangdong Province 510700, China. [2]Department of Anesthesiology, The First Affiliated Hospital of Sun Yat-sen University, Huangpu East Road No. 183, Huangpu District, Guangzhou City, Guangdong Province 510700, China. [3]Ultrasonography Department, The First Affiliated Hospital of Sun Yat-sen University, Huangpu East Road No. 183, Huangpu District, Guangzhou City, Guangdong Province 510700, China. [4]Department of Orthopaedics, Jinshan Hospital, Fudan University, Longhang Road No. 1508, Jinshan District, Shanghai City 201508, China.

References

1. Yu WG, Zhang XC, Zhu XF, Yu ZC, Xu YF, Zha GQ, et al. Proximal femoral nails anti-rotation versus dynamic hip screws for treatment of stable intertrochanteric femur fractures: an outcome analyses with a minimum 4 years of follow-up. BMC Musculoskelet Disord. 2016;17. doi:10.1186/s12891-016-1079-7.
2. Shi X, Zhou Z, Yang J, Shen B, Kang P, Pei F. Total hip arthroplasty using Non-modular cementless long-stem distal fixation for salvage of failed internal fixation of intertrochanteric fracture. J Arthroplasty. 2015;30(11):1999–2003. doi:10.1016/j.arth.2015.05.041.
3. Harrington P, Nihal A, Singhania AK, Howell FR. Intramedullary hip screw versus sliding hip screw for unstable intertrochanteric femoral fractures in the elderly. Injury. 2002;33(1):23–8. doi:10.1016/s0020-1383(01)00106-1.
4. Hak DJ, Bilat C. Avoiding varus malreduction during cephalomedullary nailing of intertrochanteric hip fractures. Arch Orthop Trauma Surg. 2011;131(5):709–10. doi:10.1007/s00402-010-1182-4.
5. Estrera K, Russell RD, Huo MH. Total hip arthroplasty after failed internal fixation of intertrochanteric hip fractures. J Am Geriatr Soc. 2014;62:S88–S9.
6. Kawasaki M, Hasegawa Y, Sakano S, Masui T, Ishiguro N. Total hip arthroplasty after failed transtrochanteric rotational osteotomy for avascular necrosis of the femoral head. J Arthroplasty. 2005;20(5):574–9. doi:10.1016/j.arth.2005.01.018.
7. Pui CM, Bostrom MP, Westrich GH, Della Valle CJ, Macaulay W, Mont MA, et al. Increased complication rate following conversion total hip arthroplasty after cephalomedullary fixation for intertrochanteric hip fractures a multi-center study. J Arthroplasty. 2013;28(8):45–7. doi:10.1016/j.arth.2013.04.048.

8. O'Malley MJ, Kang KK, Azer E, Siska PA, Farrell DJ, Tarkin IS. Wedge effect following intramedullary hip screw fixation of intertrochanteric proximal femur fracture. Arch Orthop Trauma Surg. 2015;135(10):1343–7. doi:10.1007/s00402-015-2280-0.
9. Diwanji SR, Kim SK, Seon JK, Park SJ, Yoon TR. Clinical results of conversion total hip arthroplasty after failed bipolar hemiarthroplasty. J Arthroplasty. 2008;23(7):1009–15. doi:10.1016/j.arth.2007.09.006.
10. Zha G-C, Chen Z-L, Qi X-B, Sun J-Y. Treatment of pertrochanteric fractures with a proximal femur locking compression plate. Injury. 2011;42(11):1294–9. doi:10.1016/j.injury.2011.01.030.
11. Spinnickie A, Goodman SB. Dissociation of the femoral head and trunion after constrained conversion total hip arthroplasty for poliomyelitis. J Arthroplasty. 2007;22(4):634–7. doi:10.1016/j.arth.2006.05.011.
12. Bercik MJ, Miller AG, Muffly M, Parvizi J, Orozco F, Ong A. Conversion total hip arthroplasty a reason not to use cephalomedullary nails. J Arthroplasty. 2012;27(8):117–21. doi:10.1016/j.arth.2012.04.009.
13. Park K-S, Tumin M, Peni I, Yoon T-R. Conversion total hip arthroplasty after previous transtrochanteric rotational osteotomy for osteonecrosis of the femoral head. J Arthroplasty. 2014;29(4):813–6. doi:10.1016/j.arth.2013.09.012.
14. von Roth P, Abdel MP, Harmsen WS, Berry DJ. Total hip arthroplasty after operatively treated acetabular fracture a concise follow-up, at a mean of twenty years, of a previous report. J Bone Joint Surg Am. 2015;97A(4):288–91. doi:10.2106/jbjs.n.00871.
15. Stambough JB, Nunley RM, Curry MC, Steger-May K, Clohisy JC. Rapid recovery protocols for primary total hip arthroplasty can safely reduce length of stay without increasing readmissions. J Arthroplasty. 2015;30(4): 521–6. doi:10.1016/j.arth.2015.01.023.
16. Merle C, Streit MR, Innmann M, Gotterbarm T, Aldinger PR. Long-term results of cementless femoral reconstruction following intertrochanteric osteotomy. Int Orthop. 2012;36(6):1123–8. doi:10.1007/s00264-011-1396-2.
17. Inal S, Taspinar F, Gulbandilar E, Gok K. Comparison of the biomechanical effects of pertrochanteric fixator and dynamic hip screw on an intertrochanteric femoral fracture using the finite element method. Int J Med Robot. 2015;11(1):95–103. doi:10.1002/rcs.1584.
18. Owens JB, Ely EE, Guilliani NMF, Suarez JC, Patel PD. Removal of trabecular metal osteonecrosis intervention implant and conversion to primary total hip arthroplasty. J Arthroplasty. 2012;27(6):1251–3. doi:10.1016/j.arth.2012.01.025.
19. Chen DW, Lin C-L, Hu C-C, Tsai M-F, Lee MS. Biomechanical consideration of total hip arthroplasty following failed fixation of femoral intertrochanteric fractures - a finite element analysis. Med Eng Phys. 2013;35(5):569–75. doi: 10.1016/j.medengphy.2012.06.023.
20. Roerdink WH, Aalsma AMM, Nijenbanning G, van Walsum ADP. The dynamic locking blade plate, a new implant for intracapsular hip fractures: biomechanical comparison with the sliding hip screw and twin hook. Injury. 2009;40(3):283–7. doi:10.1016/j.injury.2008.08.041.
21. Ramiah RD, Baker RP, Bannister GC. Conversion of failed proximal femoral internal fixation to total hip arthroplasty in osteopetrotic bone. J Arthroplasty. 2006;21(8):1200–2. doi:10.1016/j.arth.2006.05.031.
22. Unnanuntana A, Goodman SB. Conversion total hip replacement after malunited intertrochanteric fracture: a technical note. Am J Orthop (Belle Mead NJ). 2008;37(10):506–9.
23. Riesgo AM, Hochfelder JP, Adler EM, Slover JD, Specht LM, Iorio R. Survivorship and complications of revision total hip arthroplasty with a Mid-modular femoral stem. J Arthroplasty. 2015;30(12):2260–3. doi:10.1016/j.arth.2015.06.037.
24. Mohanty SS, Agashe MV, Sheth BA, Dash KK. Outcome of total hip arthroplasty as a salvage procedure for failed infected internal fixation of hip fractures. Indian J Orthop. 2013;47(1):87–92. doi:10.4103/0019-5413.106921.
25. Suarez JC, Slotkin EM, Szubski CR, Barsoum WK, Patel PD. Prospective, randomized trial to evaluate efficacy of a bipolar sealer in direct anterior approach total hip arthroplasty. J Arthroplasty. 2015;30(11):1953–8. doi:10.1016/j.arth.2015.05.023.
26. Schairer WW, Sing DC, Vail TP, Bozic KJ. Causes and frequency of unplanned hospital readmission after total hip arthroplasty. Clin Orthop Relat Res. 2014;472(2):464–70. doi:10.1007/s11999-013-3121-5.
27. Best MJ, Buller LT, Klika AK, Barsoum WK. Increase in perioperative complications following primary total hip and knee arthroplasty in patients with hepatitis C without cirrhosis. J Arthroplasty. 2015;30(4):663–8. doi:10.1016/j.arth.2014.11.013.

Femur first surgical technique: a smart non-computer-based procedure to achieve the combined anteversion in primary total hip arthroplasty

Mattia Loppini[1,2*], Umile Giuseppe Longo[3], Emanuele Caldarella[1], Antonello Della Rocca[1], Vincenzo Denaro[3] and Guido Grappiolo[1]

Abstract

Background: The relevance of prosthetic component orientation to prevent dislocation and impingement following total hip arthroplasty (THA) has been widely accepted. We investigated the use of a non-computer-based surgery to address the reciprocal orientation of the acetabular and femoral components.

Methods: In the femur first technique, the cup is positioned relative to the stem. When the definitive antetorsion of femoral component is fixed, the cup is positioned in a compliant anteversion to the stem. Clinical and radiographic assessments were performed before and 3 months after THA. Radiographic assessment was performed in standing position with the EOS 2D/3D radiography system. 3D images were used to preoperative anterior pelvic plane (APP) angle, postoperative acetabular inclination (AI) and anteversion (AA), and postoperative stem antetorsion. Clinical assessment was performed with Harris Hip Score (HHS).

Results: Forty patients (40 hips) underwent primary THA with an average age of 61 years (range, 36–84). Average HHS increased from 43 ± 5 (range, 37–52) preoperatively to 97 ± 6 (range, 86–100) at the last follow-up ($P < 0.0001$). Average combined anteversion value of cup with liner and stem was 38° ± 9° (range, 12°-55°). Average AI value of cup with liner was 39° ± 6° (range, 30°-55°) in the group with standard stem and 45° ± 7° (range, 39°-58°) in the group with varized stem ($P = 0.007$). Relationship analysis showed no correlation between the combined anteversion values of the cup with liner and stem with APP angle values ($r = 0.26$, $P = 0.87$).

Conclusions: Femur first technique allows the surgeon to achieve a combined anteversion ranging from 25° to 50° with a cup inclination ranging from 30° to 50°. The cup is positioned according to the functional plane of the patient regardless the preoperative pelvic tilt.

Keywords: Combined anteversion, Acetabular inclination, Femur first, Hip, Arthroplasty

* Correspondence: mattia.loppini@gmail.com
[1]Hip Diseases and Joint Replacement Surgery Unit, Humanitas Clinical and Research Centre, Via Alessandro Manzoni 56, 20089 Rozzano, Milan, Italy
[2]Humanitas University, Via Alessandro Manzoni 113, 20089 Rozzano, Milan, Italy
Full list of author information is available at the end of the article

Background

Over the last two decades, a growing relevance has been recognized to the prosthetic component orientation to prevent dislocation and impingement following total hip arthroplasty (THA).

In 1978, Lewinnek et al. [1] identified the orientation of the acetabular cup associated with the lower rate of dislocation. The suggested "safe zone" was included between 30°-50° of inclination in the coronal plane, and 5°-25° of anteversion in the axial plane. Although malpositioning of the acetabular component has been demonstrated to affect significantly the range of motion (ROM), joint stability, wear and loosening [2–5], the relative orientation of the acetabular and femoral components seems to be as important as the absolute positioning based on the bony landmarks.

The concept of combined anteversion was introduced by Ranawat et al. [6] in 1991, suggesting that the sum of the cup anteversion and stem antetorsion should be 45° for women and between 20° and 30° for men. Subsequently, several mathematical models were developed to determine the combination of cup inclination and anteversion, and stem antetorsion providing the greater ROM and lower risk of cup-neck impingement [7–9]. Among these studies, the authors recommended a cup inclination between 40° and 45°, combined with cup anteversion and stem antetorsion determined by the following formula: cup anteversion + (0.7 x stem antetorsion) = X°, where the value of X ranged from 37° to 42°. On the other hand, clinical use of combined anteversion has determined it should be between 25° up to 50° [10].

Combined anteversion technique demonstrated to reduce of 6 times the dislocation rate in cementless total hip arthroplasty [11]. Some authors suggested the intraoperative navigation to achieve a proper combined anteversion [10, 12]. In this respect, computer-based systems can detect malpositioning of the first component, and correct accordingly the second component to restore the reciprocal orientation of both components. However, the setup and application of conventional navigation systems are time- and cost-consuming, and smart non-computer-based devices should be developed to allow the surgeon to achieve the proper combined anteversion [13].

In the present study, we investigated a non-computer-based surgical technique to obtain a proper orientation of both acetabular and femoral components during a primary THA procedure, according with the concept of combined anteversion. In the femur first technique, the cup is positioned relative to the stem after the trial stem has been implanted [14]. Therefore, the definitive antetorsion of femoral component is fixed, and the cup is positioned in a compliant anteversion to the first component. Moreover, because of a relation between cup inclination and the neck-to-shaft angle of straight stems has been described [15], we also hypothesized that the femur first technique could provide the coverage of the cup accordingly with the neck-to-shaft angle of the stem. Finally, because the present technique is based on the combined anteversion concept, we hypothesized that proper functional orientation of both cup and stem components should not be affected by the preoperative value of pelvic tilt.

Although previous studies evaluated the effectiveness of femur first technique to achieve a proper combined anteversion [10, 11, 16], none investigated its role to determine the coverage of the cup, and the relationship of the combined anteversion values with pelvic tilt. The null hypotheses of the study were: 1) the femur first technique did not allow the surgeon to achieve a combined anteversion ranging from 25° to 50°, and a cup inclination ranging from 30° to 50°; and 2) there was no correlation between preoperative pelvic tilt and postoperative combined anteversion values if the femur first technique is performed.

Methods

Sample

Forty patients (40 hips) who underwent primary total hip arthroplasty from November 2014 to February 2015 were enrolled. Patients included 17 men and 23 women, with an average age of 61 years (range, 36–84) at the time of the index procedure. The average body mass index at the surgery was 27 kg/cm^2 (range, 18–39). The preoperative diagnosis included: primary osteoarthritis in 33 patients, osteoarthritis secondary to mild development dysplasia of the hip in 6 patients, and post-trauma osteoarthritis in one patient. Exclusion criteria included: patients eligible for partial or total THA revision, THA associated with other procedures (i.e. femoral osteotomy), previous pelvic and/or femoral osteotomy, severe hip dysplasia (Crowe III or IV), primitive or metastatic tumors of hip joint, previous spine and/or sacroiliac joint instrumentation, previous or current hip joint infection.

A minimum follow-up of 1 year was achieved in all patients.

Surgical procedure

In all patients, the digital preoperative radiograph in AP view was used to perform preoperative planning with the software Hip Arthroplasty Templating 2.4.3 running with OsiriX v.5.8.1 64-bit [17].

Surgery was performed by one experienced surgeon with the patient in the lateral position, through a posterolateral approach in all cases. After the release of short external rotators tendons at the insertion to greater trochanter, the capsule was incised, and the femur was dislocated. After the neck osteotomy, the femur was prepared by holding the knee flexed with the tibia in a vertical position. The starter device was introduced with the planned version for the definitive stem. The femoral rasps were inserted gradually increasing the size until proper fit was achieved. The definitive antetorsion of the stem was related with the native anatomy of the proximal femur. The type of neck, standard or varized, was defined according with the native value of caput-collum-diaphyseal angle (CCD), as measured with the radiographic assessment.

Maintaining the proper sized rasp in situ to protect the femoral shaft, the acetabulum was exposed, the labrum was removed, and the acetabulum was sequentially reamed. The definitive position of the acetabular component, in terms of anteversion and inclination angle, was identified basing of femoral stem anteversion and CCD angle. The femur was reduced with the proper sized rasp in situ by using a 44 mm trial plastic head with a long neck to compensate the absence of the acetabular component. By using a large head, it was possible to avoid an eccentric position of the head in the native acetabulum. After reduction, with the hip in neutral position at 0° of flexion and abduction, the femur was internally rotated to obtain an angle of 35°, measured with a sterile goniometer, between the longitudinal axis of the tibia and the operating table which is parallel with the floor. Because of the degree of internal rotation to produce a coplanar head and cup is the combined anteversion [6], the definitive cup should be placed parallel with the horizontal line on the trial head in both axial and coronal plane. The parallelism in the axial plane provided the proper degree of cup anteversion to obtain a combined anteversion of 35°. On the other hand, the parallelism in the coronal plane provided the proper degree of cup inclination angle. The peripheral rim of the determined position of the cup was marked with a dermographic pen on the bony surface of the acetabulum. After the femur dislocation, the definitive acetabular cup was implanted, and osteophytes surrounding the acetabulum were removed when indicated. Then, the femur was reduced with the trial components in situ without the liner, and it was placed in internal rotation of 35° with the hip in neutral position at 0° of flexion and abduction. Therefore, the coplanarity of head and cup in both axial and coronal plane was checked, and the position of the liner with the elevated rim was determined in order to optimize the joint congruency. Previous joint dislocation, the femoral rasp was removed, the definitive liner was implanted with the elevated rim in planned position, and the definitive stem was implanted. Finally, the proper length of the neck was chosen to restore the native vertical and lateral offsets. At the end, the internal rotation with hip flexion and the free ROM were performed to assess the stability of the hip [18]. No impingement, dislocation and lower limb discrepancy were observed in any patient.

In all patients, uncemented cup and stem were implanted. The acetabular system was: G7 cup (Zimmer Biomet) in 31 hips and Trabecular Metal Acetabular Shell (Zimmer Biomet) in 9. The stem system was: GTS stem (Zimmer Biomet) in 23 hips and CLS stem (Zimmer Biomet) in 17. The stem was standard in 29 hips (21 GTS with CCD of 136° and 8 CLS with CCD of 135°) and varized in 11 (2 GTS with CCD of 123° and 9 CLS with CCD of 125°).

In all patients, the bearing surface consisted in ceramic head and polyethylene liner with 10° elevated rim. The location of the elevated rim of the liner was reported by using a clock-face description where 12 o'clock indicated the side towards the head of patient, and 6 o'clock was the side towards the obturator foramen [17]. To clarify the data presentation, the site of the elevated rim was standardized to the right hip. The location of the elevated rim of the liner was: 12 o'clock in 1, 11 o'clock in 12, 9 o'clock in 6, 7 o'clock in 17, and 3 o'clock in 4 hips.

Clinical assessment

The Harris Hip Score (HHS) was performed to evaluate the clinical picture of the patient before and 3 months after surgery. The questionnaire assigns up to 91 points for the domains of pain and hip function, and up to 9 points for the domain of range of motion. The final score ranges from 0 to 100 points, with the higher scores indicating the better clinical picture. The HHS has been considered excellent for values between 90 and 100 points, good for values between 80 and 89, fair for values between 70 and 79, and poor for values under 70 [19].

The intraoperative and postoperative complications, and the occurrence of hip dislocation were also evaluated.

Radiographic assessment

All patients had a radiographic assessment in standing position before and 3 months after THA with the EOS 2D/3D radiography system (Biospace Med, Paris, France).

EOS system allows to achieve an AP and lateral radiographic view of the whole skeletal system [20–22]. The 2D images were used to perform a 3D reconstruction of skeletal system and prosthetic components with a dedicated software (sterEOS 3D, versione 1.5.3.7947, Biospace Med, Paris, France). 3D images were used to measure preoperative CCD angle and femoral antetorsion [23], preoperative anterior pelvic plane (APP) angle, postoperative acetabular inclination (AI) and anteversion (AA), and postoperative stem antetorsion [24].

The CCD angle was defined as the angle between the femoral neck axis and femoral long axis [25]. The APP angle was defined as the angle subtented by a vertical reference line and a line tangent to the anterosuperior iliac spines and the pubic symphysis [22]. The combined anteversion was determined by the following formula:

cup anteversion + (0.7 x stem antetorsion) [8]. The AI and AA were measured in the patient frame based on a vertical plane passing through the centre of the acetabular cup, which avoids the effect of a potential axial rotation of the pelvis during acquisition. On the other hand, the stem antetorsion was measured relative to posterior bi-condylar plane.

The AI and AA values measured with EOS system were also adjusted according the location of the liner's elevated rim. The 12 o'clock position was considered to reduce the AI value of 10°. The 3 o'clock and 9 o'clock positions were considered to reduce and increase the AA value of 10°, respectively. Finally, the 11 o'clock and 7 o'clock positions were not considered able to influence AI and AA values as measured with EOS system.

The outliers were the values out of the targeted ranges of combined anteversion (from 25° to 50°) and AI (from 30° to 50°).

Statistics

All the analyses were performed using SPSS for Mac (version 23.0, SPSS Inc., Chicago, Illinois). Descriptive statistics were calculated. The categorical variables were expressed as frequency with percentage. Continuous variable data were expressed as mean with standard deviation and range as minimum and maximum values.

The Wilcoxon signed-rank test with two tails was used to compare the preoperative and postoperative values of HHS. It was also used to compare the preoperative femoral antetorsion and postoperative stem antetorsion. The U Mann-Whitney test with two tails was used to compare the AI and combined anteversion values measured without liner and values recorded taking account the location of elevated rim of the liner. It was also used to compare the AI values of cup with liner in the group with standard stem and those in the group with varized stem. Finally, it was used to compare the combined anteversion values of the cup with liner and stem in the group with antetorsion of the stem ≤9° and those in the group with ≥10° of antetorsion of the stem.

The Spearman rank correlation matrix was used to assess the relationship between the combined anteversion values of the cup with liner and stem with APP angle values. For this relationship, a linear regression model was also performed and the coefficient of determination was calculated (R^2). The P was considered significant for values less than 0.05.

Results

Clinical outcome

The average HHS increased from 43 ± 5 (range, 37–52) preoperatively to 97 ± 6 (range, 86–100) at the last follow-up ($P < 0.0001$). The final scores were good in 13, and excellent in 27.

No patients reported intraoperative or postoperative complications neither dislocation of the prosthesis at the last follow-up.

Radiographic outcome

The average combined anteversion value with and without taking account the location of elevated rim of the liner was 38° ± 9° (range, 12°-55°) and 37° ± 13° (range, 2°-65°) respectively ($P = 0.88$). In the cup with liner group, there were 3 (7.5%) outliers up to 13°, whereas there were 11 (27.5%) outliers up to 23° in the cup without liner group (Fig. 1).

The average AI value with and without taking account the location of elevated rim of the liner was 40° ± 6° (range, 30°-58°) and 41° ± 7° (range, 30°-58°) respectively ($P = 0.8$). In both groups, there were 3 (7.5%) outliers up to 8°. In the subgroup analysis, the average AI value of cup with liner was 39° ± 6° (range, 30°-55°) in the group with standard stem and 45° ± 7° (range, 39°-58°) in the group with varized stem ($P = 0.007$) (Fig. 2).

The average preoperative femoral antetorsion was 11° ± 14° (range, 21° of retrotorsion - 45° of antetorsion), whereas the average postoperative stem antetorsion was 9° ± 10° (range, 23° of retrotorsion - 31° of antetorsion) ($P = 0.71$). The average combined anteversion value of the cup with liner and stem was 34° ± 8° (range, 23°-51°) in the group with antetorsion of the stem ≤9° and 41° ± 9° (range, 12°–55°) in the group with ≥10° of antetorsion of the stem ($P = 0.002$) (Fig. 3). Thirteen out of 19 (68%) patients with a preoperative femoral antetorsion ≥10° reported a postoperative antetorsion of the stem ≥10° as well.

The relationship analysis showed no correlation between the combined anteversion values of the cup with liner and stem with APP angle values ($r = 0.26$, $P = 0.87$) and no linear regression between these variables ($R^2 = 0.004$, $P = 0.71$) (Fig. 4).

Discussion

In the present study, we rejected the first null hypothesis and we accepted the second null hypothesis: 1) the femur first technique allowed to achieve a combined anteversion ranging from 25° to 50° with a cup inclination ranging from 30° to 50°; and 2) there was no correlation between preoperative pelvic tilt and postoperative combined anteversion values.

About the first hypothesis, the combined anteversion value was within the targeted range in 92.5% of hips with an average value of 38° ± 9°. The results achieved with our non-computer-based procedure were similar to those reported by Dorr et al. [10] with intraoperative computer navigation. The authors found a combined anteversion within the targeted range from 25° to 50° in 96% hips with an average value of 35.9° ± 6.7°. On the

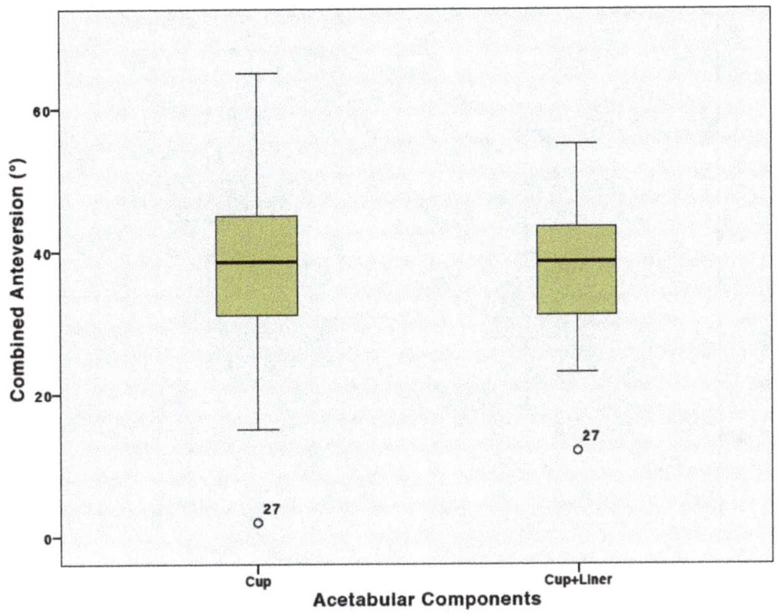

Fig. 1 Box plots showing the combined anteversion values measured in the cup with and without liner groups. Angles are expressed in degrees

other hand, Nakashima et al. [11] reported with their manual technique a combined anteversion within the targeted range from 40° to 60° in 73% hips with an average value of 50.3 ± 6.2°. Although the manual placement of the cup was associated with 27% of outliers, the combined anteversion technique significantly reduced the dislocation after primary THA.

In our current practice, we prefer to use a liner with 10° elevated rim if polyethylene is implanted to increase the hip stability [26, 27]. Therefore, we would suggest to use the elevated rim to improve the joint congruency even if the combined anteversion is within the targeted range. In our series, in 29 (72.5%) hips, the elevated rim was not used to change the combined anteversion and it was placed in the posterosuperior quadrant (11 o'clock) or posteroinferior quadrant (7 o'clock) to further increase the hip stability in internal rotation or flexion of the femur respectively. In the remaining hips (27.5%) we used the elevated rim to improve the combined anteversion as required by the intraoperative assessment with

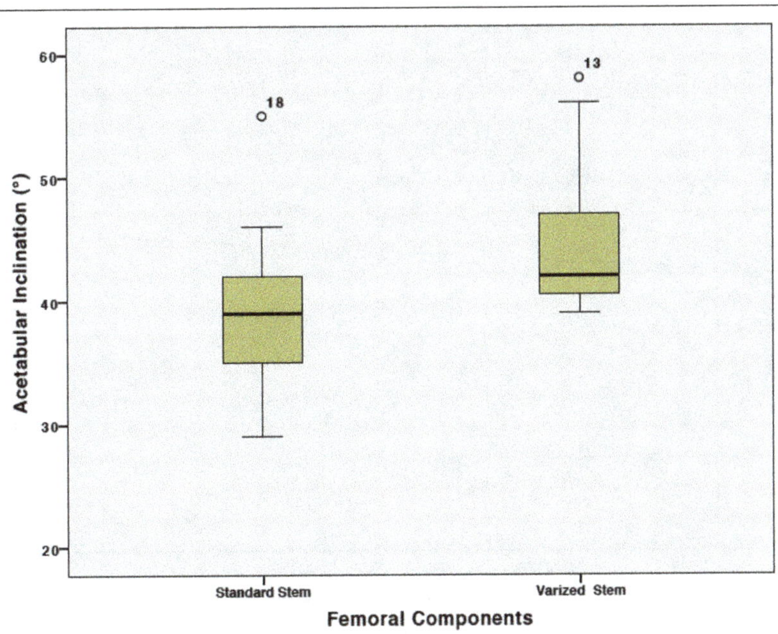

Fig. 2 Box plots showing the acetabular inclination values measured in the standard stem and varized stem groups. Angles are expressed in degrees

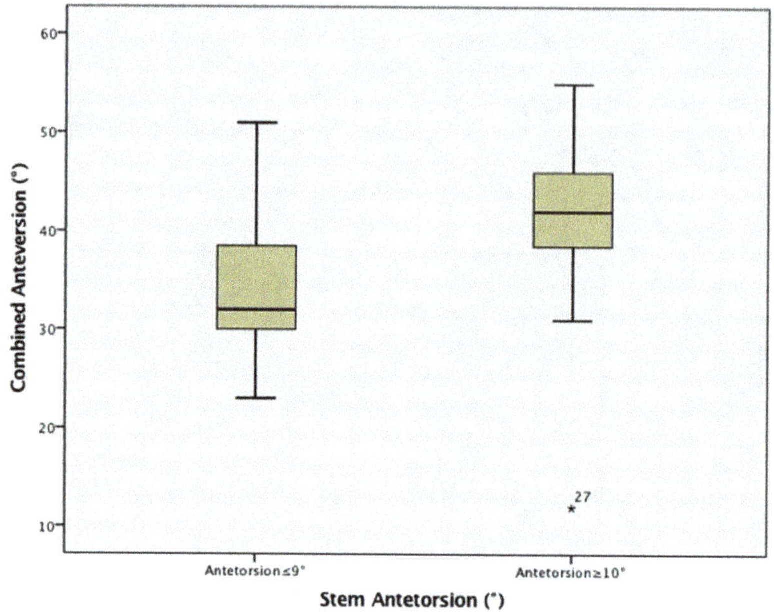

Fig. 3 Box plots showing the combined anteversion values measured with the cup-liner system in the group with ≤9° and ≥10° of antetorsion of the stem. Angles are expressed in degrees

the femur at 35° of internal rotation. Because there was no impingement or hip subluxation or dislocation, the position of the cup was not changed in these patients, but the combined anteversion was improved by positioning the elevated rim anteriorly (3 o'clock) or posteriorly (9 o'clock).

The analysis of the combined anteversion values according with the antetorsion values of the stem showed that the combined anteversion values in the group with ≥10° of stem antetorsion were significantly higher than those in the group with stem antetorsion ≤9° (P = 0.002). These findings demonstrated that the combined anteversion is strongly affected by the femoral antetorsion suggesting morphotype plays a critical role in the position of the definitive prosthetic components.

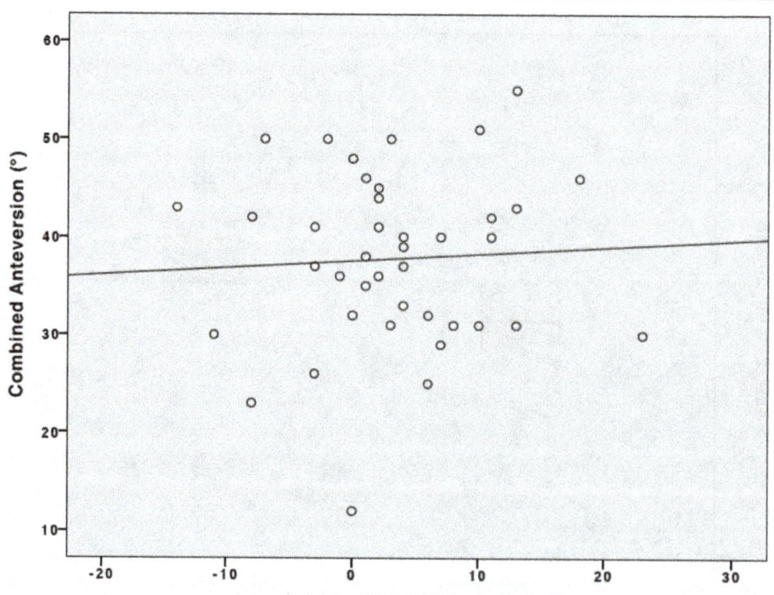

Fig. 4 Scatter plot between combined anteversion values measured with the cup-liner system and anterior pelvic plane values. Linear regression: y = 37.55 + 0.07 * x (R^2 = 0.004, P = 0.71)

In our series, the average postoperative stem antetorsion was 9° ± 10° ranging from 23° of retrotorsion to 31° of antetorsion. These results are similar to those reported in previous studies. Dorr et al. [10] showed with the computer navigation a wide range of positions of uncemented femoral stems ranging from 17° of retroversion to 28° of antetorsion. Pierchon et al. [28] and Wines et al. [29] used a postoperative CT scans reporting a range from 30° of retroversion to 45° of antetorsion of both cemented and uncemented stems. The wide range of position of the stem in terms of torsion is related with the high variability in the geometry of the proximal femur. Because the stem should have the best fit in the bone its position is affected by the patient-specific femoral anatomy.

In our series, we reported an AI value within the targeted range in 92.5% of hips with an average value of 40° ± 6°. Although we reported 3 outliers, two of them were included in the group with varized stem. The range of AI from 30° to 50° suggested by Lewinnek et al. [1] was not related with the value of CCD angle of the stem. However, we believe that cup inclination should be congruent with the neck of the stem [15]. For this reason, we would suggest to use the femoral component to determine intraoperatively the proper AI. The definitive cup should be placed parallel with the horizontal line on the trial head in both axial and coronal plane. Thus, the surgeon is able to provide the coverage of the cup according with the CCD angle of the femoral stem. Our results demonstrated that the group with varized stem had AI values significantly higher than those reported in the group with standard stem (P = 0.007). In this respect, the two outliers of 56° and 58° respectively are acceptable values if associated with a varized stem. In the present study, we did not evaluate the effect of pelvic obliquity in the frontal plane on postoperative AI. However, because of the AI was determined by the CCD angle of the femoral stem, we believe that postoperative AI is not affected by pelvic obliquity.

About the second hypothesis, the combined anteversion value achieved with femur first technique was not affected by preoperative pelvic tilt. Because of the anteversion and inclination of the cup are strongly related with the patient-specific pelvic tilt and spine sagittal balance [20, 30], some authors suggested to use intraoperative navigation taking into account the preoperative pelvic tilt of the patient [31–34]. The "safe zone" suggested by Lewinnek et al. [1] was referred to bony landmarks assuming no tilt of the pelvis. However, in the most of patients the pelvic tilt is not neutral. For this reason, the navigation systems referring to anatomical bony landmarks need to consider the pelvic tilt and correct for their measurements to avoid inaccurate position of the cup. In the present technique, the surgeon did not need to consider the pelvic tilt. The patient was in the lateral position with the pelvis hold without change the patient-specific pelvic tilt and sagittal balance. After the femoral component was fixed in terms of antetorsion and CCD angle, the cup was positioned in a compliant fashion to the stem with the hip in neutral position at 0° of flexion and abduction. Therefore, the cup was positioned according to the stem without tacking into account the preoperative pelvic tilt. In this respect, the cup was positioned according to the functional plane without changing the patient-specific pelvic tilt and spinal sagittal balance. Indeed, our results demonstrated that preoperative APP angle values did not correlate with the combined anteversion values after surgery.

During a THA procedure, the vast majority of surgeons place the prosthetic cup with the native acetabular anteversion and then place the stem achieving the best fit in the femur. Disadvantages of this approach include higher risk of hip dislocation and reduced ROMs due to a suboptimal combined anteversion [35, 36]. To overcome these complications, some authors advocated the use of femur first technique to obtain an optimal combined anteversion. Dorr et al. [10] proposed to perform a cementless THA preparing the femur first with the estimation of antetorsion, and then implanting the cup with computer navigation. Authors recommended a mean combined anteversion of 35° (range, 25° to 45°). On the other hand, Unlu et al. [16] proposed a femur first procedure using the lesser trochanter as a landmark to estimate the femoral component antetorsion. They suggested to estimate intraoperatively the antetorsion of the femoral component by the formula: operative collo-trochanteric angle (defined as the angle between the collo-femoral axis and the lesser trochanter axis) minus 34° (mean lesser trochanteric version). Finally, the position of the cup should be adjusted to provide a mean combined anteversion of 37° (range, 25° to 50°) by internal rotation without hip flexion with patient in lateral decubitus. Finally, Nakashima et al. [11] proposed to measure the stem antetorsion intraoperatively with a goniometer as the angle between the perpendicular to the axis of the tibia hold in vertical position and the neck of the stem. The cup was positioned with 20° of anteversion by using the manufacturer's jig and then it was adjusted according the stem antetorsion to achieve the targeted combined anteversion.

Although previous studies evaluated the effectiveness of femur first technique to achieve a proper combined anteversion [10, 11, 16], to our knowledge, this is the first study demonstrating that a non-computer-based femur first technique could be also used to obtain a proper inclination of the acetabular cup according with the CCD angle of the stem. Indeed, previous studies focused only to achieve a proper combined anteversion trough the femur first procedure. Moreover, we also demonstrated that the postoperative combined anteversion values achieved with this technique are not affected by preoperative APP angle values.

We are aware that the present study is affected by some limitations. First, this case series had no control cases who underwent primary THA with conventional surgical procedure. Therefore, we were not able to ascertain the superiority of femur first technique over a conventional procedure characterized by the implantation of the cup first according anatomical bony landmarks. Further studies should be performed to address this comparison. Second, all patients were operated by a single experienced surgeon. Therefore, further studies should be performed to compare in standardized fashion the outcomes achieved by junior and senior surgeons with this technique. However, in our current practice, this procedure is easily performed by all surgeons of the unit with reliable results. Third, the fixation of uncemented stem requires a stable press fit into the bone, and the implant must adapt to the variable femoral geometry. Therefore, to achieve the desired stem antetorsion could be difficult, and the present findings of antetorsion may not be referred to all commercial designs. For this reason, only two straight femoral stems were used. Moreover, the optimum range for combined anteversion is still controversial. In clinical setting, some authors proposed a range from 25° to 50° [10, 16], whereas others suggested a range form 40° to 60° [11, 37]. The present technique may allow the surgeon to adjust the orientation of the cup basing on stem antetorsion in order to provide a reliable combined antiversion within the range between 25° to 50°. Forth, we used a liner with 10° elevated rim and the definitive combined anteversion was based on the anteversion of the cup-liner system and stem. However the position of the elevated rim was collected in a systematic fashion and the radiographic measurements of AA were corrected for. Fifth, we did not compare the intraoperative estimation of the stem antetorsion by the surgeon with the postoperative radiographic measurements. However, previous studies demonstrated the low accuracy of surgeon's estimation of the stem torsion. Dorr et al. [10] reported that intraoperative estimation by the surgeon had outliers between 6° to 10° and than 10° in 23% of the hips respectively. Hirata et al. [38] demonstrated that the average value of error for the surgeon's intraoperative estimation of the stem anteversion was 7.3° ranging from 11° underestimation to 25° overestimation. Moreover, the aim of the study was to evaluate the combined anteversion and AI values achieved with the femur first procedure.

Conclusions

The femur first technique is a non-computer-based procedure that allows the surgeon to achieve a combined anteversion ranging from 25° to 50° with a cup inclination ranging from 30° to 50°. Moreover, the cup is positioned according to the functional plane of the patient regardless the preoperative pelvic tilt.

Abbreviations

AA: acetabular anteversion; AI: acetabular inclination; APP: anterior pelvic plane; CCD: caput-collum-diaphyseal; HHS: Harris Hip Score; ROM: range of motion; THA: total hip arthroplasty

Acknowledgements

We would thank the Livio Sciutto Foundation for Medical Research (www.fondazione.it). This is a Non-profit Social Organisation that recorded in its database the data of the patients included in the study, with the previous consent of the patients and respecting the current law on the privacy.

Funding

No external funding was received for this study. Livio Sciutto Foundation for Medical Research (www.fondazione.it) provided the payment for the publication fee.

Authors' contributions

GG, ML and VD designed the study protocol. EC and ADR collected the data. Analyses were planned by GG, ML, and UGL and were carried out by ML and UGL. ML and VD wrote the initial draft of the manuscript, which was critically revised by VD and GG. All authors read and approved the final manuscript.

Consent for publication

Not applicable.

Competing interests

One author (GG) is a paid consultant for Zimmer Biomet. Two authors (ML and UGL) are members of the Editorial Board of BMC Musculoskeletal Disorders. None of the other authors have any competing interests.

Author details

[1]Hip Diseases and Joint Replacement Surgery Unit, Humanitas Clinical and Research Centre, Via Alessandro Manzoni 56, 20089 Rozzano, Milan, Italy. [2]Humanitas University, Via Alessandro Manzoni 113, 20089 Rozzano, Milan, Italy. [3]Department of Orthopaedic and Trauma Surgery, Campus Bio-Medico University, Via Alvaro del Portillo 200, 00128 Trigoria, Rome, Italy.

References

1. Lewinnek GE, Lewis JL, Tarr R, Compere CL, Zimmerman JR. Dislocations after total hip-replacement arthroplasties. J Bone Joint Surg Am. 1978;60(2):217–20.
2. Del Schutte H, Jr., Lipman AJ, Bannar SM, Livermore JT, Ilstrup D, Morrey BF. Effects of acetabular abduction on cup wear rates in total hip arthroplasty. J Arthroplast 1998;13(6):621-626.
3. Kennedy JG, Rogers WB, Soffe KE, Sullivan RJ, Griffen DG, Sheehan LJ. Effect of acetabular component orientation on recurrent dislocation, pelvic osteolysis, polyethylene wear, and component migration. J Arthroplast. 1998;13(5):530–4.
4. Kummer FJ, Shah S, Iyer S, DiCesare PE. The effect of acetabular cup orientations on limiting hip rotation. J Arthroplast. 1999;14(4):509–13.

5. Biedermann R, Tonin A, Krismer M, Rachbauer F, Eibl G, Stockl B. Reducing the risk of dislocation after total hip arthroplasty: the effect of orientation of the acetabular component. J Bone Joint Surg Br. 2005;87(6):762–9.
6. Maynard MJ, Ranawac CS. Modern techniques of cemented total hip arthroplasty. Tech Orthop. 1991;6:17-25.
7. Widmer KH, Zurfluh B. Compliant positioning of total hip components for optimal range of motion. J Orthop Res. 2004;22(4):815–21.
8. Yoshimine F. The safe-zones for combined cup and neck anteversions that fulfill the essential range of motion and their optimum combination in total hip replacements. J Biomech. 2006;39(7):1315–23.
9. Hisatome T, Doi H. Theoretically optimum position of the prosthesis in total hip arthroplasty to fulfill the severe range of motion criteria due to neck impingement. J Orthop Sci. 2011;16(2):229–37.
10. Dorr LD, Malik A, Dastane M, Wan Z. Combined anteversion technique for total hip arthroplasty. Clin Orthop Relat Res. 2009;467(1):119–27.
11. Nakashima Y, Hirata M, Akiyama M, Itokawa T, Yamamoto T, Motomura G, et al. Combined anteversion technique reduced the dislocation in cementless total hip arthroplasty. Int Orthop. 2014;38(1):27–32.
12. Sendtner E, Muller M, Winkler R, Worner M, Grifka J, Renkawitz T. Femur first in hip arthroplasty–the concept of combined anteversion. Z Orthop Unfall. 2010;148(2):185–90.
13. Widmer KH. Containment versus impingement: finding a compromise for cup placement in total hip arthroplasty. Int Orthop. 2007;31(Suppl 1):S29–33.
14. Widmer KH, Majewski M. The impact of the CCD-angle on range of motion and cup positioning in total hip arthroplasty. Clin Biomech (Bristol, Avon). 2005;20(7):723–8.
15. Sarmiento A, Ebramzadeh E, Gogan WJ, McKellop HA. Cup containment and orientation in cemented total hip arthroplasties. J Bone Joint Surg Br. 1990;72(6):996–1002.
16. Unlu MC, Kesmezacar H, Kantarci F, Unlu B, Botanlioglu H. Intraoperative estimation of femoral anteversion in cementless total hip arthroplasty using the lesser trochanter. Arch Orthop Trauma Surg. 2011;131(9):1317–23.
17. Grappiolo G, Loppini M, Longo UG, Traverso F, Mazziotta G, Denaro V. Trabecular metal augments for the Management of Paprosky Type III defects without pelvic discontinuity. J Arthroplast. 2015;30(6):1024–9.
18. Harris WH. Advances in surgical technique for total hip replacement: without and with osteotomy of the greater trochanter. Clin Orthop Relat Res. 1980;146:188–204.
19. Zini R, Longo UG, de Benedetto M, Loppini M, Carraro A, Maffulli N, et al. Arthroscopic management of primary synovial chondromatosis of the hip. Arthroscopy. 2013;29(3):420–6.
20. Lazennec JY, Brusson A, Rousseau MA. Hip-spine relations and sagittal balance clinical consequences. Eur Spine J. 2011;20(Suppl 5):686–98.
21. Lazennec JY, Brusson A, Dominique F, Rousseau MA, Pour AE. Offset and anteversion reconstruction after cemented and uncemented total hip arthroplasty: an evaluation with the low-dose EOS system comparing two- and three-dimensional imaging. Int Orthop. 2015;39(7):1259–67.
22. Lazennec JY, Rousseau MA, Rangel A, Gorin M, Belicourt C, Brusson A, et al. Pelvis and total hip arthroplasty acetabular component orientations in sitting and standing positions: measurements reproductibility with EOS imaging system versus conventional radiographies. Orthop Traumatol Surg Res. 2011;97(4):373–80.
23. Than P, Szuper K, Somoskeoy S, Warta V, Illes T. Geometrical values of the normal and arthritic hip and knee detected with the EOS imaging system. Int Orthop. 2012;36(6):1291–7.
24. Lazennec JY, Rousseau MA, Brusson A, Folinais D, Amel M, Clarke I, et al. Total hip prostheses in standing, sitting and squatting positions: an overview of our 8 years practice using the EOS imaging technology. Open Orthop J. 2015;9:26–44.
25. Boese CK, Dargel J, Oppermann J, Eysel P, Scheyerer MJ, Bredow J, et al. The femoral neck-shaft angle on plain radiographs: a systematic review. Skelet Radiol. 2016;45(1):19–28.
26. Sultan PG, Tan V, Lai M, Garino JP. Independent contribution of elevated-rim acetabular liner and femoral head size to the stability of total hip implants. J Arthroplast. 2002;17(3):289–92.
27. Cobb TK, Morrey BF, Ilstrup DM. The elevated-rim acetabular liner in total hip arthroplasty: relationship to postoperative dislocation. J Bone Joint Surg Am. 1996;78(1):80–6.
28. Pierchon F, Pasquier G, Cotten A, Fontaine C, Clarisse J, Duquennoy A. Causes of dislocation of total hip arthroplasty. CT study of component alignment. J Bone Joint Surg Br. 1994;76(1):45–8.
29. Wines AP, McNicol D. Computed tomography measurement of the accuracy of component version in total hip arthroplasty. J Arthroplast. 2006;21(5):696–701.
30. Loppini M, Longo UG, Ragucci P, Trenti N, Balzarini L, Grappiolo G. Analysis of the pelvic functional orientation in the Sagittal plane: a radiographic study with EOS 2D/3D technology. J Arthroplast. 2017;32(3):1027–32.
31. Babisch JW, Layher F, Amiot LP. The rationale for tilt-adjusted acetabular cup navigation. J Bone Joint Surg Am. 2008;90(2):357–65.
32. DiGioia AM, Hafez MA, Jaramaz B, Levison TJ, Moody JE. Functional pelvic orientation measured from lateral standing and sitting radiographs. Clin Orthop Relat Res. 2006;453:272–6.
33. Lembeck B, Mueller O, Reize P, Wuelker N. Pelvic tilt makes acetabular cup navigation inaccurate. Acta Orthop. 2005;76(4):517–23.
34. Parratte S, Argenson JN. Validation and usefulness of a computer-assisted cup-positioning system in total hip arthroplasty. A prospective, randomized, controlled study. J Bone Joint Surg Am. 2007;89(3):494–9.
35. D'Lima DD, Chen PC, Colwell CW Jr. Optimizing acetabular component position to minimize impingement and reduce contact stress. J Bone Joint Surg Am. 2001;83(Suppl 2 Pt 2):87–91.
36. D'Lima DD, Urquhart AG, Buehler KO, Walker RH, Colwell CW Jr. The effect of the orientation of the acetabular and femoral components on the range of motion of the hip at different head-neck ratios. J Bone Joint Surg Am. 2000;82(3):315–21.
37. Jolles BM, Zangger P, Leyvraz PF. Factors predisposing to dislocation after primary total hip arthroplasty: a multivariate analysis. J Arthroplast. 2002;17(3):282–8.
38. Hirata M, Nakashima Y, Ohishi M, Hamai S, Hara D, Iwamoto Y. Surgeon error in performing intraoperative estimation of stem anteversion in cementless total hip arthroplasty. J Arthroplast. 2013;28(9):1648–53.

The risk factors of failed reimplantation arthroplasty for periprosthetic hip infection

Shun-Wun Jhan[1,3], Yu-Der Lu[1,3], Mel S. Lee[1,3], Chen-Hsiang Lee[2,3], Jun-Wen Wang[1,3] and Feng-Chih Kuo[1,3*]

Abstract

Background: Two-stage reimplantation arthroplasty is one of the standard treatments for chronic periprosthetic joint infection (PJI). Scanty data exist regarding the risk factors for failure after two-stage reimplantation for periprosthetic hip infection. The purpose of this study was to investigate and identify the risk factors associated with failure after two-stage reimplantation hip arthroplasty.

Methods: Sixty-two patients with hip PJI treated with a two-stage reimplantation protocol at our institution from 2005 to 2012 were reviewed. Patients requiring medical treatment or reoperation for recurrent infection were defined as treatment failure. A multivariate Cox proportional hazards model was used to analyze the risk factors associated with treatment failure.

Results: Of the 62 patients, 11 (17.7%) patients had developed reinfection after the two-stage reimplantation with a mean follow-up of 5.7 years. The implant survival was 82.2% (95% confidence interval [CI] 75.19–92.55) at 10 years. Multivariate analysis revealed BMI ≥30 kg/m^2 (hazard ratio [HR] 9.16; 95% CI 1.51–55.3; $p = 0.0158$), liver cirrhosis (HR 6.39; 95% CI 1.09–37.4; $p = 0.0398$), gram-negative organism (HR 5.68; 95% CI 1.18–27.4; $p = 0.0303$), and presence of sinus tract (HR 18.2; 95% CI 2.15–153; $p = 0.0077$) as the independent risk factors for treatment failure.

Conclusions: We found obesity, liver cirrhosis, gram-negative organism, and the presence of sinus tract were significantly related to the risks of failure after reimplantation arthroplasties.

Keywords: Reimplantation, Hip arthroplasty, Periprosthetic joint infection, Risk factor

Background

Infection is the third leading cause for revision after total hip arthroplasty (THA) [1] and the most common cause of failure after revision THA [2]. The incidence of periprosthetic joint infection (PJI) following THA varied from 0.5 to 2.2% [3]. Hip PJI also result in huge economic burden and medical resource utilization in the United States and other countries [4].

The two-stage reimplantation arthroplasty is one of the standard treatments for chronic infected hip prosthesis in the United States and many countries [5]. The goals of successful treatment included eradication of infection and restoration of function. Usually it can reach more than 90% successful rate of infection eradication [6]. However, recurrence and repetitive infections may cause troublesome complications such as bone loss, poor soft tissue integrity, prolonged and complex operation, and physical and psychological disabilities.

Several risk factors related to PJI in THA and revision THA have been well documented in previous literatures, including age [7], male [8], obesity [9], comorbidities with rheumatoid arthritis [10], diabetes [11] liver cirrhosis [12]. However, few studies have been done to analyze the risk factors of failed reimplantation protocol [6, 13]. The purpose of this study was to investigate the patient-related risk factors associated with treatment failure following the reimplantation protocol in hip PJI.

Methods

After Institutional Review Board approval, we retrospectively reviewed patients who underwent two-staged reimplantation arthroplasties for periprosthetic joint infection (PJI) of hips between January 2005 and December 2012. Eligible patients with a minimum follow-up for 2 years

* Correspondence: fongchikuo@cgmh.org.tw
[1]Department of Orthopaedic Surgery, Kaohsiung Chang Gung Memorial Hospital, No. 123, Ta Pei Road, Niao Sung Dist, Kaohsiung City 833, Taiwan
[3]Chang Gung University College of Medicine, Kaohsiung, Taiwan
Full list of author information is available at the end of the article

were included. The exclusion criteria were patients with incomplete medical data, unconfirmed diagnosis of PJI, or less than 2 years follow-up.

PJI was confirmed according to the Musculoskeletal Infection Society (MSIS) guidelines [14] with one major criteria or three out of five minor criteria. All procedures were performed through a posterolateral approach. At the first stage, it included excision of sinus tracts, removal of prosthesis, radical surgical debridement, and implantation of antibiotic-loaded cement beads. The regimen of antibiotics in the bone cement was determined according the culture results from preoperative joint aspiration or previous culture report. If the infecting microorganism could not be known at the time of resection arthroplasty, empirical combination of 2–4 g vancomycin and 2–4 g piperacillin per 40 g package of bone cement was used. During surgery, at least three sets of tissue specimens were sent for culture. Further debridement or exchange to sensitive antibiotic-loaded cement beads may be needed if the infection could not be controlled during the interim stage. According to an infectious disease specialist suggestion, culture-specific parenteral antibiotics were given postoperatively for 4 weeks, followed by oral antibiotics for 2 weeks. The timing of the second stage reimplantation was based on clinical condition and laboratory data. Reimplantation was performed after an at least 2-week antibiotic holiday without elevation of erythrocyte sedimentation rate (ESR) and C-reactive protein (CRP). In patients with other underlying diseases such as gout, autoimmune disease or other chronic diseases, the ESR and serum CRP level may not return to normal. In these patients, we performed the second reimplantation according to the clinical condition combined with a trend of decreased ESR and CRP levels after discontinuing oral antibiotics.

We divided our patients into successful and reinfection groups. The successful group was defined as functioning and stable joints without any evidence of reinfection. The reinfection group included patients who had recurrent infection, needed antibiotics suppression, or required reoperation for PJI.

Multiple potential predictive variables were collected from medical record, including patients' characteristics, comorbidities, causative organism and the operation-related factors. Minimal follow-up was at least 2 years after reimplantation.

Statistical analysis

Categorical variables are expressed as count and percentage, and continuous data as mean ± standard deviation (SD) and range. Proportional hazard regression univariate and multivariate analysis were performed to assess the association of clinically interesting covariates with the risk of recurrent infection. Hazard ratios and 95% confidence intervals (CIs) for the risk of recurrent infection of the exposure variables were reported. The survival rate free of infection was estimated with the use of Kaplan-Meier survival curve. The survival end point was defined as recurrent infection when repeated operations were necessary after definite reimplantation. Log-rank test was performed for Kaplan-Meier survival analysis between significant variables. P values < 0.05 were considered statistically significant. Statistical analysis was completed by using software (version 14.12.0; MedCalc, Ostend, Belgium).

Results

A total of 62 PJI in 62 patients (43 males and 19 females) were included. The mean age at the time of first stage operation was 57 ± 14 years (range: 27–86 years). The mean BMI was 25.3 ± 4.6 kg/m^2 (range: 17.7–39.8 kg/m^2). The mean interim period before reimplantation was 20 ± 15.8 weeks (range: 8–104 weeks). The mean follow-up was 5.7 ± 2.4 years (range: 2–10 years). The overall successful rate was 82.3%. Eleven hips (17.7%) had recurrence of PJI and required subsequent surgeries. Two of them underwent repeated two-stage reimplantation. One patient received debridement-antibiotic-implant retention. Eight patients had permanent resection arthroplasty procedures, including two patients with HIV (human immunodeficiency virus) and continuous use of drug abuse after reimplantation.

Table 1 presented univariate risk factors for treatment failure. Significant risk factors were BMI≥30 kg/m^2 (HR 4.92; 95% CI 1.50–16.1; $p = 0.0085$), illicit drug abuse (HR 10.1; 95% CI 2.11–48.0; $p = 0.0037$), liver cirrhosis (HR 7.94; 95% CI 2.39–26.2; $p = 0.0007$), gram-negative organism (HR 4.83; 95 CI 1.40–16.6; $p = 0.0124$), the presence of a sinus tract (HR 9.24; 95% CI 2.66–32.0; $p = 0.0005$), repeated debridement between stage (HR 13.7; 95% CI 1.75–107; $p = 0.0125$) and operation time>4 h (HR 8.47; 95% CI 1.08-66.3; $p = 0.0419$). In the multivariate Cox regression analysis, the following factors were independent risks for treatment failure: BMI≥30 kg/m^2 (HR 9.16; 95% CI 1.51–55.3; $p = 0.0158$), liver cirrhosis (HR 6.39; 95% CI 1.09–37.4; $p = 0.0398$), gram-negative organism (HR 5.68; 95% CI 1.18–27.4; $p = 0.0303$), and presence of sinus tract (HR 18.2; 95% CI 2.15–153; $p = 0.0077$) (Table 2).

Among the reinfection group, one patient was considered a relapse case because of the same pathogenic organism with initial microbiology. One patient still had had a negative culture result at the interim stage and the reinfection period. The other 9 patients in the reinfection group had different culture results from initial microorganisms (Table 3).

Table 4 showed the drug susceptibilities of the gram-negative microorganisms. Among the success group, two patients had *Escherichia coli* infection. One was treated

Table 1 Univariate analysis for risk factors associated with reinfection of two-stage revision THAData are mean (range) or number (%) of episodes

	Variable	Success ($N = 51$)		Reinfection ($N = 11$)		HR (95% CI)	*p* value
	Age (years)	57.8	(27–86)	53.2	(42–79)	0.97 (0.93–1.02)	0.3621
	Male	36	(70%)	7	(63%)	1.44 (0.42–4.93)	0.5587
Patient characteristics	BMI (kg/m^2)						
	<30	43	(84%)	5	(46%)	–	
	≥30	8	(16%)	6	(54%)	4.92 (1.50–16.1)	0.0085*
	Smoking	17	(33%)	5	(45%)	1.55 (0.47–5.11)	0.4641
	ASA						
	2	28	(55%)	3	(27%)	–	
	3	23	(45%)	8	(73%)	2.97 (0.78–11.2)	0.1077
	Diabetes mellitus	8	(16%)	2	(18%)	1.24 (0.26–5.78)	0.7764
	Hepatitis	10	(20%)	4	(36%)	2.16 (0.63–7.40)	0.2176
Medical diseases	Gout	6	(12%)	3	(27%)	2.27 (0.60–8.57)	0.2257
	CKD	5	(10%)	1	(9%)	1.00 (0.12–7.86)	0.9987
	ESRD	1	(2%)	1	(9%)	3.96 (0.50–31.2)	0.1910
	Drug abuse	0	(0%)	2	(18%)	10.1 (2.11–48.0)	0.0037*
	Liver cirrhosis	4	(9%)	6	(54%)	7.94 (2.39–26.2)	0.0007*
	Autoimmune disease	3	(6%)	1	(9%)	1.81 (0.22–14.4)	0.5579
	Staphylococcus aureus	7	(13.7%)	2	(18.1%)	1.43 (0.31–6.67)	0.6425
	Coagulase-negative Staphylococcus	1	(1.9%)	1	(9%)	3.46 (0.43–27.7)	0.2413
Microbiology	Methicillin-resistant organism	10	(19.6%)	1	(9%)	0.43 (0.05–3.40)	0.4287
	Gram-negative organism	4	(9%)	4	(36.3)	4.83 (1.40–16.6)	0.0124*
	Polymicrobial organism	4	(9%)	1	(9%)	1.57 (0.20–12.3)	0.6651
	Culture-negative	16	(31.3%)	2	(18.1%)	0.49 (0.10–2.28)	0.3671
	Presence of sinus tract	6	(12%)	7	(63%)	9.24 (2.66–32.0)	0.0005*
	Interim period less than 3 months	9	(17%)	3	(27%)	1.78 (0.47–6.74)	0.3949
Operation-related factors	Repeated debridement between stage	18	(35%)	10	(91%)	13.7 (1.75–107)	0.0125*
	Perioperative Blood loss >1500 ml	18	(35%)	5	(45%)	1.37 (0.41–4.49)	0.6031
	Revision operative time >4 h	26	(51%)	10	(91%)	8.47 (1.08–66.3)	0.0419*
	Allograft use in revision	42	(82%)	9	(82%)	1.04 (0.22–4.83)	0.9586

BMI body mass index, *ASA* American Society of Anesthesiologist, *ESRD* end stage renal disease, *CKD* chronic kidney disease, *HR* hazard ratio, *CI* confidence interval
*A *p* value of <0.05 was considered to be statistically significant

Table 2 Multivariate analysis for risk factors associated with reinfection after two-stage revision THA

Variables	Adjusted HR	95% CI	*p* value
Body mass index ≥30 kg/m^2	9.16	1.51–55.3	0.0158*
Drug abuse	1.66	0.14–19.4	0.6832
Liver cirrhosis	6.39	1.09–37.4	0.0398*
Gram-negative organism	5.68	1.18–27.4	0.0303*
Presence of sinus tract	18.2	2.15–153	0.0077*
Repeated debridement between stage	5.64	0.59–53.1	0.1303
Revision operative time >4 h	1.00	0.08–12.5	0.9957

HR hazard ratio, *CI* confidence interval
*A *p* value of <0.05 was considered to be statistically significant

Table 3 Microbiology of the reinfection group

Case	Initial	Reinfection
1	*Coagulase-negative Staphylococcus*	MSSA
2	Culture-negative	*Viridans streptococcus*
3	Polymicrobial	MSSA
4	MSSA	*Klebsiella pneumonia*
5	MRSA	Polymicrobial
6	Culture-negative	Culture-negative
7	*Enterobacter Cloacae*	MRSA
8	*E. coli*	*Pseudomonas aeruginosa*
9	MSSA	*Pseudomonas aeruginosa*
10	*E. coli*	*E. coli*
11	ESBL-producing *E. coli*	*E. coli*

MSSA Methicillin-sensitive *Staphylococcus aureus*, *MRSA* Methicillin-resistant Staphylococcus aureus, *E. coli Escherichia coli*, *ESBL* extended-spectrum β-lactamase

with cefazolin and the other was treated with cefuroxime. In the patient with *Pseudomonas aeruginosa* infection, piperacillin was administrated during hospitalization and oral ciprofloxacin was prescribed after discharge. The patient with *Klebsiella pneumoniae* infection was treated with piperacillin/tazobactam. Among the reinfection group, one patient with *Escherichia coli* infection was treated with cefazolin. Two patients with *Enterobacter Cloacae* and *E. coli* infection showed resistance to cefazolin and were treated with ceftazidime. In a patient with extended-spectrum beta-lactamase-producing *Escherichia coli* infection, imipenem was administrated.

The 10-year survivorship of the implant with infection-free after two-stage reimplantation was 82.2% (95% CI 75.19–92.55) (Fig. 1). The Log-rank test for Kaplan-Meier survival analysis for risk factor of treatment failure showed a significantly lower survival rate in obese patients (55.1%; $p = 0.0034$, Fig. 2), liver cirrhosis (30%; $p = 0.0001$, Fig. 3), gram-negative bacillus (50%; $p = 0.0050$, Fig. 4) and presence of sinus tract (43.1%; $p < 0.0001$, Fig. 5).

Discussion

In this representative cohort of 62 patients who underwent two-stage reimplantation arthroplasties for PJI, the 10-year survival rate for implant with infection-free was 82.2 % (95% CI 75.19–92.55). After considering risk factors for reinfection, we found patients with BMI≥30 kg/m^2, liver cirrhosis, gram-negative bacteria and the presence of sinus tract had significantly higher risks for treatment failure.

The infection eradication of two-stage exchange arthroplasty has been reported to be around 90 % in other literatures. Sanchez-Sotelo et al. reviewed 168 patients with infected THA who underwent two-staged revision THA and found the rate of reinfection was 7.1% at a mean follow-up of 7 years [15]. Haddad et al. followed up 50 patients treated according to a two-staged protocol and found the rate of reinfection was 8% at a mean follow-up of 5.8 years [16]. Chen et al. retrospectively reviewed 155 patients (157 hips) who received two-staged revision THA for hip PJI and the infection-free successful rate was 91.7% at an average of 9.7 years [6]. In our study, the reinfection rate was 17.7% at a mean follow-up of 5.7 years, which was relative high than previous studies.

Obesity had been associated with PJI following THA and revision THA [7, 17]. Spiegl et al. reported the risk factors for failed two-stage procedure after chronic hip PJI in 26 patients. They found a high BMI was one of risk factors for treatment failure [18]. In another matched-control

Table 4 The drug susceptibilities of gram-negative microorganisms

	Cefazolin	Cefuroxime	Ceftazidime	Ciprofloxacin	Gentamicin	Piperacillin	Piperacillin/ tazobactam	Imipenem	Sulfamethoxazole-Trimethoprim
Success group									
E. coli	S[a]	S	S	S	S	S	S	S	S
E. coli	I	S[a]	S	S	R	R	S	S	R
Pseudomonas aeruginosa	R	R	S	S[a]	S	S[a]	S[a]	S	R
Klebsiella pneumoniae	S	S	S	S	S	S	S	S	S
Reinfection group									
Enterobacter Cloacae	R	R	S[a]	S	S	S	S	S	R
E. coli	R	S	S[a]	S	S	R	S	S	S
E. coli	S[a]	S	S	S	S	R	S	S	S
E. coli – ESBL	R	R	R	R	R	R	S	S[a]	R

E. coli Escherichia coli, *ESBL extended-spectrum β-lactamase*
[a]means the systemic antibiotic treatment

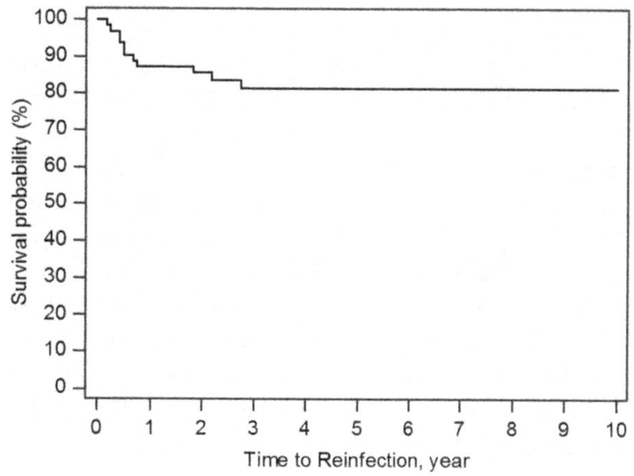

Fig. 1 Kaplan-Meier survival for implant from two-stage revision total hip arthroplasty to reinfection. The 10-year survivorship with infection-free was 82.2% (95% CI 75.19–92.55)

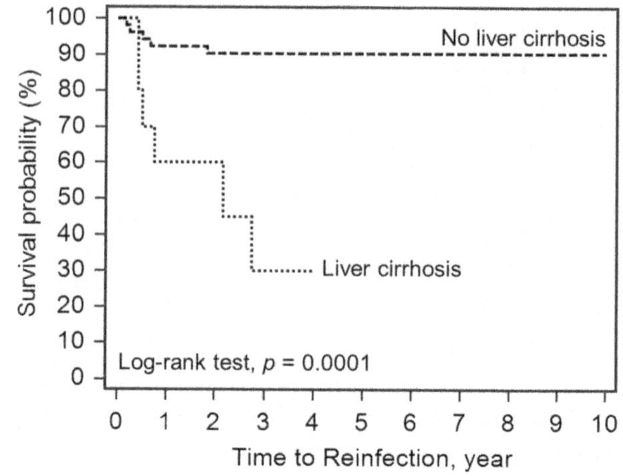

Fig. 3 Log-rank test for Kaplan-Meier survival analysis in liver cirrhosis. The 10-year survivorship with infection-free was 90.4% in patients without liver cirrhosis and 30% in liver cirrhotic patients

study compared with non-obese patients (BMI<30 kg/m^2), morbidly obese patients (BMI≥40 kg/m^2) had increased rate of reinfection following revision THA for periprosthetic joint infection [19]. In these studies, they used univariate variables for risk factor analysis. It may be interfered by other confounding factors. Tikhilov et al. used total risk score to calculate the risk of infection recurrence after two-stage procedure. They found BMI was identified as one of main factors related to infection recurrence [13]. Our study agreed with Tikhilov et al. We used multivariate analysis and found BMI≥30 kg/m^2 was associated with an increased risk for treatment failure following two-stage reimplantation.

Liver cirrhosis was another significant risk factor of treatment failure in this study. In a retrospective study of 38 cirrhotic patients after hip arthroplasties, liver cirrhosis had been associated with PJI, which was the most common cause of treatment failure [20]. In another cohort of 20 cirrhotic patients with PJI undergoing two-stage reimplantation, a higher risk of recurrent infection was noted in these cirrhotic patients with decompensated liver function [12] Chen et al. also mentioned liver cirrhosis was an independent risk factor of recurrent infection [6]. Patients with liver cirrhosis had decreased ability to activate reticuloendothelial system, neutrophil mobilization and phagocytic activity [21]. Thus, their bactericidal activity is diminished. The immune compromised status of liver

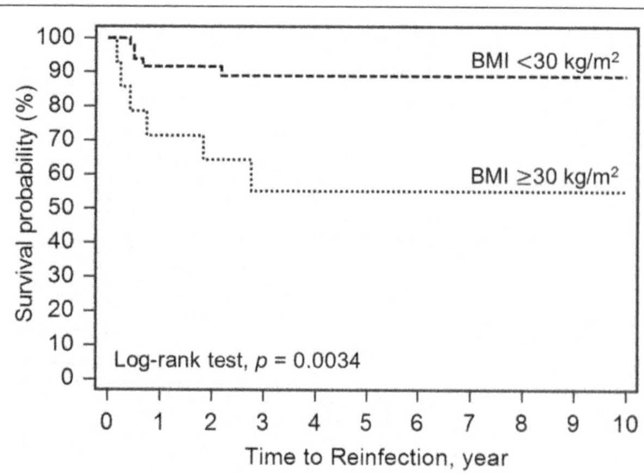

Fig. 2 Log-rank test for Kaplan-Meier survival analysis in BMI. The 10-year survivorship with infection-free was 55.1% in the patients with BMI ≥30 kg/m^2 versus 88.9% in those with BMI <30 kg/m^2

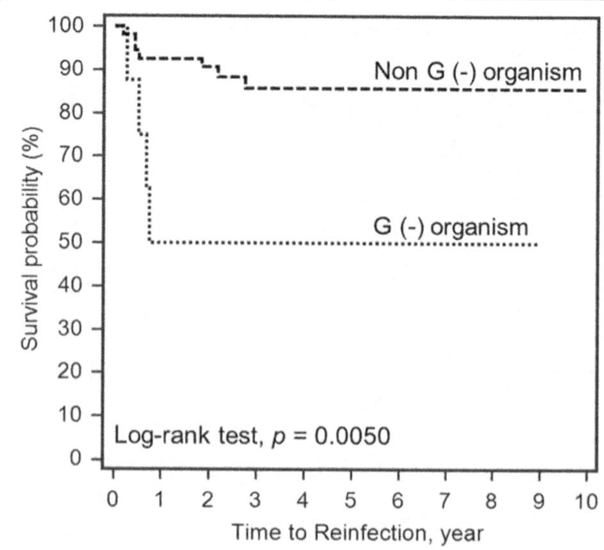

Fig. 4 Log-rank test for Kaplan-Meier survival analysis in PJI caused by Gram-negative organisms. The 10-year survivorship with infection-free was 85.8% in patients without gram negative PJI and 50% in patients with gram negative PJI

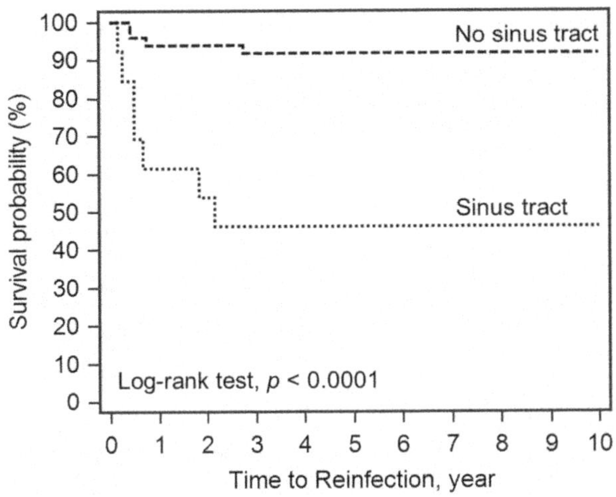

Fig. 5 Log-rank test for Kaplan-Meier survival analysis in presence of sinus tract. The 10-year survivorship with infection-free was 43.1 and 91.2% in patients with and without sinus tract

cirrhosis patients should be more stringently monitored before reimplantation to decrease chance of treatment failure.

Little literature exists with regard to the outcome of PJI caused by gram-negative organisms. Hsieh et al. reported 16 patients with GN-PJI underwent two-stage exchanged arthroplasty. The 2-year survival rate free of treatment failure for patients with GN PJI was 87% (95% CI 80–99) for two-stage exchange. They also found a similar outcome to those patients treated for gram-positive PJI [22]. Zmistowski et al. reported a 52% overall success in treating GN-PJI, which was consistent with our findings [23]. We had 8 GN-PJI with a 50% failure rate by the two-stage reimplantation protocol. In the success group, two patients had *Escherichia coli*, one had *Pseudomonas aeruginosa* and one had *Klebsiella pneumoniae*. In the reinfection group, two patients had *Escherichia coli*, one had *Enterobacter cloacae* and one had extended-spectrum β-lactamases (ESBL)-producing *Escherichia coli*. Patients with GN organism PJI had 5.8 times of treatment failure as compared with other organisms. We thought the low successful rate might be related to antibiotics in the bone cement. In our study, we used 2–4 g piperacillin in a 40–g bone cement. But three patients in the reinfection group had the drug susceptibilities showing resistance to piperacillin. Piperacillin-loaded bone cement was unable to provide antibacterial duration more than 24 h against the gram-positive and gram-negative microorganisms in vitro study [24]. Therefore, we have used ceftazidime instead of piperacillin for better local antibiotic release from the bone cement for the treatment of gram-negative PJI in our institute since January 2015. Further studies should be conducted to compare the ceftazidime and piperacillin as the local antibiotic regimen in the treatment of periprosthetic hip infection.

Presence of sinus tract as an independent risk factor for treatment failure in two-stage revision is scanty reported. Betsch et al. found presence of sinus tract was a risk factor for treatment failure in univariate analysis (HR 2.35; 95 % CI 1.10–5.0; $p = 0.02$) but not an independent risk factor in multivariate analysis [25]. In our study, we found presence of sinus tract was an independent risk factor for treatment failure (HR 18.2; 95% CI 2.15–153; $p = 0.0077$) after multivariate analysis and had lower 10-year survival rate than patients without sinus tract. In this series, sinus tracts and the superficial contaminated layers were excised at the first-stage surgery and all the surgical wounds could be closed by primary suture. No further plastic surgery was involved to perform soft tissue coverage and dead space management. The discharge sinus and fistula tract are often combined with abscess cavity and scarred tissue that are difficult to heal and collapse. If the dead space is not treated by plastic surgeons, patients with liver disease or gram negative rods infection will have wound healing problems and haematoma after surgery. It is becoming evident that adequate soft tissue coverage, usually with muscle flaps to occult the dead space after radical debridement, is paramount to the success of two stage revisions for periprosthetic joint infection [26]. The suboptimal management of dead space could explain the high percentage of repeated debridement (up to 45%) and an increased reinfection rate in relation to the average in our patients.

There were limitations of our study. First, this was a retrospective study. Second, our cohort is small and is derived from a tertiary referral medical center. The complexity of our cases may be higher than other reports. Third, the mean follow-up was 5.7 years (range: 2–10 years) that the reinfection rate might be accumulated with longer term of follow up. Fourth, the choice and the duration of parenteral and local antibiotics were not standardized. Another limitation to keep in mind is that most medical centers use gentamicin containing cement, rather than piperacillin or ceftazidime in bone cement, as their local antibiotic regimen and may produce a different outcome.

Conclusions

The 10-year survivorship of implant with infection-free after two-stage revision THA was 82.2%, which was inferior to that of previous reports. Patients with obesity, liver cirrhosis, gram-negative organism and presence of sinus tract had a significant impact of the risk of reinfection.

Abbreviations

BMI: Body mass index; CIs: Confidence intervals; CRP: C-reactive protein; *E. coli*: *Escherichia coli*; ESBL: Extended-spectrum β-lactamases; ESR: Erythrocyte sedimentation rate; GN: Gram-negative; HIV: Human immunodeficiency virus; HR: Hazard ratios; MRSA: Methicillin-resistant *Staphylococcus aureus*; MSSA: Methicillin-sensitive *Staphylococcus aureus*; PJI: Periprosthetic joint infection; SD: Standard deviation; THA: Total hip arthroplasty

Acknowledgements

The authors would like to acknowledge Prof. Hsueh-Wen Chang for help with the statistical analyses.

Funding

None.

Authors' contributions

SWJ have participated in drafting the manuscript and collecting data. FCK have been involved in designing this study and analyzing data. YDL and CHL have contributed to conception of the study. MSL and JWW have provided critical revisions of the manuscript. All authors read and approved the final manuscript.

Competing interests

The authors declare that they have no competing interests.

Consent for publication

Not applicable.

Author details

[1]Department of Orthopaedic Surgery, Kaohsiung Chang Gung Memorial Hospital, No. 123, Ta Pei Road, Niao Sung Dist, Kaohsiung City 833, Taiwan. [2]Division of Infectious Diseases, Department of Internal Medicine, Kaohsiung Chang Gung Memorial Hospital, Kaohsiung, Taiwan. [3]Chang Gung University College of Medicine, Kaohsiung, Taiwan.

References

1. Ulrich SD, Seyler TM, Bennett D, Delanois RE, Saleh KJ, Thongtrangan I, et al. Total hip arthroplasties: what are the reasons for revision? Int Orthop. 2008; 32(5):597–604.
2. Jafari SM, Coyle C, Mortazavi SM, Sharkey PF, Parvizi J. Revision hip arthroplasty: infection is the most common cause of failure. Clin Orthop Relat Res. 2010;468(8):2046–51.
3. Ong KL, Kurtz SM, Lau E, Bozic KJ, Berry DJ, Parvizi J. Prosthetic joint infection risk after total hip arthroplasty in the Medicare population. J Arthroplast. 2009;24(6 Suppl):105–9.
4. Kasch R, Assmann G, Merk S, Barz T, Melloh M, Hofer A, et al. Economic analysis of two-stage septic revision after total hip arthroplasty: what are the relevant costs for the hospital's orthopedic department? BMC Musculoskelet Disord. 2016;17:112.
5. Hanssen AD, Spangehl MJ. Treatment of the infected hip replacement. Clin Orthop Relat Res. 2004;420:63–71.
6. Chen SY, Hu CC, Chen CC, Chang YH, Hsieh PH. Two-stage revision Arthroplasty for Periprosthetic hip infection: mean follow-up of ten years. Biomed Res Int. 2015;2015:345475.
7. Kurtz SM, Lau E, Schmier J, Ong KL, Zhao K, Parvizi J. Infection burden for hip and knee arthroplasty in the United States. J Arthroplast. 2008;23(7):984–91.
8. Prokopetz JJ, Losina E, Bliss RL, Wright J, Baron JA, Katz JN. Risk factors for revision of primary total hip arthroplasty: a systematic review. BMC Musculoskelet Disord. 2012;13:251.
9. Malinzak RA, Ritter MA, Berend ME, Meding JB, Olberding EM, Davis KE. Morbidly obese, diabetic, younger, and unilateral joint arthroplasty patients have elevated total joint arthroplasty infection rates. J Arthroplast. 2009;24(6 Suppl):84–8.
10. Moucha CS, Clyburn TA, Evans RP, Prokuski L. Modifiable risk factors for surgical site infection. Instr Course Lect. 2011;60:557–64.
11. Maradit Kremers H, Lewallen LW, Mabry TM, Berry DJ, Berbari EF, Osmon DR. Diabetes mellitus, hyperglycemia, hemoglobin A1C and the risk of prosthetic joint infections in total hip and knee arthroplasty. J Arthroplast. 2015;30(3):439–43.
12. Hsieh PH, Ueng SW, Lee MS, Shih HN, Huang KC. Prosthetic hip infection in patients with liver cirrhosis: an outcome analysis. Int J Infect Dis. 2010;14(12): e1054–9.
13. Tikhilov R, Bozhkova S, Denisov A, Labutin D, Shubnyakov I, Razorenov V, et al. Risk factors and a prognostic model of hip periprosthetic infection recurrence after surgical treatment using articulating and non-articulating spacers. Int Orthop. 2016;40(7):1381–7.
14. Parvizi J, Gehrke T. Definition of periprosthetic joint infection. J Arthroplast. 2014;29(7):1331.
15. Sanchez-Sotelo J, Berry DJ, Hanssen AD, Cabanela ME. Midterm to long-term followup of staged reimplantation for infected hip arthroplasty. Clin Orthop Relat Res. 2009;467(1):219–24.
16. Haddad FS, Muirhead-Allwood SK, Manktelow AR, Bacarese-Hamilton I. Two-stage uncemented revision hip arthroplasty for infection. J Bone Joint Surg Br. 2000;82(5):689–94.
17. Bozic KJ, Kurtz SM, Lau E, Ong K, Vail TP, Berry DJ. The epidemiology of revision total hip arthroplasty in the United States. J Bone Joint Surg Am. 2009;91(1):128–33.
18. Spiegl U, Friederichs J, Patzold R, Militz M, Josten C, Buhren V. Risk factors for failed two-stage procedure after chronic posttraumatic periprosthetic hip infections. Arch Orthop Trauma Surg. 2013;133(3):421–8.
19. Houdek MT, Wagner ER, Watts CD, Osmon DR, Hanssen AD, Lewallen DG, et al. Morbid obesity: a significant risk factor for failure of two-stage revision total hip arthroplasty for infection. J Bone Joint Surg Am. 2015;97(4):326–32.
20. Hsieh PH, Chen LH, Lee MS, Chen CH, Yang WE, Shih CH. Hip arthroplasty in patients with cirrhosis of the liver. J Bone Joint Surg Br. 2003;85(6):818–21.
21. Garcia-Tsao G, Wiest R. Gut microflora in the pathogenesis of the complications of cirrhosis. Best Pract Res Clin Gastroenterol. 2004;18(2):353–72.
22. Hsieh PH, Lee MS, Hsu KY, Chang YH, Shih HN, Ueng SW. Gram-negative prosthetic joint infections: risk factors and outcome of treatment. Clin Infect Dis. 2009;49(7):1036–43.
23. Zmistowski B, Fedorka CJ, Sheehan E, Deirmengian G, Austin MS, Parvizi J. Prosthetic joint infection caused by gram-negative organisms. J Arthroplast. 2011;26(6 Suppl):104–8.
24. Chang Y, Tai CL, Hsieh PH, Ueng SW. Gentamicin in bone cement: a potentially more effective prophylactic measure of infectionin joint arthroplasty. Bone Joint Res. 2013;2(10):220–6.
25. Betsch BY, Eggli S, Siebenrock KA, Tauber MG, Muhlemann K. Treatment of joint prosthesis infection in accordance with current recommendations improves outcome. Clin Infect Dis. 2008;46(8):1221–6.
26. Bejon P, Berendt A, Atkins BL, Green N, Parry H, Masters S, et al. Two-stage revision for prosthetic joint infection: predictors of outcome and the role of reimplantation microbiology. J Antimicrob Chemother. 2010;65(3):569–75.

25

Developmental hip dysplasia treated by total hip arthroplasty using a cementless Wagner cone stem in young adult patients with a small physique

Ping Zhen[1,2*†], Jun Liu[2†], Hao Lu[2], Hui Chen[2], Xusheng Li[2] and Shenghu Zhou[2]

Abstract

Background: Developmental hip dysplasia (DDH) may lead to severe acetabular and femoral abnormalities that can render total hip arthroplasty (THA) challenging, especially in DDH patients with a small physique. Most conventional cemented or cementless femoral components are often difficult to implant in the narrow femoral canal and require slight version correction during surgery. The aim of this study was to present the mid-term results of THA in the treatment of DDH patients with a small physique using a cementless Wagner cone prosthesis (Zimmer®, US).

Methods: Between January 2006 and March 2010, we retrospectively reviewed 50 patients who were treated at our center. A total of 50 patients (52 hips; 45 women, five men; mean age 32.5 years; range 27 to 38 years) who underwent THA were observed. The mean femoral medullary canal dimension at the isthmus was 7.6 mm (range 6. 0 to 8.7). According to the Crowe classification, 19 hips presented dysplasia of grade I, while 33 presented dysplasia of grade II. All patients were treated with THA using a cementless Wagner cone prosthesis. Clinical and radiologic evaluations were performed on all patients.

Results: The mean duration of follow-up was 7.7 years (range 5.4 to 10.5). The Harris hip score (HHS) improved from 63 ± 9 (range 55 to 70) pre-operatively to 92 ± 8 (range 88 to 100) at the last follow-up. The HHS at the most recent follow-up was excellent in 66% of patients (34 hips), good in 26% (14 hips), fair in 6% (3 hips), and poor in 2% (1 hip). Radiographic evaluation demonstrated excellent osteointegration of the implants. Stem subsidence was present in three stems, and the range of stem subsidence was 2 mm in two stems (3.9%) and 3 mm in one stem (1.9%). Femoral osteolysis was observed in nine hips (18%) in the proximal zones, and no distal osteolysis was noted. Heterotopic ossification was observed in three hips (5.8%); of these, two were classified as Brooker's grade 1, and one was classified as Brooker's grade 2 at the most recent follow-up. None of the implants were revised.

Conclusions: Based on the tapered shape and free setting of anteversion, the Wagner cone femoral stem facilitates its implantation in dysplastic hips. Therefore, this series of short stems with a smaller diameter can ensure safe implantation in narrow medullary canals, especially in young DDH patients with a small physique.

(Continued on next page)

* Correspondence: zhenpingok@163.com
†Equal contributors
[1]Department of Orthopedics, The Second Affiliated Hospital of Lanzhou University, Cuiying Door, No. 82, Chengguan District, Lanzhou City, Gansu Province 730030, People's Republic of China
[2]Department of Orthopaedics, Lanzhou General Hospital of PLA, South Binhe Road, No. 333, Lanzhou City, Gansu Province 730050, People's Republic of China

(Continued from previous page)

Keywords: Total hip arthroplasty, Cementless femoral stem, Wagner cone stem, Developmental hip dysplasia, Small physique

Background

Developmental hip dysplasia (DDH) consists of abnormal development of the hip joint that is characterized by anatomical alterations involving both the acetabulum and the femur [1, 2]. In DDH, significant deformities, such as dysplastic acetabulum, deformity of the femoral head and a shortened femoral neck with excessive anteversion, may be present [2–5]. Especially in some Asian DDH patients with a small physique, the femur usually presents with a short skeleton and an excessive narrow canal [6]. Total hip arthroplasty (THA) is technically difficult in such small-proportioned patients because most conventional cemented or cementless femoral components are often difficult to implant in the narrow femoral canal and require slight version correction of the femoral stem [6–9].

The Wagner stem was originally designed in 1987 [10] to treat patients with severe proximal femoral bone loss in revision surgery [11, 12]. The Wagner cone prosthesis hip stem was designed for uncemented fixation in challenging bone conditions at the proximal femur, such as proximal femoral deformities, especially in DDH patients [1]. The circular cross-section of this implant facilitates unimpeded rotation during implantation and enables the free setting of anteversion to restore normal anteversion in dysplastic hips [7, 8, 13]. Meanwhile, a series of short stems are available in 12 diameters from 6.4 to 15.4 mm to appropriately fit the intramedullary canal in DDH patients with a small physique [14].

Since 2006, we have performed total hip replacements for 52 joints in 50 young adult patients with DDH (Crowe I and II). Forty-eight patients underwent a unilateral procedure, and two underwent a bilateral staged procedure. The aim of this study was to present the clinical and radiological outcomes of THA in the treatment of DDH patients with a small physique by cementless Wagner cone prosthesis in our center after a minimum follow-up of 5.4 years.

Methods

Patient demographics

Between January 2006 and March 2010, 50 patients (52 hips) with osteoarthritis secondary to hip dysplasia types I and II according to the Crowe classification underwent THA in our center. The average age of the 45 females and five males at the time of surgery was 32.5 years (27–38). The patients' mean height, body weight, and body mass index (BMI) were 156 ± 2.5 cm (160 ± 5.6 cm), 50 ± 3.2 kg (53 ± 6.3 kg), and 21.8 ± 3.8 (23.1 ± 2.8), respectively. All operations were performed by one of the members of our institution's hip team (Ping Zhen or Xusheng Li).

Pre-operatively, all patients were evaluated clinically and radiographically. The Harris hip score (HHS) was used for clinical evaluation. For all patients, standard radiographs of the pelvis in anteroposterior view and of the affected hip in axial view were obtained. On radiographs, the degree of dysplasia was determined using the Crowe system [15], based on which 19 hips presented dysplasia grade I and 33 presented grade II. The transverse diameter of the medullary canal was also measured on an anteroposterior view of the femur using a custom-programmed, semi-automated analysis software module within ImagePro Plus (Mediacybernetics, Silver Springs, MD) [16]. The femoral medullary canal dimensions at the isthmus ranged from 6.0 to 8.7 mm (mean, 7.6 mm) in this study. In addition, computed tomography (CT scans) were performed on 38 patients to evaluate the structure of the dysplastic acetabulum and antetorsion of the femur head. The mean antetorsion angle of the femur head was 52° (range 46° to 62°) in these patients. Based on radiographs, thorough pre-operative planning was conducted for all patients, including assessment of the available bone stock and determination of the position and choice of the femoral and acetabular implants. The appropriate implant and femoral offset were chosen by pre-operative templating. Patient demographics are listed in Table 1.

Surgical technique and implantation

THA was performed in patients under general or spinal anesthesia. A posterolateral approach was used, with the patient placed on the contralateral side. After capsulotomy, we confirmed the position of the femoral head in relation to the acetabulum. The hip was then dislocated, and osteotomy of the femoral neck was performed at the designated level. The primitive acetabulum was reamed, and an uncemented, press-fit cup was applied in or close to the anatomical position. A box osteotome, trochanteric reamer or a burr was used to remove bone from

Table 1 Patient demographics

Demographic	Data
Gender	5 male (5 hips), 45 female (47 hips)
Mean age	32.5 years (range 27 to 38)
Mean height	156 ± 2.5 cm (160 ± 5.6 cm)
Mean weight	50 ± 3.2 kg (53 ± 6.3 kg)
BMI	21.8 ± 3.8 (23.1 ± 2.8)
Classification of Crowe	19 hips of grade I, 33 hips of grade II
Mean antetorsion angle	52° (range 46° to 62°)
Mean dimension of the femoral medullary canal (at the isthmus)	7.6 mm (range 6.0 to 8.7 mm)
Stem length	18 stems in 100.5 mm, 34 in 110 mm
Distal diameter of the stem	18 stems in 6.4 mm, 16 in 7.4 mm, 7 in 8.4 mm, 6 in 9.4 mm, 5 in 10.4 mm
Mean follow-up	7.7 years (range 5.4 to 10.5)

the medial portion of the greater trochanter and the lateral portion of the femoral neck. The femoral medullary canal was progressively reamed with tapered reamers in the longitudinal direction of the femur until noticeable resistance was felt. A Wagner cone prosthesis uncemented stem was inserted by guiding it with its appropriate device, aiming to obtain approximately 10–20° of anteversion. The prosthesis was rotated into the desired anteversion and was impacted into its definitive position with a few moderate mallet blows. The correct depth of penetration as per the pre-operative planning was verified. After the hip was reduced, the stability and range of motion were assessed, and the appropriate limb length was verified in comparison to the contralateral limb. In this series of patients, a ceramic-polyethylene bearing was used in 27 hips, and a ceramic-ceramic bearing was used in 25 hips.

Considering that the main problem regarding the femur, as noted previously, is excessive anteversion of the femoral neck and the small femoral canal in DDH [7], the use of the uncemented Wagner cone prosthesis hip stem (Zimmer ®, US) allowed us to correct the femoral head version and to ensure safe implantation of the femoral stem. Based on a 5° tapered stem with a circular cross-section (Fig. 1), the Wagner cone prosthesis stem can be placed in any anteversion orientation by the surgeon (Fig. 2). The new Wagner cone prosthesis stem is available in two different neck angles (125° and 135°) and provides good options to facilitate appropriate restoration of biomechanical parameters, including the center of rotation, offset and leg length. This series of cone stems is available in lengths from 100.5 to 110 mm and in diameters from 6.4 to 10.4 mm (distal section distance: at 96 mm distance from the shoulder of the prosthesis). In this study, in 18 THAs, the inserted femoral

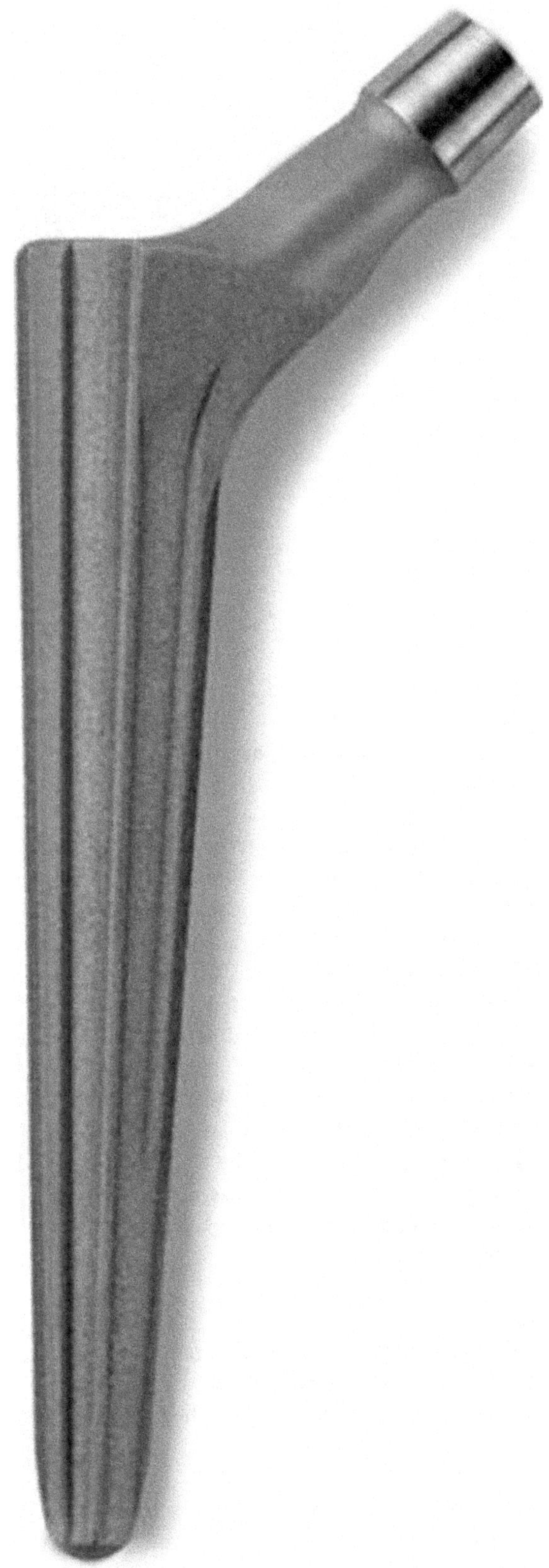

Fig. 1 The Wagner cone prosthesis has a tapered shape with a cone angle of 5°, and the 8 sharp longitudinal ribs of the stem are beneficial for bony apposition and optimum rotational stability

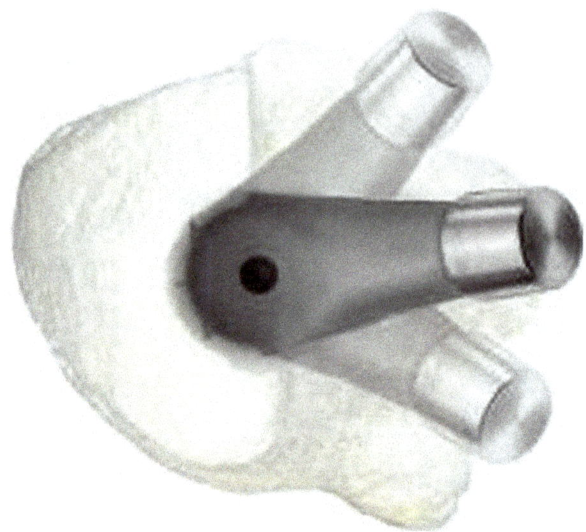

Fig. 2 The circular cross-section facilitates unimpeded rotation during implantation to enable the free setting of anteversion

cone stem had a diameter of 6.4 mm; in 16 cases, the stem diameter was 7.4 mm; in seven cases, the diameter was 8.4 mm; in six cases, the diameter was 9.4 mm; and in five cases, the diameter was 10.4 mm.

Follow-up and radiographic analysis

Clinical and radiographic follow-up were performed every 2 years postoperatively. Clinical evaluation was carried out using the HHS. Routine radiographs comprising an anteroposterior view of the pelvis as well as anteroposterior and lateral views of the affected hip were performed and compared to the initial postoperative radiographs. Radiographs were evaluated by two fellowship-trained hip arthroplasty surgeons (MD and NR) for evidence of biological fixation (using the fixation/stability score of Engh [17]), subsidence (as described by Pelligrini et al [18]), osteolysis (based on Gruen modes of failure [19]), and heterotopic ossification (graded according to Brooker's classification [20]).

Results

The mean duration of follow-up was 7.7 years (range 5.4–10.5 years). Two patients with two THAs were lost to follow-up, one after six and the other after 8 years.

Clinical outcome

The HHS improved between the pre-operative evaluation and the last follow-up in this group. The average HHS was 63 ± 9 (range 55–70) pre-operatively, 90 ± 7 (range 82–98) 12 months after surgery, and 92 ± 8 (range 88–100) at the final follow-up. The HHS at the most recent follow-up was excellent in 66% of the patients (34 hips), good in 26% (14 hips), fair in 6% (3 hips), and poor in 2% (1 hip). Twenty-eight patients (30 hips) had no limp (60%), 16 patients (16 hips) had a mild limp (32%), three patients (3 hips, 6%) had a moderate limp, and one patient (1 hip) had a severe limp (2%). Mild thigh pain was described in association with three hips (6%) within 1 year; this pain typically occurred only with prolonged activity, was not disabling, and did not require medication. One patient reported mild pain in the groin. The mean correction of limb length (comparing the pre-operative length with that at the last radiological follow-up) was 2.2 cm (range 1.5 to 3.2 cm). The mean pre-operative and postoperative discrepancies were 2.29 ± 1.05 cm and 0.67 ± 1.13 cm, respectively.

Radiographic assessment of the femoral component

Press-fit of the stem was achieved in 49 joints (94.2%) immediately after surgery. Three stems were shown to be slightly undersized immediately after surgery. Anatomical reconstruction of the correct antetorsion was achieved in all cases (Figs. 3, 4, 5 and 6). Based on the Engh classification, stable osseous ingrowth was confirmed in 48 joint stems (92.3%) and was suspected in two stems (3.9%); in the remaining two stems (3.9%), stable fibrous fixation was evident. There were no unstable stems (Figs. 7, 8 and 9). Stem subsidence was present in three stems; the stem subsidence ranged from 2 mm, in two stems (3.9%), to 3 mm, in one stem (1.9%). Nonprogressive radiolucent lines were found in Gruen's zone 1 in nine patients, in zone 7 in one patient, in zones 1 and 7 in seven patients, in zones 1, 2, and 7 in one patient, and in zones 1, 2, 6, and 7 in one patient. Femoral osteolysis was observed in nine hips (18%) in the proximal zones (zone 1 and 7 in five hips, zone 1 alone in three hips, and zone 7 alone in one hip). No distal osteolysis was noted. No femoral prosthesis developed varus or a valgus tilt over time. Heterotopic ossification was observed in three hips (5.8%): of these, two showed Brooker's grade 1 and one showed Brooker's grade 2 at the most recent follow-up. No stem revisions occurred in this study.

There were no cases of intraoperative femoral fracture or femoral perforation during rasping of the canal or stem implantation, nor did deep infections or wound-healing problems occur postoperatively. One dislocation developed within 1 month after the procedure. This patient was treated with a closed reduction and a hip brace without the need for further surgery. No recurrence was observed.

Discussion

DDH routinely presents as hip incongruence secondary to low or high dislocation. The associated anatomical deformities of the hip include hypoplastic acetabulum and deformity of the proximal femur [1–3, 7–9]. If not

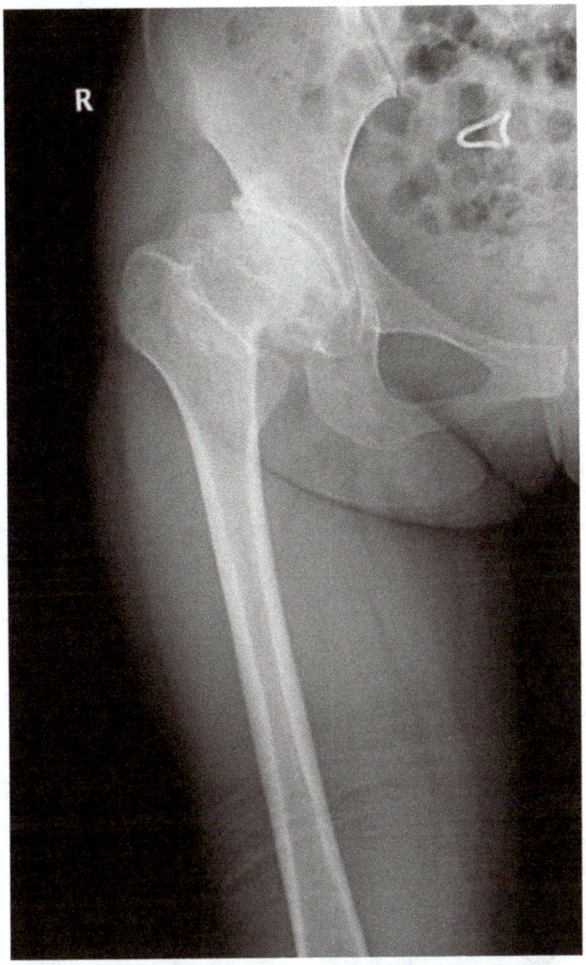

Fig. 3 Pre-operative radiographic aspect in an anteroposterior view of a 32-year-old female with Crowe grade II developmental hip dysplasia on her right side. The patient presented with a narrow femoral canal and excessive anteversion of the femoral neck

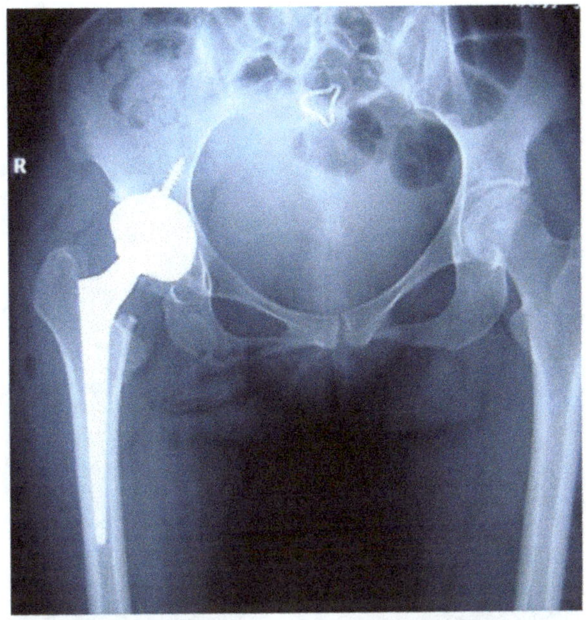

Fig. 4 Immediate postoperative anteroposterior radiographs demonstrating correct placement of the implant and normal anteversion

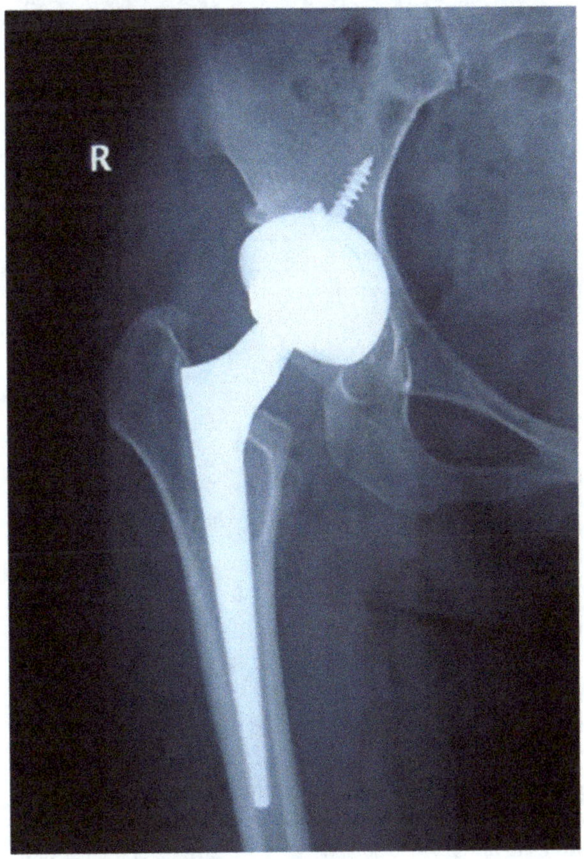

Fig. 5 Radiographic aspect in the anteroposterior view at 8 years of follow-up: the implant is stable, and no signs of bone resorption are noticeable

diagnosed and adequately treated during childhood, DDH may lead to early functional impairment and anatomical alterations of the hip joint in young adults [1]. Many surgical strategies, including acetabular reconstruction, femoral osteotomy and hip arthroplasty, have been proposed for the treatment of DDH in adolescents [1]. Based on good-to-excellent hip-joint congruency in joint-preserving surgery, periacetabular and femoral osteotomies have been recommended if degeneration of the articular cartilage is minimal [8], especially in patients <30 years of age [21].

As a progressive treatment, THA in young DDH patients remains widely debated [7–9] because the young age of the patient raises the issue of the long-term survival of the implant [1, 22, 23]. However, THA is the optimum therapy in such patients with severe subluxation or late coxarthrosis [22–24].

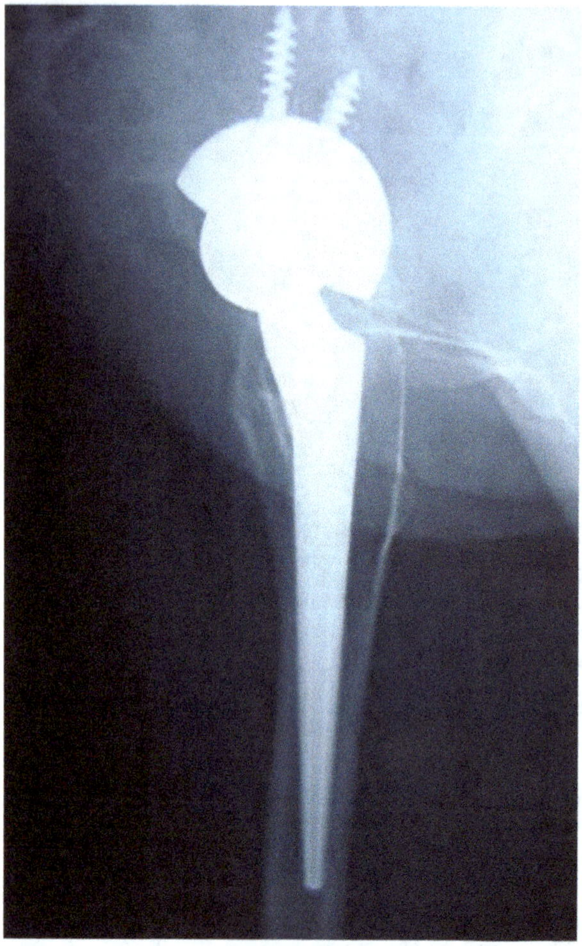

Fig. 6 Frog-leg lateral radiograph on the right side at 8 years of follow-up

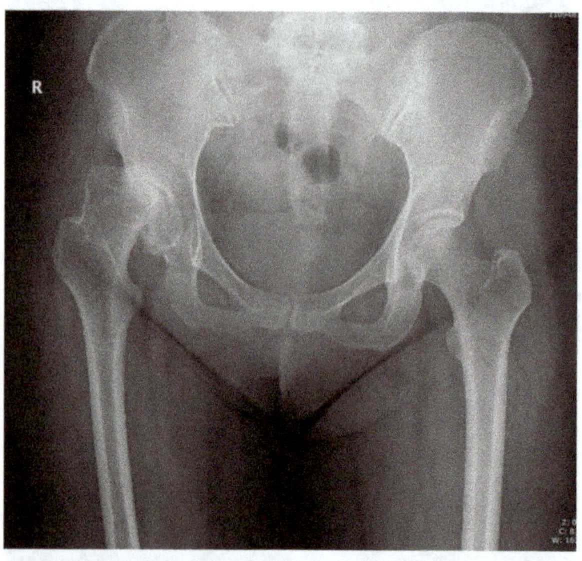

Fig. 7 Pre-operative radiographic aspect in an anteroposterior view of a 40-year-old female with Crowe grade II hip dysplasia on her right side. The patient presented with a narrow femoral canal

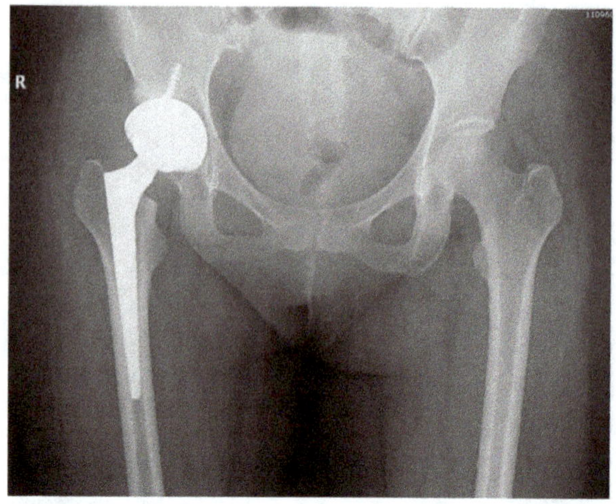

Fig. 8 Immediate postoperative anteroposterior radiographs demonstrating correct placement of the implant. Press-fit of the stem was achieved

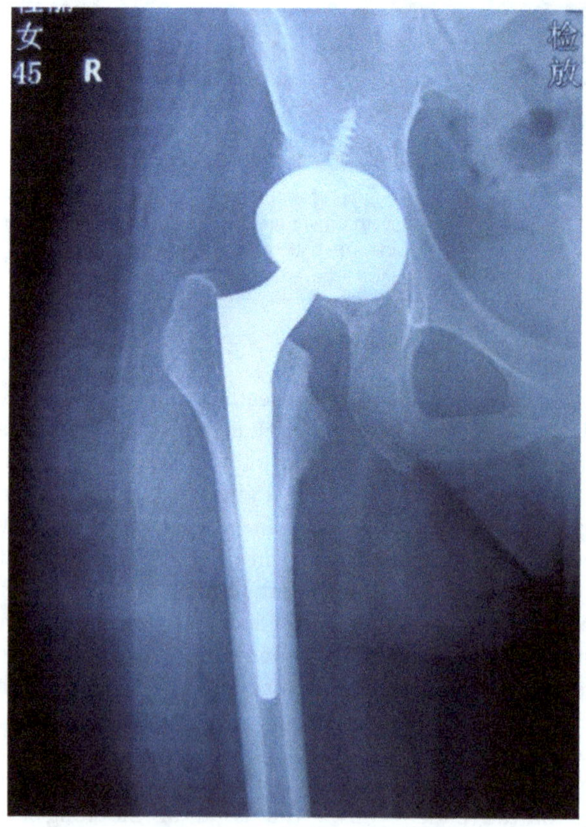

Fig. 9 Radiographic aspect in the anteroposterior view at 5 years of follow-up: the implant is stable, and no signs of bone resorption are noticeable

DDH may lead to severe acetabular and femoral abnormalities, including small acetabular and femoral dimensions, soft tissue contracture, inadequate acetabular bone stock, and excessive femoral anteversion [1, 3, 7–9]. These anatomical alterations increase the difficulty of THA and may also threaten the long-term survival of the prosthetic implant [1, 6–9, 25–27]. The main problems associated with the femur are a deformed head, a short neck with excessive anteversion and a narrow femoral canal [2, 3]. DDH patients can have small physiques [25–28], especially in Asian patients [6]. Some narrow femoral canals are too small to accommodate many standard femoral components during THA [25]. In early studies, the treatment of hip disease in such patients often required the use of miniature or micro-miniature femoral components, and a cemented technique was preferred [25, 28]; however, significant problems have been encountered in these situations, including intraoperative femoral fracture, instability, poor femoral cement mantle and component loosening due to the smaller femoral anatomy [25]. Meanwhile, the young age of DDH patients increases the importance of the long-term survival of the cemented implants [1]. Although no precise definition of a small physique and narrow femoral canal have been developed in previous studies [6, 25–28], most cementless standard stems in small-proportioned patients are also limited [26] because current cementless stems are designed to extend to the isthmus of the medullary canal to stabilize component alignment and prevent varus migration [7]. When such patients undergo hip arthroplasty, standard cementless femoral stems always encounter this difficulty in insertion, and extensive reaming and rasping are used to obtain safe implantation [29]; however, more vigorous reaming may easily cause perforation or fracture during the operation. Meanwhile, dysplastic hips usually present with excessive anteversion of the femoral head, and anatomical reconstruction of the correct antetorsion should be achieved by rotating the stem in the medullary canal. However, most conventional cementless stems that are designed with rectangular cross-sections generally fill the metaphysis of the proximal femur. Consequently, there is little opportunity to alter the stem version after insertion [26, 30–32]. Thus, for this abnormality in proximal femoral anatomy, an alternative to the use of a nonmodular femoral component is often needed [26]. Modular implants, such as the S-ROM prosthesis [26, 32] and custom-made prostheses [33], allow for variable versions, thus providing the ability to alter the version to help balance the hip with respect to internal and external rotation [2, 6, 10–12]. Moreover, S-ROM cementless femoral stems are available in a variety of distal diameters from 9 to 23 mm (in Japan, S-ROM stems as small as 6 mm are available) [26] that can fit in small femoral canals. In fact, modular prostheses are always accompanied by a subtrochanteric shorting osteotomy procedure for hips with high dislocation [26, 32, 34] or an atypical femoral geometry [34]. Moreover, modular femoral components also raise concerns about fretting, corrosion, and mechanical failure [35, 36], and an increasing number of reports have described the failure of modular implants due to fracture at the modular junctions [37, 38].

Although several prostheses have been used for treating DDH [8, 26, 28, 29, 31–33], only a few studies have considered the Wagner stem as a possibility [1, 7, 13, 30]. Based on its 5° tapered stem with a circular cross-section, the Wagner cone prosthesis stem can be placed in any anteversion orientation by the surgeon. Moreover, as a relatively short stem with a small diameter, the Wagner cone prosthesis can easily be implanted in narrow medullary canals, comparable to conventional cemented or uncemented stems [1, 7, 14, 39, 40]. The conical stem used in these cases allows good correction of the over-anteverted neck, and the eight-rib design provides good rotational stability, In this study, indications for the Wagner cone prosthesis are femurs with slim and narrow canals (medullary canal diameter at isthmus <10 mm) or combined with excessive anteversion of the neck (femoral anteversion of >40°) in young DDH patients, in which the femoral shortening osteotomy is not needed in Crowe type I and II dysplastic hips. In this series, excellent survival of the stem was accomplished (a mean of 7.7 years), and minimal complications were observed. Despite the small size of the titanium alloy femoral components, no bending or fracture of the femoral stem was observed. Thus, this cone prosthesis is a good and inexpensive solution for cases of Crowe type I and II dysplastic hips.

This study should be interpreted in light of several important limitations. First, this study did not compare the results of THA using Wagner cone stems and some standard cementless stems. However, by comparing the present cohort with our historical control, we concluded that the Wagner-based procedure resulted in satisfactory outcomes. Second, this was a retrospective study with all the problems inherent with this methodology. Third, this study was unable to separately analyze bilateral and unilateral cases.

Conclusion

Based on its free setting of anteversion and small diameter, the new Wagner cone femoral stem facilitates its implantation in dysplastic hips with narrow femoral canals and excessive anteversion. Further studies aimed at better defining the indications for this procedure will lead to even better results. Further follow-up is also needed to confirm whether these results will be maintained over a longer term.

Abbreviations

BMI: Body mass index; THA: Total hip arthroplasty

Funding

This work was supported by the National Natural Science Foundation of China (81371983); the Social Development of Technology Research Projects of Gansu Province (S04671); and the Youth Science and Technology Foundation of Gansu province (1606RJYA300).

Authors' contributions

PZ performed the data collection and analysis and participated in writing the manuscript. JL and CH performed the database setup and statistical analysis. PZ and XSL performed the operations. HL participated in the study design and coordination and helped draft the manuscript. All authors have read and approved the final manuscript.

Competing interests

The authors declare that they have no competing interests.

Consent for publication

Not applicable, as no identifying personal information is included in this manuscript.

References

1. Faldini C, Miscione MT, Chehrassan M, Acri F, Pungetti C, d'Amato M, Luciani D, Giannini S. Congenital hip dysplasia treated by total hip arthroplasty using cementless tapered stem in patients younger than 50 years old: results after 12-years follow-up. J Orthop Traumatol. 2011;12(4):213–8.
2. Sugano N, Noble PC, Kamaric E, Salama JK, Ochi T, Tullos HS. The morphology of the femur in developmental dysplasia of the hip. J Bone Joint Surg (Br). 1998;80(4):711–9.
3. Noble PC, Kamaric E, Sugano N, Matsubara M, Harada Y, Ohzono K, Paravic V. Three-dimensional shape of the dysplastic femur: implications for THR. Clin Orthop Relat Res. 2003;417:27–40.
4. Casper DS, Kim GK, Parvizi J, Freeman TA. Morphology of the proximal femur differs widely with age and sex: relevance to design and selection of femoral prostheses. J Orthop Res. 2012;30(7):1162–6.
5. Noble PC, Alexande JW, Lindah LJ, Yew DT, Granbrry WM, Tullos HS. The anatomic basis of femoral component design. Clin Orthop Relat Res. 1988; 235:148–65.
6. Nakamura Y, Mitusui H, Kikuchi A, Toh S, Katano H. Total hip arthroplasty using a cylindrical cementless stem in patients with a small physique. J Arthroplasty. 2011;26(1):77–81.
7. Claramunt RT, Marqués F, León A, Vilà G, Mestre C. Total hip replacement with an uncemented Wagner cone stem for patients with congenital hip dysplasia. Int Orthop. 2011;35(12):1767–70.
8. Rogers BA, Garbedian S, Kuchinad RA, Backstein D, Safir O. Total hip arthroplasty for adult hip dysplasia. J Bone Joint Surg Am. 2012;94(19):1809–21.
9. Paavilainen T. Total hip replacement for developmental dysplasia of the hip. Acta Orthop Scand. 1997;68(1):77–84.
10. Wagner H. Revision prosthesis for the hip joint in severe bone loss. Orthopade. 1987;16(2):295–300.
11. Böhm P, Bischel O. Femoral revision with then Wagner SL revision stem, evaluation of one hundred and twenty-nine revisions followed for a mean of 4.8 years. J Bone Joint Surg Am. 2001;83(9):1023–31.
12. Regis D, Sandri A, Bonetti I, Bartolozzi P, Braggion M. Femoral revision with the Wagner tapered stem. A 10-to 15-year follow-up study. J Bone Joint Surg (Br). 2011;93(10):1320–6.
13. Schuh A, Schraml A, Hohenberger G. Long-term results of the Wagner cone prosthesis. Int Orthop. 2009;33(1):53–8.
14. Pak P, de Steiger R. Cone femoral prosthesis for osteoarthritis of the hip femoral dysplasia. J Orthop Surg. 2008;16(2):206–10.
15. Crowe JF, Mani VJ, Ranawat CS. Total hip replacement in congenital dislocation and dysplasia of the hip. J Bone Joint Surg Am. 1979;61(1):15–23.
16. Husmann O, Rubin PJ, Leyvraz PF, De RB, Argenson JN. Three-dimensional morphology of the proximal femur. J Arthroplasty. 1997;12(4):444–50.
17. Engh CA, Massin P, Suthers KE. Roentgenographic assessment of the biologic fixation of porous-surfaced femoral components. Clin Orthop Relat Res. 1990;257:107–28.
18. Pellegrini VD, Hughes SS, Evarts CM. A collarless cobalt-chrome femoral component in uncemented total hip arthroplasty. Five- to eight-year follow-up. J Bone Joint Surg (Br). 1992;74(6):814–50.
19. Gruen TA, McNelce GM, Amstutz HC. "Modes of failure" of cemented stem-type femoral components: a radiographic analysis of loosening. Clin Orthop Relat Res. 1979;141:17–27.
20. Sierra RJ, Schoeniger SR, Millis M, Ganz R. Periacetabular osteotomy for containment of the nonarthritic dysplastic hip secondary to poliomyelitis. J Bone Joint Surg Am. 2010;92(18):2917–23.
21. Thawrani D, Sucato DJ, Podeszwa DA, DeLaRocha A. Complications associated with the Bernese periacetabular osteotomy for hip dysplasia in adolescents. J Bone Joint Surg Am. 2010;92(8):1707–14.
22. Sanchez-Sotelo J, Trousdale RT, Berry DJ, Cabanela ME. Surgical treatment of developmental dysplasia of the hip in adults: I. Nonarthroplasty options. J Am Acad Orthop Surg. 2002;10(5):334–44.
23. Flecher X, Aubaniac JM, Parratte S, Argenson JN. Is there a need for conservative surgery in DDH adult patients? Lessons learned after 30 years experience. Hip Int. 2007;17 Suppl 5(2):S83–90.
24. Karachalios T, Hartofilakidis G. Congenital hip disease in adults: terminology, classification, pre-operative planning and management. J Bone Joint Surg (Br). 2010;92(7):914–21.
25. Rahimtoola ZO, Finger S, Imrie S, Goodman SB. Outcome of total hip arthroplasty in small-proportioned patients. J Arthroplasty. 2000;15(1):27–34.
26. Drexler M, Dwyer T, Marmor M, Abolghasemian M, Chakravertty R, Chechik O, Cameron HU. Nineteen year results of THA using modular 9 mm S-ROM femoral component in patients with small femoral canals. J Arthroplasty. 2013;28(9):1667–70.
27. Cameron HU, Lee OB, Chou H. Total hip arthroplasty in patients with deficient bone stock and small femoral canals. J Arthroplasty. 2003;18(1):35–40.
28. Chiu KH, Shen WY, Cheung KW, Cheung KW, Tsui HF. Primary Exeter total hip arthroplasty in patients with small femurs: a minimal of 10 years follow-up. J Arthroplasty. 2005;20(3):275–81.
29. Jun Oh K, Imrie S, Hwang K, Ramachandran R, Shegog M, Goodman SB. Total hip arthroplasty using the miniature anatomic medullary locking stem. Clin Orthop Relat Res. 2006;447:85–91.
30. Wagner H, Wagner M. Cone prosthesis for the hip joint. Arch Orthop Trauma Surg. 2000;120(1):88–95.
31. Perka C, Fischer U, Taylor WR, Matziolis G. Developmental hip dysplasia treated with total hip arthroplasty with a straight stem and a threaded cup. J Bone Joint Surg Am. 2004;86-A(2):312–9.
32. Takao M, Ohzono K, Nishii T, Miki H, Nakamura N, Sugano N. Cementless Modular total hip arthroplasty with subtrochanteric shortening osteotomy for hips with developmental dysplasia. J Bone Joint Surg Am. 2011;93:548–55.
33. McCarthy JC, Bono JV, O'Donnell PJ. Custom and modular components in primary total hip replacement. Clin Orthop Relat Res. 1997;344:162–71.
34. Park MS, Kim KH, Jeong WC. Transverse subtrochanteric shortening osteotomy in primary total hip arthroplasty for patients with severe hip developmental dysplasia. J Arthroplasty. 2007;22(7):1031–6.
35. Ellman MB, Levine BR. Fracture of the modular femoral neck component in total hip arthroplasty. J Arthroplasty. 2013;28(1):196e1–5.
36. Dangles CJ, Altstetter CJ. Failure of the modular neck in a total hip arthroplasty. J Arthroplasty. 2010;25:1169e5–7.
37. Parisi T, Burroughs B, Kwon YM. Modular Hip Implant Fracture at the Stem-Sleeve Interface. Orthopedics. 2015;38(3):234–9.

Which patient-specific and surgical characteristics influence postoperative pain after THA in a fast-track setting?

Yvon M. den Hartog[1*], Gerjon Hannink[2], Nick T. van Dasselaar[3], Nina M. Mathijssen[1] and Stephan B. Vehmeijer[1]

Abstract

Background: In our hospital a fast-track setting including a multimodal pain protocol is used for total hip arthroplasty (THA). Despite this multimodal pain protocol there is still a large range in reported postoperative pain between patients, which hinders mobilization and rehabilitation postoperatively. The goal of this study was to identify which patient-specific and surgical characteristics influence postoperative pain after THA in a fast-track setting.

Methods: All 74 patients with osteoarthritis of the hip who underwent primary THA procedure by anterior supine intermuscular approach between November 2012 and January 2014 were included in this prospective cohort study. The protocol for pain medication was standardized.
Postoperative pain determined with the Numeric Rating Score was collected at 17 standardized moments. Linear mixed models were used to examine potential patient-specific and surgical factors associated with increased postoperative pain.

Results: Pain patterns differed substantially across individuals. Adjusted for other variables in the model, preoperative use of pain medication (regression coefficient 0.78 (95% CI 0.28–1.26); $p = 0.005$) and preoperative neuropathic pain scored by DN4 (regression coefficient 0.68 (95% CI 0.15–1.20); $p = 0.02$) were the only factors significantly associated with higher postoperative pain scores.

Conclusions: The knowledge of which factors are associated with higher postoperative pain scores after THA in a fast-track setting may help optimizing perioperative postoperative pain management and preoperative education of these patients.

Keywords: Total hip arthroplasty, Fast-track, Multimodal pain protocol, Pain management, Postoperative pain

Background

Total hip arthroplasty (THA) is associated with considerable postoperative pain [1]. Almost all pain after surgery arises as a result of tissue damage at the surgical site [2]. This postoperative pain hinders early mobilization and rehabilitation with subsequent consequences on mobility and overall recovery [3]. In the last few years fast-track protocols have been introduced worldwide for elective primary THA. These are partly based on pain management protocols and include a rigorous perioperative pain management program, which allow for an optimized perioperative period [4, 5]. In 2009, a fast-track protocol including a multimodal pain protocol was successfully introduced in our teaching hospital [6]. The multimodal pain protocol, developed to reduce acute postoperative pain to enable quick mobilization and rehabilitation included paracetamol, celecoxib, gabapentine, dexamethasone and esketamine [7–12]. Furthermore, we use the anterior supine intermuscular (ASI) approach for THA procedures in our hospital. Since this approach uses both an intermuscular and internervous plane and causes less surgical trauma, lower postoperative pain scores and less pain medication consumption have been described for this approach [13–18]. Despite the introduction of a multimodal pain protocol and use of the

* Correspondence: yvondenhartog@hotmail.com
[1]Department of Orthopaedic Surgery, Reinier de Graaf Hospital, Delft, the Netherlands
Full list of author information is available at the end of the article

ASI approach, there is still a large range in reported postoperative pain between patients.

Previous studies have shown that specific patient- and provider characteristics could influence postoperative pain [19–27]. Only one of these studies reported solely on postoperative pain after primary THA [21]. None of these studies were performed in a fast-track setting and no multimodal pain protocols developed to reduce acute postoperative pain were included in these studies.

The proper identification of patients who are at risk to experience more postoperative pain directly after primary THA might provide details for further optimization of postoperative pain management and preoperative education of these patients. Therefore, the goal of this study was to identify which patient-specific and surgical characteristics influence postoperative pain after primary THA by ASI approach in a fast-track setting including a multimodal pain protocol.

Methods

All 74 patients with osteoarthritis (72 patients with primary osteoarthritis, 2 patients with secondary osteoarthritis) of the hip who underwent primary THA procedure by ASI approach between November 2012 and January 2014 were included in this prospective cohort study. All procedures were performed in a fast-track setting, by one experienced orthopedic hip surgeon (SBV). Patients with neurological conditions which potentially influence pain perception; American Society of Anaesthesiologists (ASA) classification III/IV; medical contra-indication for spinal anesthesia; cardiovascular impairment in the present or past; known allergy against any element of the medication that is given for the multimodal pain protocol; abuse of alcohol or drugs; rheumatoid arthritis; BMI > 40 kg/m^2; and patients with cognitive impairment were excluded.

As part of the fast-track setting, all patients joined a patient education program prior to surgery. All patients received spinal anesthesia with a low dose of bupivacaine (6–8 mg intrathecally). Propofol was administered for sedation and to allow a single shot of esketamine. The multimodal protocol for perioperative pain medication was standardized (Table 1). Before discharge, adequate pain relief had to be achieved by oral pain medication: the Numeric Rating Scale (NRS) for pain had to be below 3 in rest and below 5 during mobilization (NRS; 0 to 10, best to worst).

Postoperative pain determined with the NRS was collected at 17 standardized moments, from 1 h after surgery until the afternoon of the second day after surgery (Fig. 1). The study protocol was approved by our local Ethics Committee (2012–000989-37/NL39970.098.12). The study was retrospectively registered in the ISRCTN registry under identifier ISRCTN15422220 (date of registration: July 25, 2017).

Table 1 The standardized multimodal protocol for perioperative pain medication

Timing	Medication
2 h before surgery	Paracetamol (acetaminophen) 1000 mg per os.
	Celecoxib (Celebrex®) [a] 400 mg per os.
	Gabapentin 600 mg per os.
Just before surgery	Dexamethasone 0.15 mg/kg iv. [b]
	Esketamine 15 mg iv.
4 h after surgery	Paracetamol (acetaminophen) 1000 mg per os.
8 h after surgery	Paracetamol (acetaminophen) 1000 mg per os.
	Gabapentin 300 mg per os.
Before the night	Tramadol 100 mg supp.
Day 1	Paracetamol (acetaminophen) 1000 mg per os 4 times a day.
	Celecoxib (Celebrex®) [a] 200 mg per os in the morning.
	Gabapentin 300 mg per os in the morning.
After day 1	Paracetamol (acetaminophen) 1000 mg per os 4 times a day (with a maximum of 2 weeks).
	Celecoxib (Celebrex®) [a] 200 mg per os in the morning (until 2 weeks after surgery).
Rescue medication	Celecoxib (Celebrex®) [a] 200 mg per os extra after the first night Piritramid (Dipidolor®) 10 mg im, which could be repeated every 4 h.

The standardized multimodal protocol for perioperative pain medication was determined based on literature [7–12]

[a]In combination with celecoxib (Celebrex®) all patients will receive omeprazol 20 mg per os once a day as prophylaxis. When the patient was already using a proton pomp inhibitor before admittance no omeprazol was administered

[b]Dexamethasone solution in 50cm^3 saline is administered slowly to avoid adverse side effects like severe perianal pain

Potential factors associated with increased postoperative pain (gender; ASA classification; age; BMI; diabetes mellitus (DM); surgery time; incision length; living situation; preoperative pain determined with the NRS, preoperative use of pain medication; use of antidepressants; as well as preoperative scores of the neuropathic pain diagnostic questionnaire (DN4), and Amsterdam Preoperative Anxiety and Information Scale (APAIS) for anxiety and information requirements) were examined with univariable linear mixed models for repeated measures. Decision to include these variables was based on guidance from directed acyclic graphs [28]. Based on the criteria in the original article about the APAIS by Moerman and others [29], the APAIS anxiety scale was dichotomized (4–10: no, 11–20: yes), and the APAIS

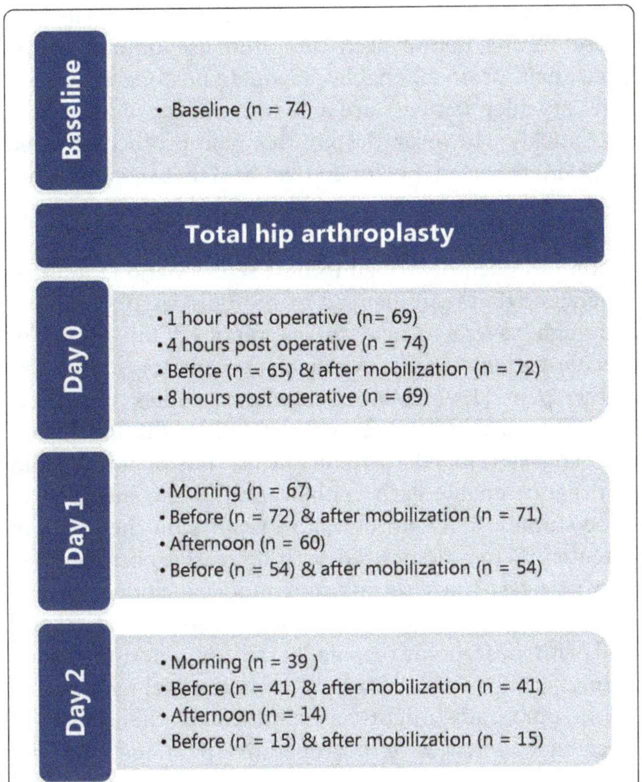

Fig. 1 Overview of pre- and postoperative pain measurements. Postoperative pain determined with the NRS was collected at 17 standardised moments, from 1 h after surgery until the afternoon of the second day after surgery

need-for-information scale was divided into three categories (2–4: no or little, 5–7: average, and 8–10: high). The DN4 questionnaire score was dichotomized (1–3 unlikely; 4–7 likely) [30, 31].

Factors that were associated with the outcome in univariable analyses (*p*-values <0.20) were included in multivariable analyses. In the multivariable analyses *p*-values less than 0.05 were considered significant. Missing data were assumed to be missing at random. Regression coefficients are presented with their 95% confidence intervals. The statistical analyses were performed using R version 3.1.2 with package 'nlme' [32, 33].

Results

Mean age of all patients was 67.1 year (range 42.7–84.6) and mean BMI was 27.1 kg/m^2 (range 20.1–38.9). Mean LOS was 1.8 nights (range 1–7). Most patients lived together with cohabitants (n = 58; 78.4%) and were discharged to their own home (n = 72; 97.3%). Patient characteristics are listed in Table 2.

Seventy-three patients received an uncemented protheses (Taperloc® femoral prosthesis and an Universal® cup, both Biomet, Warsaw, In, USA), one patient received a cemented prosthesis because of inferior bone quality due to severe osteoporosis. (Exceed Muller® cup and a Taperloc® femoral prosthesis, both Biomet, Warsaw, In, USA).

Table 2 Patient characteristics for the total group of 74 patients undergoing primary total hip arthroplasty

		Total n (%) *n* = 74
Age (year)		67.1 (42.7–84.6) [a]
BMI (kg/m^2)		27.1 (20.1–38.9) [a]
Gender	male	36 (48.6%)
ASA classification	ASA2	47 (63.5%)
Surgery time (minutes)		79.2 (49–116) [a]
Diabetes Mellitus		7 (9.5%)
Incision length (cm)		9.97 (7.5–12.0) [a]
Living situation	with cohabitants	58 (78.4%)
Preoperative antidepressants use		4 (5.4%)
Preoperative pain medication use		50 (67.6%)
Preoperative pain (NRS) [b]		5.26 (0–9) [a]
DN4	likely	16 (21.6%)
APAIS anxiety	yes	15 (23.1%)
APAIS information	no/little	24 (37.5%)
	average	24 (37.5%)
	high	16 (25.0%)

[a]mean (range)
[b]*n* = 72 patients

Pain patterns differed substantially across individuals. Moreover, pain varied across the standardized moments (Table 3). Adjusted for the other factors in the model, preoperative use of pain medication (regression coefficient 0.78 (95% CI 0.28–1.26); p = 0.005) and preoperative neuropathic pain scored by DN4 (regression coefficient 0.68 (95% CI 0.15–1.20); p = 0.02) were the only factors that were significantly associated with higher postoperative pain scores (Table 4).

Discussion

The aim of this study was to identify which patient-specific and surgical characteristics influence postoperative pain after primary THA by ASI approach in a fast-track setting, using a multimodal pain protocol which was developed to reduce acute postoperative pain to enable quick mobilization and rehabilitation. The only two factors associated with increased postoperative pain adjusted for the other factors in the model, were preoperative use of pain medication (regression coefficient 0.78 (95% CI 0.28–1.26); p = 0.005) and preoperative neuropathic pain scored by DN4 (regression coefficient 0.68 (95% CI 0.15–1.20); p = 0.02).

In our study, we used a multimodal pain protocol, including paracetamol, celecoxib, gabapentin, dexamethasone and esketamine [7–12]. This pain protocol is part

Table 3 Pain scores determined with the NRS at the standardized moments

NRS		N	mean (range)
Preoperative		72	5.26 (0.0–9.0)
Day of surgery	1 h	69	1.51 (0.0–8.0)
	4 h	74	2.97 (0.0–9.0)
	Before mobilization	69	2.62 (0.0–6.0)
	After mobilization	65	2.93 (0.0–10.0)
	8 h	72	2.40 (0.0–8.0)
Day 1	Morning	67	1.63 (0.0–5.0)
	Before mobilization	72	1.71 (0.0–7.0)
	After mobilization	71	2.25 (0.0–9.0)
	Afternoon	60	1.57 (0.0–6.0)
	Before mobilization	54	1.26 (0.0–4.0)
	After mobilization	54	1.73 (0.0–6.0)
Day 2	Morning	39	2.00 (0.0–7.0)
	Before mobilization	41	1.54 (0.0–6.0)
	After mobilization	41	1.84 (0.0–4.5)
	Afternoon	14	1.82 (0.0–3.0)
	Before mobilization	15	1.27 (0.0–3.0)
	After mobilization	15	1.93 (0.0–4.0)

of a fast-track setting and is developed to reduce acute postoperative pain to enable patients to quickly mobilize and rehabilitate in an optimized and safe perioperative period [4, 5]. Mean postoperative pain score determined with the NRS collected at 17 standardized moments, varied from 1.51 (range 0.0–8.0) to 2.97 (range 0.0–9.0). These results demonstrate that the use of our multimodal pain protocol enables adequate postoperative pain relief in which patients are able to mobilize and rehabilitate quickly. However, despite this pain protocol, a large range in reported postoperative pain between patients still exists, including some outliers with high postoperative pain scores.

Pain has been described to be a sensory and emotional experience that is influenced by multiple factors [34, 35]. Although several other studies reported on effects of specific patient- and provider characteristics on postoperative pain [19–27], none of these studies were performed in a fast-track setting with a multimodal pain protocols developed to reduce acute postoperative pain (and hence enable early mobilization), were included in these studies. Since no literature reports on the effect of potential factors associated with increased postoperative pain in a fast-track setting, our model included various potential factors that have been described to be associated with postoperative pain based on a non-fast-track setting [19–27, 36]. The use of a multimodal pain protocol in our study might have influenced the effects of these characteristics on postoperative pain and could be a reason for discrepancy between our results and results of these other studies.

Preoperative use of pain medication provides information on the preoperative pain levels of patients and has been shown to be associated with more severe postoperative pain [26, 27]. Our study supports these findings. In contrast,

Table 4 Regression coefficients with 95% CIs for potential factors associated with increased postoperative pain after THA in a fast-track setting

		Univariable analyses		Multivariable analysis	
		coefficient (95% CI)	*p*-value	coefficient (95% CI)	*p*-value
Age		0.006 (−0.02–0.03)	0.66	–	–
BMI		0.03 (−0.03–0.09)	0.28	–	–
Gender	male vs. female	−0.31 (−0.79–0.18)	0.22	–	–
ASA classification	ASA2 vs. ASA1	0.30 (−0.21–0.80)	0.25	–	–
Surgery time		−0.01 (−0.03–0.0005)	0.06	0.0004 (−0.01–0.01)	0.96
Diabetes Mellitus		−0.05 (−0.88–0.78)	0.92	–	–
Incision length		0.02 (−0.26–0.31)	0.89	–	–
Living situation	with cohabitants vs. alone	0.53 (−0.05–1.10)	0.08	0.50 (−0.08–1.07)	0.11
Preoperative antidepressants use	yes vs. no	0.66 (−0.39–1.71)	0.22	–	–
Preoperative pain medication use	yes vs. no	0.68 (0.18–1.18)	0.009	0.78 (0.28–1.26)	0.005
Preoperative pain		0.10 (−0.01–0.21)	0.08	−0.02 (−0.13–0.09)	0.73
DN4	likely vs. unlikely	0.70 (0.13–1.28)	0.02	0.68 (0.15–1.20)	0.02
APAIS anxiety	yes vs. no	−0.06 (−0.67–0.54)	0.84	–	–
APAIS information	average vs. no/little	−0.02 (−0.61–0.56)	0.93	−0.21 (−0.74–0.31)	0.45
	high vs. no/little	0.50 (−0.16–1.15)	0.15	0.45 (−0.12–1.02)	0.15

Factors that were associated with the outcome in univariable analyses (*p*-values <0.20) were included in a multivariable linear mixed model for repeated measures. In the multivariable analyses *p*-values <0.05 were considered significant

another study on postoperative pain 12 to 24 h after elective abdominal surgery, demonstrated no effect of preoperative use of pain medication on postoperative pain [23].

Our multimodal protocol for postoperative pain medication was standardized for all patients. The effect of this pain protocol might therefore not be sufficient for single patients who are used to pain medication. On the other hand, in a study on postoperative pain after thoracic surgery a decrease in postoperative pain medication use for patients who used pain medication preoperatively was found [37].

DN4 [30, 31] is a validated questionnaire for neuropathic pain, which was preoperatively scored for all patients in our study. The differences between neuropathic pain and non-neuropathic (nociceptive) pain have been described in literature [30]. Osteoarthritis, the main indication for THA in our study, causes non-neuropathic pain [30]. Patients who experience non-neuropathic pain from osteoarthritis preoperatively, are more likely to benefit from THA and will experience less pain postoperatively. Since preoperative neuropathic pain is not caused by osteoarthritis of the hip [30], THA will probably not resolve this neuropathic pain. As a consequence, these patients will be more likely to experience more postoperative pain after primary THA.

In the present study, none of the other factors were significantly associated with postoperative pain. All of these potential factors have been described to be associated with postoperative pain in non-fast-track setting studies [19–27, 36]. Contrasting results on the effect of age on postoperative pain have been reported in literature, including an association between younger age and a higher level of postoperative pain [20, 23, 24, 27] as well as a lack of effect of age on the level of postoperative pain [26, 38].

BMI has been shown to be associated with an increased inflammatory response [38], which is related to higher levels of postoperative pain [39], whereas others demonstrated no effect of BMI on postoperative pain scores [24, 39, 40]. In our study we excluded patients with BMI > 40 kg/m^2, which might be a reason for lack of effect of BMI on postoperative pain.

Regarding gender, contrasting results on the effect on postoperative pain have been reported in literature as well. These results include both higher postoperative pain for female patients [24, 27, 38] and no effect of gender on postoperative pain [22, 23, 25, 26].

Higher ASA classification has also been shown to be associated with increased postoperative pain [23]. However, in our study we only included patients with ASA classification I or II, which might be a reason for lack of effect of ASA classification on postoperative pain.

An increased incision length results in increased tissue damage, and might subsequently result in increased postoperative pain. This relation has been described in literature [24]. In our study the ASI approach was used. Since this approach uses both an intermuscular and internervous plane, less surgical trauma and hence lower postoperative pain scores and less pain medication consumption have been described [13–18].

Use of antidepressants provides information on patients' mental state, which could be predictive for the patients' response on pain medication and pain experience [25]. Moreover, in literature depression symptoms have been mentioned to be related to higher level of postoperative pain [23, 38, 41].

Furthermore, we used different validated questionnaires preoperatively for all patients to define preoperative pain and pain characteristics, including the APAIS [29]. Anxious patients respond differently to anesthesia and pain than non-anxious patients and therefore require larger doses of anaesthetics [19, 20, 25, 42, 43]. It has been reported that the anxiety/'worry' component of the APAIS is positively associated with the occurrence of early postoperative pain, whereas a strong information seeking behavior reduces the incidence of severe postoperative pain [24]. This is in contrast to others who report that patients who require more information about impending discomforts preoperatively may sensitize the individual to the experience [19].

Some potential limitations of our study should be discussed. First, although only 74 patients were included in the present study, a strength of the study is that we used linear mixed models. These do not only model the correlation between repeated measures of the same patient, they also assess fluctuations in postoperative pain over time. Second, although others investigated effects of occupation and/or level of education [19, 23, 40, 41], SF-36 [24], and heart rate and blood pressure [36] on postoperative pain, we were not able to include these variables in our model, because these variables were not reported in a consistent way in the patient files. Third, one single orthopaedic surgeon performed all surgical procedures which reduces variation in operative technique, however, could potentially mask systematic faults in surgical technique or surgical approach. Fourth, the indication of THA could be questioned in patients who do not need any preoperative pain medication. In our study, 50 out of 76 reported to use preoperative pain medication. National and international evidence-based guidelines for hip and knee OA recommend to start with (a combination of) conservative treatments. Despite the recommendation in guidelines to start with conservative treatments and only use surgical intervention if a patient does not respond sufficiently to conservative treatment options, the use of conservative treatments in daily practice is suboptimal [44–47]. It has been shown that conservative treatments were not fully exploited in 81%

of the patients who were referred to specialized knee/hip OA outpatient clinics [44]. Even worse, a recent study showed that only 10% of the patients in orthopaedic practice received all recommended non-surgical treatments before surgery [48].

A qualitative systematic review of Ip and others [36] identified factors associated with postoperative pain and analgesic consumption. Type of surgery was an important predictive factor for postoperative pain. This suggests that results of our study are applicable for primary THA. Furthermore, this could be another reason for the discrepancy between different studies describing postoperative pain after different types of surgery, besides differences in the pain protocol used.

Conclusion

Only preoperative use of pain medication and preoperative neuropathic pain were associated with increased postoperative pain after primary THA in a fast-track setting, including a multimodal pain protocol which was developed to reduce acute postoperative pain to enable quick mobilization and rehabilitation. This knowledge provides further details for optimization of postoperative pain management and preoperative patient education.

Abbreviations

APAIS: Amsterdam preoperative anxiety and information scale; ASA: American Society of Anaesthesiologists; ASI: Anterior supine intermuscular; BMI: Body mass index; DM: Diabetes mellitus; DN4: Douleur neuropathique en 4 questions; LOS: Length of hospital stay; NRS: Numeric rating scale; THA: Total hip arthroplasty

Acknowledgements

We would like to show our gratitude to the patients who made this study possible.

Funding

No funding was received.

Authors' contributions

All authors (YMdH, GH, NTvD, NMM, SBV) designed the study and interpreted data. YMdH and GH made the statistical analyses. YMdH, GH and NMM wrote the first version of the manuscript. All authors critically revised different versions of the manuscript. YMdH is the corresponding author. All authors read and approved the final manuscript.

Consent for publication

Written consent for publication of the results was obtained from all study participants.

Competing interests

The authors declare that they have no competing of interests.

Author details

[1]Department of Orthopaedic Surgery, Reinier de Graaf Hospital, Delft, the Netherlands. [2]Orthopaedic Research Lab, Department of Orthopaedics, Radboud university medical center, Nijmegen, the Netherlands. [3]Department of Anaesthesiology and Pain Medicine, Reinier de Graaf Hospital, Delft, the Netherlands.

References

1. Busch CA, Whitehouse MR, Shore BJ, MacDonald SJ, McCalden RW, Bourne RB. The efficacy of periarticular multimodal drug infiltration in total hip arthroplasty. Clin Orthop Relat Res. 2010;468(8):2152–9.
2. Kerr DR, Kohan L. Local infiltration analgesia: a technique for the control of acute postoperative pain following knee and hip surgery: a case study of 325 patients. Acta Orthop. 2008;79(2):174–83.
3. Kehlet H, Andersen LØ. Local infiltration analgesia in joint replacement: the evidence and recommendations for clinical practice. Acta Anaesthesiol Scand. 2011;55(7):778–84.
4. Kehlet H, Wilmore DW. Multimodal strategies to improve surgical outcome. Am J Surg. 2002;183(6):630–41.
5. Husted H, Jensen CM, Solgaard S, Kehlet H. Reduced length of stay following hip and knee arthroplasty in Denmark 2000–2009: from research to implementation. Arch Orthop Trauma Surg. 2012;132(1): 101–4.
6. den Hartog YM, Mathijssen NM, Vehmeijer SB. Reduced length of hospital stay after the introduction of a rapid recovery protocol for primary THA procedures. Acta Orthop. 2013;84(5):444–7.
7. Rasmussen ML, Mathiesen O, Dierking G, Christensen BV, Hilsted KL, Larsen TK. Multimodal analgesia with gabapentin, ketamine and dexamethasone in combination with paracetamol and ketorolac after hip arthroplasty: a preliminary study. Eur J Anaesthesiol. 2010;27(4):324–30.
8. de Oliviera GS Jr, Almeida MD, Benzon HT, RJ MC. Perioperative single dose systemic dexamethasone for postoperative pain: a meta-analysis of randomized controlled trials. Anesthesiology. 2011;115(3):575–88.
9. Lunn TH, Husted H, Solgaard S, Kristensen BB, Otte KS, Kjersgaard AG, Gaarn-Larsen L, Kehlet H. Intraoperative local infiltration analgesia for early analgesia after total hip arthroplasty: a randomized, double-blind, placebo-controlled trial. Reg Anesth Pain Med. 2011;36(5):424–9.
10. Lunn TH, Andersen LØ, Kristensen BB, Husted H, Gaarn-Larsen L, Bandholm T, Ladelund S, Kehlet H. Effect of high-dose preoperative methylprednisolone on recovery after total hip arthroplasty: a randomized, double-blind, placebo-controlled trial. Br J Anaesth. 2013;110(1):66–73.
11. Carmichael NM, Katz J, Clarke H, Kennedy D, Kreder HJ, Gollish J, McCartney CJ. An intensive perioperative regimen of pregabalin and celecoxib reduces pain and improves physical function scores six weeks after total hip arthroplasty: a prospective randomized controlled trial. Pain Res Manag. 2013;18(3):127–32.
12. Schmidt PC, Ruchelli G, Mackey SC, Carroll IR. Perioperative gabapentinoids: choice of agent, dose, timing, and effects on chronic postsurgical pain. Anesthesiology. 2013;119(5):1215–21.
13. Alecci V, Valente M, Crucil M, Minerva M, Pellegrino CM, Sabbadini DD. Comparison of primary total hip replacements performed with a direct anterior approach versus the standard lateral approach: perioperative findings. J Orthop Traumatol. 2011;12(3):123–9.
14. Goebel S, Steinert AF, Schillinger J, Eulert J, Broscheit J, Rudert M, Nöth U. Reduced postoperative pain in total hip arthroplasty after minimal-invasive anterior approach. Int Orthop. 2012;36(3):491–8.
15. Pogliacomi F, Paraskevopoulos A, Costantino C, Marenghi P, Ceccarelli F. Influence of surgical experience in the learning curve of a new approach in hip replacement: anterior mini-invasive vs. standard lateral. Hip Ints. 2012;22(05):555–61.
16. Barrett WP, Turner SE, Leopold JP. Prospective randomized study of direct anterior vs postero-lateral approach for total hip arthroplasty. J Arthroplast. 2013;28(9):1634–8.
17. Ilchmann T, Gersbach S, Zwicky L, Clauss M. Standard transgluteal versus minimal invasive anterior approach in hip arthroplasty: a prospective, consecutive cohort study. Orthop Rev (Pavia). 2013;5(4):e31.
18. Zawadsky MW, Paulus MC, Murray PJ, Johansen MA. Early outcome comparison between the direct anterior approach and the mini-incision

posterior approach for primary total hip arthroplasty: 150 consecutive cases. J Arthroplast. 2014;29(6):1256–60.
19. Scott LE, Clum GA, Peoples JB. Preoperative predictors of postoperative pain. Pain. 1983;15(3):283–93.
20. Perry F, Parker RK, White PF, Clifford PA. Role of psychological factors in postoperative pain control and recovery with patient-controlled analgesia. Clin J Pain. 1994;10(1):57–63.
21. Slappendel R, Weber EW, Bugter ML, Dirksen R. The intensity of preoperative pain is directly correlated with the amount of morphine needed for postoperative analgesia. Anesth Analg. 1999;88(1):146–8.
22. Dahmani S, Dupont H, Mantz J, Desmonts JM, Keita H. Predictive factors of early morphine requirements in the post-anaesthesia care unit (PACU). Br J Anaesth. 2001;87(3):385–9.
23. Caumo W, Schmidt AP, Schneider CN, Bergmann J, Iwamoto CW, Adamatti LC, Bandeira D, Ferreira MB. Preoperative predictors of moderate to intense acute postoperative pain I patients undergoing abdominal surgery. Acta Anaesthesiol Scand. 2002;64(10):1265–71.
24. Kalkman CJ, Visser K, Moen J, Bonsel GJ, Grobbee DE, Moons KG. Preoperative prediction of severe postoperative pain. Pain. 2003;105(3):415–23.
25. Granot M, Ferber SG. The roles of pain catastrophizing and anxiety in the prediction of postoperative pain intensity: a prospective study. Clin J Pain. 2005;21(5):439–45.
26. Aubrun F, Valade N, Coriat P, Riou B. Predictive factors of severe postoperative pain in the postanesthesia care unit. Anest Analg. 2008;106(5):1535–41.
27. Liu SS, Buvanendran A, Rathmell JP, Sawhney M, Bae JJ, Moric M, Perros S, Pope AJ, Poultsides L, Della Vall CJ, Shin NS, McCartney CJ, Ma Y, Shah M, Wood MJ, Manion SC, Sculco TP. Predictors for moderate to severe acute postoperative pain after total hip and knee replacement. Int Orthop. 2012;36(11):2261–7.
28. Shrier I, Platt RW. Reducing bias through directed acyclic graphs. BMC Med Res Methodol. 2008;8:70.
29. Moerman N, van Dam FS, Muller MJ, Oosting H. The Amsterdam Preoperative Anxiety and Information Scale (APAIS). Anesth Analg. 1996;82(3):445–51.
30. Bouhassira D, Attal N, Alchaar H, Boureau F, Brochet B, Bruxelle J, Cunin G, Fermanian J, Ginies P, Grun-Overdyking A, Jafari SChluep H, Lantéri-Minet M, Laurent B, Mick G, Serrie A, Valade D, Vicaut E. Comparison of pain syndromes associated with nervous or somatic lesions and development of a new neuropathic pain diagnostic questionnaire (DN4). Pain. 2005;114(1–2):29–36.
31. van Seventer R, Vos C, Giezeman M, Meerding WJ, Arnould B, Regnault A, van Eerd M, Martin C, Huygen F. Validation of the Dutch version of the DN4 diagnostic questionnaire for neuropathic pain. Pain Pract. 2013;13(5):390–8.
32. R Core Team. R: a language and environment for statistical computing. Vienna: R Foundation for Statistical Computing; 2014. http://www.R-project.org/.
33. Pinheiro J, Bates D, DebRoy S, Sarkar D, R Core Team. nlme: linear and nonlinear mixed effects models. R package version. 2014;3:1–118. http://cran.r-project.org/web/packages/nlme/.
34. Melzack R, Wall P. Pain mechanisms: a new theory. Science. 1965;150(3699):971–9.
35. Loeser J, Melzack R. Pain: an overview. Lancet. 1999;353(9164):1607–9.
36. Ip HY, Abrishami A, Peng PW, Wong J, Chung F. Predictors of postoperative pain and analgesic consumption. Anesthesiology. 2009;111(3):657–77.
37. Bachiocco V, Rucci P, Carli G. Request of analgesics in post-surgical pain. Relationships to psychological factors and pain-related variables. Pain Clinic. 1996;9(2):169–79.
38. de Cosmo G, Congedo E, Lai C, Primieri P, Dottarelli A, Aceto P. Preoperative psychologic and demographic predictors of pain perception and tramadol consumption using intravenous patient-controlled analgesia. Clin J Pain. 2008;24(5):399–405.
39. Motaghedi R, Bae JJ, Memtsoudis SG, Kim DH, Beathe JC, Paroli L, YaDeau JT, Gordon MA, Maalof DB, Lin Y, Ma Y, Cunningham-Rundless S, Liu SS. Association of obesity with inflammation and pain after total hip arthroplasty. Clin Orthop Relat Res. 2014;472(5):1442–8.
40. Chia YY, Chow LH, Hung CC, Liu K, Ger LP, Wang PN. Gender and pain upon movement are associated with the requirements for postoperative patient-controlled iv analgesia: a prospective survey of 2.298 Chinese patients. Can J Anaesth. 2002;49(3):249–55.
41. Taenzer P, Melzack R, Jeans ME. Influence of psychological factors on postoperative pain, mood and analgesic requirements. Pain. 1986;24(3):331–42.
42. Williams JGL, Jones JR. Psychophysiological responses to anesthesia and operation. JAMA. 1968;203:127–9.
43. Thyer BA, Papsdorf JD, Davis R, Vallecorsa S. Autonomic correlates of the subjective anxiety scale. J Behav Ther Exp Psychiatry. 1984;15:3–7.
44. Snijders GF, den Broeder AA, van Riel PL, Straten VH, de Man FH, van den Hoogen FH. Evidence-based tailored conservative treatment of knee and hip osteoarthritis: between knowing and doing. Scand J Rheumatol. 2011;40:225–31.
45. Shrier I, Feldman DE, Gaudet MC, Rossignol M, Zukor D, Tanzer M. Conservative non-pharmacological treatment options are not frequently used in the management of hip osteoarthritis. J Sci Med Sport. 2006;9:81–6.
46. De Haan MN, Guzman J, Bayley MT, Bell MJ. Knee osteoarthritis clinical practice guidelines – how are we doing? J Rheumatol. 2007;34:2099–105.
47. Hunter DJ. Quality of osteoarthritis care for community-dwelling older adults. Clin Geriatr Med. 2010;26:401–17.
48. Hofstede SN, Vliet Vlieland TP, van den Ende CH, Nelissen RG, Marang-van de Mheen PJ, van Bodegom-Vos L. Variation in use of non-surgical treatments among osteoarthritis patients in orthopaedic practice in the Netherlands. BMJ Open. 2015;5(9):e009117.

27

An underlying diagnosis of osteonecrosis of bone is associated with worse outcomes than osteoarthritis after total hip arthroplasty

Jasvinder A. Singh[1,2,3*], Jason Chen[4], Maria C. S. Inacio[4], Robert S. Namba[5] and Elizabeth W. Paxton[4]

Abstract

Background: Well-designed studies of complications and readmission rates in patients undergoing total hip arthroplasty (THA) with osteonecrosis are lacking. Our objective was to examine if a diagnosis of osteonecrosis was associated with complications, mortality and readmission rates after THA.

Methods: We analyzed prospectively collected data from an integrated healthcare system's Total Joint Replacement Registry of adults with osteonecrosis vs. osteoarthritis (OA) undergoing unilateral primary THA during 2001–2012, in an observational cohort study. We examined mortality (90-day), revision (ever), deep (1 year) and superficial (30-day) surgical site infection (SSI), venous thromboembolism (VTE, 90-day), and unplanned readmission (90-day). Age, gender, race, body mass index, American Society of Anesthesiologists class, and diabetes were evaluated as confounders. We used logistic or Cox regression to calculate odds or hazard ratios (OR, HR) with 95% confidence intervals (CI).

Results: Of the 47,523 primary THA cases, 45,252 (95.2%) had OA, and 2,271 (4.8%) had osteonecrosis. Compared to the OA, patients with osteonecrosis were younger (median age 55 vs. 67 years), and were less likely to be female (42.5% vs. 58.3%) or White (59.8% vs. 77.4%). Compared to the OA, the osteonecrosis cohort had higher crude incidence of 90-day mortality (0.7% vs. 0.3%), SSI (1.2% vs. 0.8%), unplanned readmission (9.6% vs. 5.2%) and revision (3.1% vs. 2.4%). After multivariable-adjustment, patients with osteonecrosis had a higher odds/hazard of mortality (OR: 2.48; 95% CI:1.31–4.72), SSI (OR: 1.67, 95%CI:1.11–2.51), unplanned 90-day readmissions (OR: 2.20; 95% CI:1.67–2.91) and a trend towards higher revision rate 1-year post-THA (HR: 1.32; 95% CI: 0.94–1.84), than OA patients.

Conclusions: Compared to OA, a diagnosis of osteonecrosis was associated with worse outcomes post-THA. A detailed preoperative discussion including the risk of complications is needed for informed consent from patients with osteonecrosis.

Keywords: Total hip replacement, Readmission, Osteoarthritis, Osteonecrosis, Arthroplasty, Joint replacement, Diagnosis, Risk factor

* Correspondence: Jasvinder.md@gmail.com
"The views expressed in this article are those of the authors and do not necessarily reflect the position or policy of the Department of Veterans Affairs or the United States government."
[1]Medicine Service, Birmingham VA Medical Center, Birmingham, AL, USA
[2]Department of Medicine at School of Medicine, and Division of Epidemiology at School of Public Health, University of Alabama, Faculty Office Tower 805B, 510 20th Street S, Birmingham, AL 35294, USA
Full list of author information is available at the end of the article

Background

Total hip arthroplasty (THA) is a successful surgical treatment for end stage arthritis [1]. The most common underlying diagnosis in patients undergoing elective THA is osteoarthritis (OA), followed by osteonecrosis, congenital hip disorders, and inflammatory arthritis [2]. A systematic review of 67 studies with 2,593 patients with 3,277 hips concluded that osteonecrosis was not associated with higher revision rates after THA compared to the other underlying diagnoses [3], with minor exceptions. A small single-site retrospective study of 31 patients with glucocorticoid-induced osteonecrosis undergoing THA reported improvement in pain and function with THA but high complication and reoperation rates [4]; however, there were no controls.

Post-THA complications and associated hospital readmissions are undesirable THA outcomes of great interest clinically, due to associated morbidity. Post-arthroplasty complications, such as surgical site infections (SSI) and thromboembolic complications, are responsible for most surgically related readmissions [5–7]. Overall, 90-day readmission rates range 7–8% after primary THA or primary total knee arthroplasty [7–9]. Readmission rate can have a significant impact on health care resources, especially given the high volume of these procedures. Mortality is rare after THA (mostly elective) and is extremely undesirable.

We recently showed that an underlying diagnosis of RA was associated with higher readmission rate compared to OA [10]. To our knowledge, studies of complications and readmission rates in patients undergoing THA with osteonecrosis are lacking. It is possible that outcomes in patients with osteonecrosis undergoing THA have improved over time due to the improvement in bearing surfaces and ubiquitous use of cementless fixation [11].

The objective of our study was to examine whether compared to OA, an underlying diagnosis of osteonecrosis was associated with a higher adjusted risk of complications and readmissions after primary THA (study hypothesis). We also performed exploratory analyses to assess the association of the cause of osteonecrosis with complications and readmissions post-primary THA.

Methods

We described study methods and results as recommended in the Strengthening of Reporting in Observational studies in Epidemiology (STROBE) statement [12].

Study design, data source, and patient sample

We performed a cohort study of patients who had undergone an elective unilateral primary THA using the Kaiser Permanente (KP) Total Joint Replacement Registry (TJRR). We identified a cohort of patients who underwent elective unilateral primary THA between 04/01/2001 and 12/31/2012. The KP is a integrated healthcare system that covers over 9.5 million members in 7 US geographical areas. We have previously reported details on the KP TJRR data collection procedures, structure, and participation [13, 14]. The KP TJRR uses paper and electronic data capture tools to collect information by surgeons and other healthcare providers at the point of care, as well as data from other databases (including the electronic medical records) using electronic screening algorithms. The information from different data sources of the registry is linked using the integrated healthcare system's unique patient identifiers. The data repository for the registry is a SQL database. A quarterly quality control check of these data ensures high accuracy. Specifically, the KP TJRR prospectively collects outcomes (i.e. readmissions, revision, SSI, venous thromboembolism (VTE)). Several outcomes including revision, SSI and VTE are adjudicated by review of charts by trained research associates [13, 14].

In a chart review of random sample of osteonecrosis and OA cases ($n = 60$; 30 cases each of osteonecrosis and OA) performed by an abstractor blinded to the database diagnosis, we found that the true positive rate of diagnoses (OA vs. osteonecrosis) was 88%. All registered cases in the KP TJRR are tracked until outcome and/or end of their lives. The voluntary participation of the KP TJRR in 2011 was 95% [14].

This study included all unilateral primary elective THA procedures, in patients aged 18 years old or older, with surgery indication for OA and/or osteonecrosis registered during the study period ($N = 47{,}523$). Patients who had a diagnosis of both OA and osteonecrosis ($N = 563$) were not included in the study. Patients who underwent revision THA, partial THA, or conversion procedures, as the index procedure, were not included in the study. This was done for two reasons: (1) the majority of THA are elective primary THA, our condition of interest; and (2) to keep the population homogeneous and allow easy interpretation of results. Cases from the geographical regions where the organization owns the hospitals (Southern California, Northern California, and Hawaii), covering 92% of the KP TJRR registered cases, were included. The final sample had cases from 50 hospitals and 362 surgeons.

Outcome measures

The outcomes of interest in this study were mortality within 90 days, SSI (30 days for superficial and 1 year for deep infections), VTE within 90 days, unplanned readmissions within 90 days of the index primary elective THA, and revision (ever and for any reason). All outcome measures were obtained from the KP TJRR using

2001–12 data; timing of outcome assessment was chosen based on clinical relevance, based on feedback from an expert surgeon (R.N.). SSIs, which can be either deep or superficial were defined according to the Centers for Disease Control and Prevention/National Healthcare Safety Network criteria [15]. Superficial and deep SSI were also combined into one measure in this study since we anticipated a small number of events for these two components individually. The VTE measure, which included symptomatic deep vein thrombosis (DVT) and pulmonary embolism (PE) in this study due to the small number of events, were identified using the Agency for Healthcare Research and Quality patient safety indicators technical specifications [16] and further confirmed by chart review validation by trained clinical research associates. Readmissions are captured by the KP TJRR using quarterly extracts from the institutional electronic medical records of all hospital readmissions post discharge from the original joint arthroplasty procedure, available from 2009. Only unplanned readmissions, which were determined based on the 2014 Centers for Medicare and Medicaid Services Procedure-Specific Readmission Measures Updates and Specification Report for Elective Primary THA [17] were included in the analysis. Planned admissions such as those likely for subsequent hip arthroplasty procedures (e.g. International Classifications of Disease, 9th Revision, code (ICD-9) 715.34, Osteoarthrosis, localized, pelvic region and thigh and ICD-9: 733.42, aseptic necrosis of head and neck of femur) were not included in the reported readmissions. Revisions were defined as any re-operation of the index procedure where a component was replaced.

Exposure of interest

An underlying diagnosis of osteonecrosis was the exposure of interest, compared with a diagnosis of OA. This information was obtained from the KP TJRR intra-operative forms completed by the surgeon at the time of surgery and does not rely on administrative data coding schemes. We also explored the associations by the cause/type of osteonecrosis, categorized as idiopathic vs. non-idiopathic, using the 2009–2012 data, the year of the beginning of prospective collection of intra-operative diagnosis and readmission data. Additional file 1 shows the sub-categories of non-idiopathic category glucocorticoid-induced vs. not glucocorticoid-induced (including hip fracture, alcohol abuse, sickle cell disease, lupus, pancreatitis, HIV, vasculitis and other autoimmune conditions).

Covariates and potential confounders

Age (<65 and ≥65 years old, based on Medicare-eligible age of 65 years and higher), gender; race (White and Others), body mass index (BMI, continuous in 5 unit increment); American Society of Anesthesiologists (ASA) class (<3 vs. ≥3), and medical comorbidities using the Elixhauser co-morbidity measure [18] were evaluated as possible confounders/covariates.

Statistical analyses

We calculated summary statistics to describe the study sample by whether the primary diagnosis was osteonecrosis vs. OA. We compared categorical variables between the two groups using 2-sided chi-square or Fisher's exact tests where appropriate. A logistic regression was used to model the relationship between osteonecrosis (OA being the reference category) and mortality, VTE, SSIs, and readmissions while accounting for the nesting of observations within the surgeon variable. We created Cox proportional hazard models to evaluate the association of osteonecrosis compared to OA and the time to revision surgery. Covariates tested as confounders, were included in the final adjusted model if they changed estimates by >10% and $p < 0.10$ or deemed clinically important for the relationship studied. Odds ratios (OR), hazard ratios (HR), 95% confidence internals (CI), and *p*-values are reported. A sensitivity analysis was conducted to evaluate the robustness of estimations accounting for missing data. We also performed sensitivity analyses that adjusted for the competing risk of death. No formal sample size calculations were done for this observational cohort study. Data were analyzed using SAS (Version 9.2, SAS Institute, Cary, NC, USA) and *p*-value <0.05 was considered statistical significant.

Results

Demographic and clinical characteristics of study sample

There were 47,523 patients included in the study from 2001 to 12. Of these, 2,271 (4.8%) had an underlying diagnosis of osteonecrosis. Demographic and clinical features of patients with osteonecrosis are shown in Table 1. Compared to the cohort of patients with OA, the osteonecrosis group was younger (median (interquartile range (IQR)): 55 (46–64) vs. 67 (59–75)) years old, had more males (1,306 (57.5%) vs. 18,875 (41.7%)), and had less White (1,358 (59.8%) vs. 35,009 (77.4%)) patients. Patients with osteonecrosis had lower BMI (<30 kg/m^2: 1,505 (66.3%) vs. 26,358 (58.3%)), slightly higher ASA scores (ASA ≥ 3: 897 (39.5%) vs. 15,827 (35.0%)), and were less likely to have diabetes (451 (19.9%) vs. 10,042 (22.2%)). Additional file 2 shows that several comorbidities were more prevalent in patients with osteonecrosis compared with those with osteoarthritis.

Between 2009 and 2012 (period of prospective collection of intra-operative diagnosis and readmission data), of a total of 670 patients, 507 (76%) had idiopathic osteonecrosis and 163 (24%) had non-idiopathic

Table 1 Study cohort characteristics by primary diagnosis at total hip arthroplasty surgery

		Total		Osteoarthritis		Osteonecrosis	
		n	%	n	%	n	%
Total N		47,523	100.0	45,252	95.2	2,271	4.8
Age, years	Median (IQR)	66.0 (58.0–74.0)		67.0 (59.0–75.0)		55.0 (46.0–64.0)	
Age category, years	<65	20,899	44.0	19,195	42.4	1,704	75.0
	≥65	26,624	56.0	26,057	57.6	567	25.0
Gender	Male	20,181	42.5	18,875	41.7	1,306	57.5
	Female	27,341	57.5	26,376	58.3	965	42.5
Race	White	36,367	76.5	35,009	77.4	1,358	59.8
	Black	3,637	7.7	3,324	7.4	313	13.8
	Hispanic	3,283	6.9	3,030	6.7	253	11.1
	Asian	1,606	3.4	1,436	3.2	170	7.5
	Other/Multi-racial	753	1.6	707	1.6	46	2.0
	Unknown	1,877	4.0	1,746	3.9	131	5.8
BMI category[a], kg/m^2	<30	27,863	58.6	26,358	58.3	1,505	66.3
	≥30 and <35	11,625	24.5	11,170	24.7	455	20.0
	≥35	7,394	15.6	7,138	15.8	256	11.3
ASA category[a]	1 and 2	29,312	61.7	28,008	61.9	1,304	57.4
	≥3	16,724	35.2	15,827	35.0	897	39.5
Diabetes		10,493	22.1	10,042	22.2	451	19.9

IQR interquartile range, *BMI* body mass index, *ASA* American Society of Anesthesiologists
[a]Missing data: BMI (1.4%), ASA (3.1%)

osteonecrosis. Among the non-idiopathic category, 40 (6%) patients had glucocorticoid-induced osteonecrosis and 123 (18%) patients had causes other than glucocorticoid-induced osteonecrosis. Additional file 3 shows that patient characteristics were similar between idiopathic vs. non-idiopathic etiology; similarly Additional file 4 shows that characteristics were similar between glucocorticoid-induced vs. not glucocorticoid-induced osteonecrosis.

Crude outcome incidence

Compared to patients with OA, patients with osteonecrosis had higher incidence of the following complications post-THA: 90-day mortality (0.7% vs. 0.3%), SSI (combined: 1.2% vs. 0.8%; 90-day deep infection: 0.6% vs. 0.5%; 30-day superficial infection: 0.6% vs. 0.3%), 90-day VTE (1.4% vs. 1.2%, DVT: 0.8% vs. 0.7%, PE: 0.6% vs. 0.5%), 90-day unplanned readmission (9.6% vs. 5.2%) and revision at any time during the follow-up (3.1% vs. 2.4%; Table 2). The median follow up time for revision outcome was 3.2 years (Interquartile range, 1.4–5.8). Unadjusted revision-free survival showed a trend favoring osteoarthritis compared to osteonecrosis (Fig. 1; $p = 0.108$).

Additional files 5 and 6 shows that the unadjusted rates of outcomes were similar by underlying cause of osteonecrosis except the following: higher 90-day readmission

Table 2 Crude incidence of outcomes by primary diagnosis at total hip arthroplasty surgery

	Osteoarthritis		Osteonecrosis	
	n	%	n	%
Death, 90 days	138	0.3	15	0.7
Surgical site infection, any	367	0.8	27	1.2
Deep, 1-year[a]	230	0.5	13	0.6
Superficial, 30-days[b]	137	0.3	14	0.6
Venous thromboembolism, 90-days	551	1.2	31	1.4
Deep vein thrombosis[c]	323	0.7	18	0.8
Pulmonary embolism[d]	228	0.5	13	0.6
Readmission, 90 days unplanned[e]	846	5.2	64	9.6
Revision, ever[f]	1,075	2.4	70	3.1

[a]Deep surgical site infection excluded patient who died or left the system within 1 year without deep SSI (1549, 3.3%), $n = 45974$ (96.7%)
[b]Superficial surgical site infection excluded patient who died or left the system within 30 days without superficial SSI (138, 0.3%), $n = 47385$ (99.7%)
[c]Deep vein thrombosis (DVT) excluded patient who died or left the system within 90 days without DVT (376, 0.8%), $n = 47147$ (99.2%)
[d]Pulmonary embolism (PE) excluded patient who died or left the system within 90 days without PE (374, 0.8%), $n = 47149$ (99.2%)
[e]Readmissions includes limited sample (operative years 2009–2012 and 3 geographical regions), $n = 17179$. Excluded patient who died or left the system within 90 days without readmission (85, 0.5%), final $n = 17094$ (99.5%)
[f]The median follow-up for revision outcome was 3.2 years (inter-quartile range, 1.4–5.8 years)

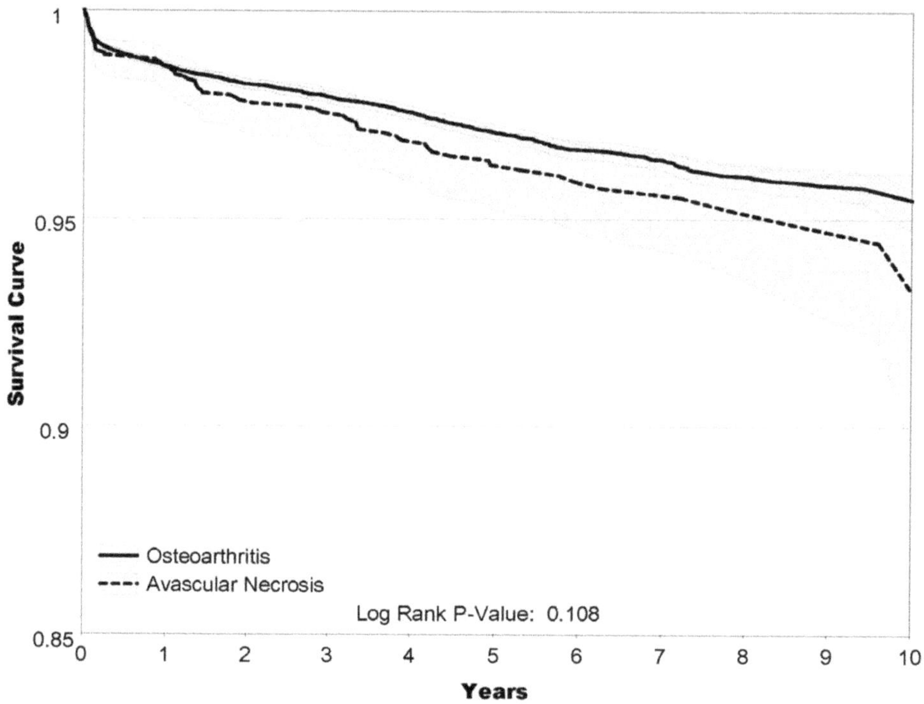

Fig. 1 Revision Free Survival Estimates for Cohorts with Osteonecrosis and Osteoarthritis. The figure shows the hip implant survival curve comparing osteoarthritis to osteonecrosis after primary total hip arthroplasty. The unadjusted revision-free survival showed a trend favoring osteoarthritis compared to osteonecrosis ($p = 0.108$)

(14.7% vs. 7.7%) and revision rates (3.1% vs. 1.2%) in non-idiopathic group vs. idiopathic group (see Additional file 5); and higher 90-day readmission rate (17.5% vs. 13.8%) in glucocorticoid-induced vs. not glucocorticoid-induced osteonecrosis (see Additional file 6),

Adjusted odds of mortality, SSI, VTE and readmission and adjusted risk of revision

After adjusting for age, race, BMI, and ASA class, the risk of 90-day mortality was significantly higher for patients with osteonecrosis than OA for the overall sample

Table 3 Unadjusted and adjusted association of osteonecrosis with death, surgical site infection (SSI), venous thromboembolism (VTE), and revision compared to osteoarthritis in patients undergoing total hip arthroplasty

Osteonecrosis vs. Osteoarthritis	Unadjusted OR (95%CI)	*p*-value	Adjusted OR (95%CI)	*p*-value
Death, 90 days[a]	2.12 (1.23–3.66)	0.007	2.48 (1.31–4.72)	0.006
SSI (deep and superficial)[b]	1.45 (0.97–2.18)	0.069	1.67 (1.11–2.51)	0.013
VTE (DVT and PE), <90 days[c]	1.16 (0.78–1.70)	0.466	1.37 (0.92–2.03)	0.118
Readmission, 90 days unplanned[d]	1.89 (1.43–2.48)	<0.001	2.20 (1.67–2.91)	<0.001
	Unadjusted HR (95%CI)	*p*-value	Adjusted HR (95%CI)	*p*-value
Revision (within 1 Year)[e]	1.00 (0.70–1.44)	0.992	0.92 (0.63–1.33)	0.652
Revision (after 1 Year)	1.44 (1.04–2.01)	0.030	1.32 (0.94–1.84)	0.109

SSI surgical site infection, as defined by the CDC, *VTE* venous thromboembolism, *DVT* deep vein thrombosis, *PE* pulmonary embolism- as defined by AHRQ, *OR* odds ratio, *HR* hazard ratio, *CI* confidence interval

All multivariable models were adjusted for covariates if they changed estimates by >10% and $p < 0.10$ in univariate analyses or deemed clinically important for the relationship studied

[a]Adjusted model excluded cases with missing BMI (641, 1.4%) and ASA (1,487, 3.1%), final $n = 45,431$ (95.6%). Multivariable-adjusted model was adjusted for age, race, BMI, and ASA

[b]The combined SSI includes 30-day superficial SSI and 1-year deep SSI. Adjusted model excluded cases with missing BMI (641, 1.4%), ad patients who died or left the system within 1 year (1,539, 3.2%), final $n = 45506$ (95.8%). Multivariable-adjusted model was adjusted for BMI

[c]The combined VTE outcome includes deep vein thrombosis and pulmonary embolism. Adjusted model excluded cases where patients either died or left the system within 90 days ($n = 370$, 0.8%), final $n = 47,153$ (99.2%). Multivariable-adjusted model was adjusted for age

[d]Readmissions includes limited sample (operative years 2009–2012 and 3 geographical regions), $n = 17,179$. Final adjusted model excluded cases where patients either died or left the system within 90 days ($n = 85$, 0.5%), final $n = 17,094$ (99.5%). Multivariable-adjusted model was adjusted for age

[e]Adjusted model had no exclusions due to missing values, $n = 47,523$ (100%). Multivariable-adjusted model was adjusted for age

(OR: 2.48; 95% CI, 1.31–4.72) (Table 3). After adjusting for BMI, the odds of SSI (deep and superficial) in patients with osteonecrosis were 1.67 (95% CI: 1.11–2.51) times higher than patients with OA (Table 3). In the age-adjusted model, the risk of VTE (DVT and PE) was not statistically significantly different between two groups (OR: 1.37; 95% CI, 0.92–2.03) (Table 3). After adjusting for age, 90-day unplanned readmission was statistically significantly higher in patients with osteonecrosis than those with OA (OR: 2.20; 95% CI, 1.67–2.91) (Table 3).

A time interaction was observed for revision after adjusting for age. While the risk estimates for revision surgery were not statistically significant overall, the direction of the risk estimates changed for patients within one year of the surgery vs. longer time, for OA vs. osteonecrosis. Specifically, compared to patients with OA, patients with osteonecrosis did not have any significantly different hazard of revision (HR = 0.92, 95% CI: 0.63–1.33) within one year of the surgery, but after one year, patients with osteonecrosis seemed to have a 1.32-times higher (95% CI: 0.94–1.84) hazard of revision surgery (Table 3).

Exploring differences by the underlying cause of osteonecrosis, the age-adjusted 90-day readmission was significantly higher in non-idiopathic vs. idiopathic group, with adjusted odds ratio of 2.13 (95% CI: 1.23–3.68). Additional file 7 shows that the revision rate seemed higher, but did not meet statistical significance. Additional file 8 shows that there was no significant difference in 90-day readmission was noted in glucocorticoid-induced vs. not glucocorticoid-induced osteonecrosis.

Reasons for readmission

The five most common principal discharge ICD-9 codes for the unplanned 90-day readmissions in patients with osteonecrosis were as follows: 996.42 (Dislocation of prosthetic joint), 038.9 (Unspecified septicemia), 486 (Pneumonia), 282.62 (Hemoglobin SS disease, sickle cell disease with crisis), and 493.22 (Chronic obstructive lung disease/asthma with exacerbation). In comparison, the five most common principal discharge ICD 9 codes for 90-day readmissions in patients with OA were as follows: 996.42 (dislocation of prosthetic joint), 996.66 (infection & inflammation reaction due to internal joint prosthesis), 998.59 (other postoperative infection), 38.9 (unspecified septicemia), and 996.44 (periprosthetic fracture around prosthetic joint). Additional file 9 shows the top 15 causes for readmission.

Sensitivity analyses: missing data and competing risk of death

The impact of the 2,092 (4.4%) missing data (1,487 (3.1%) in ASA class, 1 (0.0%) in gender, and 641 (1.3%) in BMI) was evaluated. The distribution of other patient characteristics between patients with missing data and those with complete data were not different. The crude incidence rates for all outcomes were not statistically significantly different except for 90-day mortality (1.2% in patients with missing data vs. 0.3% others). To evaluate the impact of these missing data points in the estimations, we modeled diagnoses and 90-day mortality without BMI and ASA adjustments and found 90-day mortality for patients with osteonecrosis was increased (OR: 3.39; 95% CI, 1.93–5.96, $p < 0.001$), indicating that main analyses provided conservative estimates. Sensitivity analyses that adjusted for competing risk of death showed that there were no changes in any of the above analyses (data available on request).

Discussion

In this study of 47,523 patients in KP TJRR registry undergoing primary THA, of whom 2,271 had osteonecrosis, we found that an underlying diagnosis of osteonecrosis was associated with higher risk of SSI, 90-day readmission and mortality following THA compared to OA. To our knowledge, our study is one of the most comprehensive studies to quantify the rate of several complications and unplanned 90-day readmission post-THA in a large, representative total joint registry study with validated outcomes. Our study overcomes a key limitation of previous studies, i.e., lack of a comparator group [3]. Our study also fills an important knowledge gap, i.e., are clinically important outcomes including revision surgery higher in patients with osteonecrosis? Several findings are novel and deserve further discussion.

The 90-day readmission rates following THA were 50% higher in patients with osteonecrosis compared to OA. To our knowledge, this is a novel finding of high interest to surgeons and policyholders. In absence of any previously published studies, this is the first study to demonstrate this difference. Readmission after an elective surgery such as THA can significantly influence health care utilization. Given that osteonecrosis is the second most common reason for primary THA, this excess utilization is clinically meaningful. With 332,000 THAs performed in 2010 in the US, the 90-day post-THA unplanned readmission rate of 6.8% translates into >12,000 admissions annually. Our finding of higher unplanned readmission rates in patients with osteonecrosis post-THA with an odds ratio of 2.20 adds to our recent study finding that RA was associated with 74% higher 90-day readmission compared to OA in patients undergoing THA or total knee arthroplasty [19].

We hypothesized the following potential reasons for a higher rate of readmission in patients with osteonecrosis compared to OA: (1) a higher rate of corticosteroid use or alcohol consumption, frequent causes of osteonecrosis (as noted by us, Additional file 1); (2) higher comorbidity and complexity in patients with osteonecrosis (higher ASA class in a previous study) [20]; (3) association of osteonecrosis with conditions such as trauma, autoimmune diseases and coagulation abnormalities, which are potential risk factors for poor THA outcomes; and (4) potential differences in bone structure and quality in osteonecrosis vs. OA, which might be related to implant-related complications. In fact, our data show that the prevalence of certain comorbidities (e.g. liver disease, chronic liver disease, deficiency anemia, alcohol abuse) was higher in patients with osteonecrosis.

The 90-day mortality was 2.5-times higher in patients with osteonecrosis who underwent primary THA, compared to OA. Due to the limitation of most previous studies of osteonecrosis to patients under the age of 50 years (and even smaller sample sizes), the ability to study a rare outcome, such as mortality, was previously limited. A large study sample size allowed us to assess this outcome appropriately. As noted above, a higher rate of comorbidity and potentially corticosteroid-associated complications in patients with osteonecrosis, may have contributed to higher mortality rates. Regardless of the cause, patients with osteonecrosis undergoing primary THA should be made aware of our finding of a significant difference in mortality post-THA compared to OA patients undergoing THA, providing them with relative and absolute risk. Based on our study findings, more studies into the etiology of this rare, but critical outcome are needed in patients with osteonecrosis. A better understanding of modifiable risk factors that are associated with excess mortality can allow them to be targeted for interventions aimed at reducing mortality in patients with osteonecrosis undergoing primary THA.

Another important and new clinical finding from our study was the higher risk of SSI in patients with osteonecrosis undergoing primary THA. Corticosteroid use, alcohol use or autoimmune diseases, risk factors for osteonecrosis, may also increase the risk of SSIs, due to known associations of these factors with the risk of infections [21–23]. One study of patients with glucocorticoid-induced osteonecrosis in patients undergoing THA without any controls showed a high complication rate [4]. Our study adds to this literature by showing that outcomes such as SSIs occurred more frequently in the overall cohort of patients with osteonecrosis undergoing primary THA, not just those with glucocorticoid-induced osteonecrosis.

In exploratory analyses by the underlying cause of osteonecrosis, adjusted 90-day readmission was significantly higher (2.13-times) and revision rate borderline higher, in non-idiopathic vs. idiopathic group. This is not surprising considering that comorbidities (alcohol abuse, lupus, hip fracture etc.) in the non-idiopathic are potential risk factors for poor outcomes and readmissions. Numbers for complications/outcomes by glucocorticoid-induced vs. other causes of osteonecrosis were too small to allow any meaningful comparison.

Our study has several limitations. Despite our efforts to control for several covariates and confounders in our observational study, residual confounding bias is possible. We were unable to investigate the outcomes of osteonecrosis by each underlying reason (corticosteroid, alcohol abuse, sickle cell disease, lupus etc.), due to the limitation of the number of patients with these diagnoses in our cohort, making the analyses very underpowered to perform any analyses. Larger studies in the future (perhaps data from national arthroplasty registries or data from several national registries combined) should investigate whether osteonecrosis associated with sickle cell, alcohol abuse etc. has worse outcome than other causes of osteonecrosis. These findings may not be generalizable to the U.S. general population; however, the membership of KP has been shown to be demographically and socioeconomically representative of the geographical regions it covers [24, 25]. The study strengths include a large sample size, comparison of OA to osteonecrosis and the adjustment for important covariates. Some patients may have died before having one of the outcome measures because we treated each outcome as an independent event. Therefore, it is possible that we underestimated the incidence of the other complications. However, we performed models with death as the competing risk that showed no change in analyses, indicating that the associations of osteonecrosis we noted were not affected by the competing mortality risk.

Conclusions

In summary, we found patients with osteonecrosis had higher risk of mortality, SSI and unplanned readmission post-THA, compared to patients with OA. These differences were both clinically meaningful and statistically significant. Our study findings have clinical implications. Surgeons can discuss increased rates of these complications/risks (absolute and relative) with patients with osteonecrosis before obtaining informed consent from patients undergoing THA. Our study also has implications for future research. We identified several aspects of poorer outcomes in patients with osteonecrosis compared to those with OA that need further investigation. Research into the underlying reasons for higher complication rate in patients with osteonecrosis undergoing primary THA should help understand this key clinical problem.

Additional files

Additional file 1: Diagnostic codes for subtypes of osteonecrosis. This file shows the idiopathic and non-idiopathic causes of osteonecrosis, alongside the diagnostic codes and further sub-categorization of non-idiopathic osteonecrosis into glucocorticoid-induced vs. other causes.

Additional file 2: Prevalence of Comorbidities by Primary Diagnosis at Total Hip Arthroplasty Surgery. This file shows the prevalence of various comorbidities in patients with osteoarthritis vs. osteonecrosis as the underlying reason and the primary diagnosis for the Total Hip Arthroplasty Surgery.

Additional file 3: Characteristics of patients with osteonecrosis by the underlying etiology, Idiopathic vs. Non-Idiopathic. This file shows the comparison of key characteristics between Idiopathic and Non-Idiopathic etiology of osteonecrosis.

Additional file 4: Patient characteristics for patients with Non-Idiopathic osteonecrosis only (Glucocorticoid-induced vs. Not). This file shows the comparison of key characteristics between Glucocorticoid-induced vs. Not glucocorticoid-induced among those with a non-Idiopathic etiology of osteonecrosis.

Additional file 5: Unadjusted outcomes in patients with osteonecrosis by the underlying etiology, Idiopathic vs. Non-Idiopathic. This file shows the unadjusted comparisons of the outcomes in patients with Idiopathic vs. Non-Idiopathic etiology of osteonecrosis.

Additional file 6: Unadjusted outcomes in patients with Non-Idiopathic osteonecrosis only (Glucocorticoid-induced vs. Not Glucocorticoid-induced). This file shows the unadjusted comparisons of the outcomes in patients with Glucocorticoid-induced vs. Not Glucocorticoid-induced etiology of osteonecrosis among those with a non-Idiopathic etiology of osteonecrosis.

Additional file 7: Adjusted association of Non-Idiopathic vs. idiopathic cause of osteonecrosis with outcomes, revision and 90-day unplanned readmissions. This file shows the age-adjusted association of non-Idiopathic vs. idiopathic cause of osteonecrosis for revision and 90-day unplanned readmissions.

Additional file 8: Adjusted* association of glucocorticoid-induced osteonecrosis vs. not glucocorticoid-induced osteonecrosis with outcomes. This file shows the age-adjusted association of glucocorticoid-induced osteonecrosis vs. not glucocorticoid-induced osteonecrosis for 90-day unplanned readmissions.

Additional file 9: Top 15 International Classification of Diseases, Ninth Revision (ICD-9) codes and descriptions of unplanned readmissions within 90 days of Total Hip Arthroplasty Surgery by primary diagnosis (osteoarthritis vs. osteonecrosis). This file shows the top 15 reasons for unplanned readmissions within 90 days of Total Hip Arthroplasty Surgery by primary diagnosis, osteoarthritis vs. osteonecrosis.

Abbreviations

ASA: American Society of Anesthesiologists; BMI: Body mass index; CI: Confidence internals; HR: Hazard ratio; OA: Osteoarthritis; OR: Odds ratio; THA: Total hip arthroplasty

Acknowledgments

Not applicable.

Funding

No direct funding was obtained for this study.

Authors' contributions

All authors have read and approved the manuscript. JS, MI, EP: development of study question and protocol. JS, MI, EP, RN: modification and finalization of study protocol. MI, JC: data programming, data analysis. JS, MI, EP, RN, JC: Interpretation of data analysis. JS: First Draft of manuscript. JS, MI, EP, RN, JC: Critical revisions and approval of the final version of the manuscript.

Competing interests

There are no financial conflicts related directly to this study. JAS has received research grants from Takeda and Savient and consultant fees from Savient, Takeda, Regeneron, Merz, Iroko, Bioiberica, Crealta and Allergan pharmaceuticals, WebMD, UBM LLC and the American College of Rheumatology. JAS serves as the principal investigator for an investigator-initiated study funded by Horizon pharmaceuticals through a grant to DINORA, Inc., a 501 (c)(3) entity. JAS is a member of the executive of OMERACT, an organization that develops outcome measures in rheumatology and receives arms-length funding from 36 companies; a member of the American College of Rheumatology's (ACR) Annual Meeting Planning Committee (AMPC); Chair of the ACR Meet-the-Professor, Workshop and Study Group Subcommittee; and a member of the Veterans Affairs Rheumatology Field Advisory Committee. Other authors declare no financial conflict. The authors declare that they have no competing interests.

Consent for publication

No individual person's data were presented in any form in this study and therefore no consent to publish was required.

Author details

[1]Medicine Service, Birmingham VA Medical Center, Birmingham, AL, USA. [2]Department of Medicine at School of Medicine, and Division of Epidemiology at School of Public Health, University of Alabama, Faculty Office Tower 805B, 510 20th Street S, Birmingham, AL 35294, USA. [3]Department of Orthopedic Surgery, Mayo Clinic College of Medicine, Rochester, MN, USA. [4]Department of Surgical Outcomes and Analysis, Kaiser Permanente, San Diego, CA, USA. [5]Department of Orthopaedic Surgery, Kaiser Permanente, Irvine, CA, USA.

References

1. Learmonth ID, Young C, Rorabeck C. The operation of the century: total hip replacement. Lancet. 2007;370(9597):1508–19.
2. Anderson A, Singh JA. Pegloticase for chronic gout. Cochrane Database Syst Rev. 2010;3(3):CD008335.
3. Johannson HR, Zywiel MG, Marker DR, Jones LC, McGrath MS, Mont MA. Osteonecrosis is not a predictor of poor outcomes in primary total hip arthroplasty: a systematic literature review. Int Orthop. 2011;35(4):465–73.
4. Rahman WA, Garbuz DS, Masri BA. Total hip arthroplasty in steroid-induced osteonecrosis: early functional and radiological outcomes. Can J Surg. 2013;56(1):41–6.
5. Avram V, Petruccelli D, Winemaker M, de Beer J. Total Joint Arthroplasty Readmission Rates and Reasons for 30-Day Hospital Readmission. J Arthroplasty. 2013;29(3):465-8.
6. Pugely AJ, Callaghan JJ, Martin CT, Cram P, Gao Y. Incidence of and risk factors for 30-day readmission following elective primary total joint arthroplasty: analysis from the ACS-NSQIP. J Arthroplasty. 2013;28(9):1499–504.
7. Saucedo JM, Marecek GS, Wanke TR, Lee J, Stulberg SD, Puri L. Understanding Readmission After Primary Total Hip and Knee Arthroplasty: Who's at Risk? J Arthroplasty. 2013;29(2):256-6.

8. Schairer WW, Vail TP, Bozic KJ. What Are the Rates and Causes of Hospital Readmission After Total Knee Arthroplasty? Clin Orthop Relat Res. 2013; 472(1):181-7.
9. Schairer WW, Sing DC, Vail TP, Bozic KJ. Causes and Frequency of Unplanned Hospital Readmission After Total Hip Arthroplasty. Clin Orthop Relat Res. 2013;472(2):464-70.
10. Singh JA, Inacio MC, Namba RS, Paxton EW. Rheumatoid arthritis is associated with higher 90-day hospital readmission rates compared to osteoarthritis after hip or knee arthroplasty: A cohort study. Arthritis Care Res (Hoboken). 2015;67:718-24.
11. Issa K, Pivec R, Kapadia BH, Banerjee S, Mont MA. Osteonecrosis of the femoral head: the total hip replacement solution. Bone Joint J. 2013;95-B(11 Suppl A):46–50.
12. STROBE Statement. Strengthening the reporting of observational studies in epidemiology. Link: http://www.strobe-statement.org/fileadmin/Strobe/uploads/checklists/STROBE_checklist_v4_cohort.pdf. Accessed 1 Mar 2017.
13. Paxton EW, Inacio MC, Khatod M, Yue EJ, Namba RS. Kaiser Permanente National Total Joint Replacement Registry: aligning operations with information technology. Clin Orthop Relat Res. 2010;468(10):2646–63.
14. Paxton EW, Kiley ML, Love R, Barber TC, Funahashi TT, Inacio MC. Kaiser Permanente implant registries benefit patient safety, quality improvement, cost-effectiveness. Jt Comm J Qual Patient Saf. 2013;39(6):246–52.
15. Horan TC, Andrus M, Dudeck MA. CDC/NHSN surveillance definition of health care-associated infection and criteria for specific types of infections in the acute care setting. Am J Infect Control. 2008;36(5):309–32.
16. Agency for Healthcare Research and Quality. Patient Safety Indicators Technical Specifications. http://www.qualityindicators.ahrq.gov/Downloads/Modules/PSI/V50/TechSpecs/PSI_12_Perioperative_Pulmonary_Embolism_or_Deep_Vein_Thrombosis_Rate.pdf. Accessed 3 Mar 2017.
17. Yale New Haven Health Services Corporation/Center for Outcomes Research & Evaluation (YNHHSC/CORE). 2014 Procedure-Specific Readmission Measures Updates and Specifications Report Elective Primary Total Hip Arthroplasty (THA) and/or Total Knee Arthroplasty (TKA) – Version 3.0 [March 2014]. 2014.
18. Elixhauser A, Steiner C, Harris DR, Coffey RM. Comorbidity measures for use with administrative data. Med Care. 1998;36(1):8–27.
19. Singh JA, Inacio MC, Namba RS, Paxton EW. Rheumatoid Arthritis is Associated With Higher Ninety-Day Hospital Readmission Rates Compared to Osteoarthritis After Hip or Knee Arthroplasty: A Cohort Study. Arthritis Care Res (Hoboken). 2015;67(5):718–24.
20. Singh JA, Lewallen DG. Patients with osteoarthritis and avascular necrosis have better functional outcomes and those with avascular necrosis worse pain outcomes compared to rheumatoid arthritis after primary hip arthroplasty: a cohort study. BMC Med. 2013;11:210.
21. Ismael H, Horst M, Farooq M, Jordon J, Patton JH, Rubinfeld IS. Adverse effects of preoperative steroid use on surgical outcomes. Am J Surg. 2011; 201(3):305–8. discussion 308–309.
22. Nath B, Li Y, Carroll JE, Szabo G, Tseng JF, Shah SA. Alcohol exposure as a risk factor for adverse outcomes in elective surgery. J Gastrointest Surg. 2010;14(11):1732–41.
23. Rantala A, Lehtonen OP, Niinikoski J. Alcohol abuse: a risk factor for surgical wound infections? Am J Infect Control. 1997;25(5):381–6.
24. Koebnick C, Langer-Gould AM, Gould MK, Chao CR, Iyer RL, Smith N, Chen W, Jacobsen SJ. Sociodemographic characteristics of members of a large, integrated health care system: comparison with US Census Bureau data. Perm J. 2012;16(3):37–41.
25. Karter AJ, Ferrara A, Liu JY, Moffet HH, Ackerson LM, Selby JV. Ethnic disparities in diabetic complications in an insured population. JAMA. 2002; 287(19):2519–27.

Permissions

All chapters in this book were first published in MD, by BioMed Central; hereby published with permission under the Creative Commons Attribution License or equivalent. Every chapter published in this book has been scrutinized by our experts. Their significance has been extensively debated. The topics covered herein carry significant findings which will fuel the growth of the discipline. They may even be implemented as practical applications or may be referred to as a beginning point for another development.

The contributors of this book come from diverse backgrounds, making this book a truly international effort. This book will bring forth new frontiers with its revolutionizing research information and detailed analysis of the nascent developments around the world.

We would like to thank all the contributing authors for lending their expertise to make the book truly unique. They have played a crucial role in the development of this book. Without their invaluable contributions this book wouldn't have been possible. They have made vital efforts to compile up to date information on the varied aspects of this subject to make this book a valuable addition to the collection of many professionals and students.

This book was conceptualized with the vision of imparting up-to-date information and advanced data in this field. To ensure the same, a matchless editorial board was set up. Every individual on the board went through rigorous rounds of assessment to prove their worth. After which they invested a large part of their time researching and compiling the most relevant data for our readers.

The editorial board has been involved in producing this book since its inception. They have spent rigorous hours researching and exploring the diverse topics which have resulted in the successful publishing of this book. They have passed on their knowledge of decades through this book. To expedite this challenging task, the publisher supported the team at every step. A small team of assistant editors was also appointed to further simplify the editing procedure and attain best results for the readers.

Apart from the editorial board, the designing team has also invested a significant amount of their time in understanding the subject and creating the most relevant covers. They scrutinized every image to scout for the most suitable representation of the subject and create an appropriate cover for the book.

The publishing team has been an ardent support to the editorial, designing and production team. Their endless efforts to recruit the best for this project, has resulted in the accomplishment of this book. They are a veteran in the field of academics and their pool of knowledge is as vast as their experience in printing. Their expertise and guidance has proved useful at every step. Their uncompromising quality standards have made this book an exceptional effort. Their encouragement from time to time has been an inspiration for everyone.

The publisher and the editorial board hope that this book will prove to be a valuable piece of knowledge for researchers, students, practitioners and scholars across the globe.

List of Contributors

Duan Wang, Qi Li, Hao-Yang Wang, Ze-Yu Luo, Fu-Xing Pei and Zong-Ke Zhou
Department of Orthopedics, West China Hospital/ West China School of Medicine, Sichuan University, 37# Wuhou Guoxue road, Chengdu 610041, People's Republic of China

De-Hua Li
Key Laboratory of Birth Defects and Related Diseases of Women and Children, Ministry of Education, Sichuan University, Chengdu 610041, People's Republic of China
Department of Nursing, West China Second University Hospital/West China Women's and Children's Hospital, Chengdu 610041, China

Yang Yang
State Key Laboratory of Oral Diseases, West China Hospital of Stomatology, Sichuan University, Chengdu 610041, People's Republic of China

Yvon M. den Hartog, Nina M. Mathijssen and Stephan B. Vehmeijer
Department of Orthopaedic Surgery, Reinier de Graaf Hospital, Delft, the Netherlands

Gerjon Hannink
Orthopaedic Research Lab, Department of Orthopaedics, Radboud university medical center, Nijmegen, the Netherlands

Ping Zhen
Department of Orthopedics, The Second Affiliated Hospital of Lanzhou University, Cuiying Door, No. 82, Chengguan District, Lanzhou City, Gansu Province 730030, People's Republic of China
Department of Orthopaedics, Lanzhou General Hospital of PLA, South Binhe Road, No. 333, Lanzhou City, Gansu Province 730050, People's Republic of China

Jun Liu, Hao Lu, Hui Chen, Xusheng Li and Shenghu Zhou
Department of Orthopaedics, Lanzhou General Hospital of PLA, South Binhe Road, No. 333, Lanzhou City, Gansu Province 730050, People's Republic of China

Shun-Wun Jhan, Yu-Der Lu, Mel S. Lee, Jun-Wen Wang and Feng-Chih Kuo
Department of Orthopaedic Surgery, Kaohsiung Chang Gung Memorial Hospital, No. 123, Ta Pei Road, Niao Sung Dist, Kaohsiung City 833, Taiwan
Chang Gung University College of Medicine, Kaohsiung, Taiwan

Chen-Hsiang Lee
Division of Infectious Diseases, Department of Internal Medicine, Kaohsiung Chang Gung Memorial Hospital, Kaohsiung, Taiwan
Chang Gung University College of Medicine, Kaohsiung, Taiwan

Mattia Loppini
Hip Diseases and Joint Replacement Surgery Unit, Humanitas Clinical and Research Centre, Via Alessandro Manzoni 56, 20089 Rozzano, Milan, Italy
Humanitas University, Via Alessandro Manzoni 113, 20089 Rozzano, Milan, Italy

Umile Giuseppe Longo and Vincenzo Denaro
Department of Orthopaedic and Trauma Surgery, Campus Bio-Medico University, Via Alvaro del Portillo 200, 00128 Trigoria, Rome, Italy

Emanuele Caldarella, Antonello Della Rocca and Guido Grappiolo
Hip Diseases and Joint Replacement Surgery Unit, Humanitas Clinical and Research Centre, Via Alessandro Manzoni 56, 20089 Rozzano, Milan, Italy

Xianshang Zeng, Ke Zhan and Weiguang Yu
Department of Orthopedics, The First Affiliated Hospital of Sun Yat-sen University, Huangpu East Road No. 183, Huangpu District, Guangzhou City, Guangdong Province 510700, China

Lili Zhang
Department of Anesthesiology, The First Affiliated Hospital of Sun Yat-sen University, Huangpu East Road No. 183, Huangpu District, Guangzhou City, Guangdong Province 510700, China

Dan Zeng
Ultrasonography Department, The First Affiliated Hospital of Sun Yat-sen University, Huangpu East Road No. 183, Huangpu District, Guangzhou City, Guangdong Province 510700, China

Xinchao Zhang and Mingdong Zhao
Department of Orthopaedics, Jinshan Hospital, Fudan University, Longhang Road No. 1508, Jinshan District, Shanghai City 201508, China

Shinya Hayashi, Shingo Hashimoto, Tomoyuki Matsumoto, Koji Takayama, Kotaro Nishida and Ryosuke Kuroda
Department of Orthopaedic Surgery, Kobe University Graduate School of Medicine, 7-5-1 Kusunoki-cho, Chuo-ku, Kobe 650-0017, Japan

Takayuki Nishiyama
Department of Orthopaedic Surgery, Kakogawa City Hospital, Kakogawa, Japan

Kazunari Ishida
Department of Orthopaedic Surgery, Kobe Kaisei Hospital, Kobe, Japan

Matthew Jian-Qiao Peng, Hai-Yan Chen and Bo Bai
Guangdong Orthopedics Implantation key Lab, Orthopedics Department of 1st Affiliated Hospital, Guangzhou Medical University, 151 YanJiangXi Rd, Guangzhou 510120, China

Yong Hu
Neural Electrophysiology Lab, University of Hong Kong, Room 501, Haking Wong Building, Pokfulam Road, Pok Fu Lam, Hong Kong

XiangYang Ju
Clinical Physics & Bioengineering Department, University of Glasgow, 378 Sauchiehall St., Glasgow G2 3JZ, UK
Ze-Yu Luo, Hao-Yang Wang, Duan Wang, Fu-Xing Pei and Zong-Ke Zhou Department of Orthopedics, West China Hospital/West China School of Medicine, Sichuan University, 37# Wuhou Guoxue Road, Chengdu 610041, People's Republic of China

Hui Pan
Department of Hematology, The First Affiliated Hospital of Chongqing Medical University, No. 1 Youyi Road, Yuzhong District, Chongqing 400016, People's Republic of China

Tsan-Wen Huang and Kuo-Ti Peng
Department of Orthopaedic Surgery, Chang Gung Memorial Hospital, Chiayi, Taiwan
Chang Gung University, Taoyuan, Taiwan
No. 6, West Section, Chia-Pu Road, Pu-Tzi City, Chia-Yi Hsien 613, Taiwan

Chao-Jan Wang
Chang Gung University, Taoyuan, Taiwan
Department of Diagnostic and Interventional Radiology, Chang Gung Memorial Hospital, Linkou, Taiwan
5 Fu-Hsin Street, Kweishan, Taoyuan, Taiwan

Hsin-Nung Shih and Yuhan Chang
Chang Gung University, Taoyuan, Taiwan
Department of Orthopaedic Surgery, Chang Gung Memorial Hospital, Linkou, Taiwan
5 Fu-Hsin Street, Kweishan, Taoyuan, Taiwan

Kuo-Chin Huang
Chang Gung University, Taoyuan, Taiwan
Department of Orthopaedic Surgery, Kaohsiung Chang Gung Memorial Hospital, No. 123, Dapi Rd., Niaosong District, Kaohsiung City 83301, Taiwan
No. 123, Dapi Rd., Niaosong District, Kaohsiung City 83301, Taiwan

Mel S. Lee
Chang Gung University, Taoyuan, Taiwan
Department of Orthopaedic Surgery, Kaohsiung Chang Gung Memorial Hospital, No. 123, Dapi Rd., Niaosong District, Kaohsiung City 83301, Taiwan

Maya Hürlimann, Filippo-Franco Schiapparelli, Niccolo Rotigliano and Michael T. Hirschmann
Department of Orthopaedic Surgery and Traumatology, Kantonsspital Baselland (Bruderholz, Liestal, Laufen), CH-4101 Bruderholz, Switzerland
University of Basel, Basel, Switzerland

Enrique Testa
Department of Orthopaedic Surgery and Traumatology, Kantonsspital Baselland (Bruderholz, Liestal, Laufen), CH-4101 Bruderholz, Switzerland

Felix Amsler
Amsler Consulting, CH-4059 Basel, Switzerland

Nick T. van Dasselaar
Department of Anaesthesiology and Pain Medicine, Reinier de Graaf Hospital, Delft, the Netherlands

Wei Xuan
South Western Sydney Clinical School, University of New South Wales, Liverpool Hospital, Elizabeth Drive, Liverpool, NSW 2170, Australia
Ingham Institute of Applied Medical Research, Westfields Liverpool, Liverpool, NSW 2170, Australia
Mindaugas Stravinskas, Sarunas Tarasevicius and Simonas Laukaitis Lithuanian University of Health, Kaunas, Lithuania

Seung-Chan Kim, Young-Wook Lim, Woo-Lam Jo, Dong-Chul Park, Jin-Woo Lee, Won-Woo Kang and Yong-Sik Kim
Department of Orthopaedic Surgery, Seoul St. Mary's Hospital, College of Medicine, The Catholic University of Korea, Banpodae-ro 222, Seocho-gu, Seoul 137-701, South Korea

Junichi Nakamura, Shigeo Hagiwara, Sumihisa Orita, Ryuichiro Akagi, Kazuhisa Takahashi and Seiji Ohtori
Department of Orthopaedic Surgery, Graduate School of Medicine, Chiba University, 1-8-1 Inohana, Chuo-ku, Chiba City, Chiba 260-8677, Japan

Takane Suzuki
Department of Bioenvironmental Medicine, Graduate School of Medicine, Chiba University, 1-8-1 Inohana, Chuo-ku, Chiba City, Chiba 260-8677, Japan

Masahiko Suzuki
Research Center for Frontier Medical Engineering, Chiba University, 1-33 Yayoi-cho, Inage-ku, Chiba City 263-8522, Japan

Rene Burchard
Department of Health, University of Witten/ Herdecke, Witten, Germany
Department of Trauma and Orthopaedic Surgery, Kreisklinikum Siegen, Siegen, Germany

Sabrina Braas
Department of Trauma and Orthopaedic Surgery, Kreisklinikum Siegen, Siegen, Germany
Department of Orthopaedics and Rheumatology, University of Marburg, Marburg, Germany

Christian Soost
Department of Statistics an Econometrics, University of Siegen, Siegen, Germany

Jan Adriaan Graw
Department of Anesthesiology and Operative Intensive Care Medicine (CCM, CVK), Charité - Universitätsmedizin Berlin, Freie Universität Berlin, Humboldt-Universität zu Berlin, and Berlin Institute of Health, Campus Virchow-Klinikum, Berlin, Germany

Jan Schmitt
Department of Orthopaedics and Rheumatology, University of Marburg, Marburg, Germany
Department of Orthopaedics and Trauma Surgery, Lahn-Dill-Kliniken Wetzlar, Wetzlar, Germany

Pei Zhang
Dalian Medical University, Dalian, Liaoning 116044, China

Yuan Liang, Pengtao Chen and Yongchao Fang
Department of Orthopedics, Clinical Medical College of Yangzhou University, Subei People's Hospital, Nantong West Road 98, Yangzhou 225001, China

Jinshan He
Department of Orthopedics, Clinical Medical College of Yangzhou University, Subei People's Hospital, Nantong West Road 98, Yangzhou 225001, China
Department of Orthopedics, Clinical Medical College of Yangzhou University, Subei People's Hospital of Jiangsu Province, Yangzhou, China

Jingcheng Wang
Dalian Medical University, Dalian, Liaoning 116044, China
Department of Orthopedics, Clinical Medical College of Yangzhou University, Subei People's Hospital, Nantong West Road 98, Yangzhou 225001, China
Department of Orthopedics, Clinical Medical College of Yangzhou University, Subei People's Hospital of Jiangsu Province, Yangzhou, China

Jian Zhong, Hai-bo Si, Yi Zeng, Jing Yang, Zong-ke Zhou, Peng-de Kang, Fu-xing Pei and Bin Shen
Department of orthopaedics, West China Hospital, Sichuan University, Chengdu 610041, People's Republic of China

Szilard Nemes, Erik Bülow and Ola Rolfson
Swedish Hip Arthroplasty Register, Centre of Registers Västra Götaland, Gothenburg, Sweden
Department of Orthopedics, Institute of Clinical Sciences, Sahlgrenska Academy, University of Gothenburg, Gothenburg, Sweden

Dennis Lind and Cecilia Rogmark
Swedish Hip Arthroplasty Register, Centre of Registers Västra Götaland, Gothenburg, Sweden
Department of Orthopedics, Lund University, Skane University Hospital, Malmö, Sweden

Peter Cnudde
Swedish Hip Arthroplasty Register, Centre of Registers Västra Götaland, Gothenburg, Sweden
Department of Orthopedics, Institute of Clinical Sciences, Sahlgrenska Academy, University of Gothenburg, Gothenburg, Sweden
Department of Orthopedics, Hywel Dda University Healthboard, Prince Philip Hospital, Bryngwyn Mawr, Llanelli, UK

Ronen Debi, Evyatar Slamowicz, Ornit Cohen, Omri Lubovsky and Ehud Atoun
Department of Orthopedic Surgery, Barzilai Medical Center, 2 Hahistadrut Street, 78278 Ashkelon, Israel
Affiliated to the Ben-Gurion University of the Negev, Beer sheva, Israel

Avi Elbaz
AposTherapy Research Group, Herzelyia, Israel

Dror Lakstein and Zachary Tan
Department of Orthopaedic Surgery, Wolfson Medical Center, Holon, Israel

Johannes C. Reichert and Ulrich Nöth
Department of Orthopaedic Surgery, König-Ludwig-Haus, Center for Musculoskeletal Research, Julius-Maximilians-University, Brettreichstraße 11, 97074 Würzburg, Germany
Department of Orthopaedic and Trauma Surgery, Evangelisches Waldkrankenhaus Spandau, Stadtrandstrasse 555, 13589 Berlin, Germany

Eberhard von Rottkay and Lars Rackwitz
Department of Orthopaedic and Trauma Surgery, Evangelisches Waldkrankenhaus Spandau, Stadtrandstrasse 555, 13589 Berlin, Germany

Franz Roth, Tim Renz, Johannes Hausmann, Julius Kranz and Maximilian Rudert
Department of Orthopaedic Surgery, König-Ludwig-Haus, Center for Musculoskeletal Research, Julius-Maximilians-University, Brettreichstraße 11, 97074 Würzburg, Germany

Hiromasa Tanino, Tatsuya Sato, Yasuhiro Nishida, Ryo Mitsutake and Hiroshi Ito
Department of Orthopaedic Surgery, Asahikawa Medical University, Midorigaoka-Higashi 2-1-1-1, Asahikawa 078-8510, Japan

Sun-jung Yoon and Myung-sik Park
Department of Orthopedic Surgery, Research Institute of clinical medicine of Chonbuk National University, Biomedical Research Institute of Chonbuk National University Hospital, 54907 Gunji-Ro 20, Dukjin-Gu, Chonbuk, Jeonju, South Korea

Dean K. Matsuda
DISC Sports and Spine Center, Marina del Rey, CA, USA

Yun Ho Choi
Department of Anatomy, Medical School, Institute for Medical Sciences, Chonbuk National University, Jeonju 561-180, South Korea

Pu Shao, Zhizhou Li, Modi Yang, Yuhui Yang, Lian Duan and Jianlin Zuo
Department of Orthopedics, China-Japan Union Hospital of Jilin University, 126 xiantai street, Changchun 130033, People's Republic of China

Te Liu and Jinlan Jiang
Scientific Research Centre of China-Japan Union Hospital of Jilin University, 126 xiantai street, Changchun 130033, People's Republic of China

Yuzhuo Wang
Department of Orthodontics, School and Hospital of Stomatology, Jilin University, Changchun 130021, People's Republic of China

Justine M. Naylor and Ian A. Harris
South Western Sydney Clinical School, University of New South Wales, Liverpool Hospital, Elizabeth Drive, Liverpool, NSW 2170, Australia
South West Sydney Local Health District, Liverpool, NSW 2170, Australia
Ingham Institute of Applied Medical Research, Westfields Liverpool, Liverpool, NSW 2170, Australia

Andrew Hart and Rajat Mittal
South Western Sydney Clinical School, University of New South Wales, Liverpool Hospital, Elizabeth Drive, Liverpool, NSW 2170, Australia

Malin Nilsson, Deepak Bushan Raina and Lars Lidgren
Department of Orthopedics, Lund University Hospital, Lund, Sweden

Taro Tezuka, Yutaka Inaba, Naomi Kobayashi, Hyonmin Choe, Syota Higashihira and Tomoyuki Saito
Department of Orthopedic Surgery, Yokohama City University, 3-9 Fukuura, Kanazawa-ku, Yokohama, Japan

Michael A. Heffler, Ryan Barlow and Avneesh Chhabra
Department of Orthopedic Surgery, University of Texas Southwestern Medical Center, Dallas, TX, USA
Department of Radiology, University of Texas Southwestern Medical Center, 5323 Harry Hines Blvd, Dallas, TX 75390-8896, USA

Yin Xi
Department of Radiology, University of Texas Southwestern Medical Center, 5323 Harry Hines Blvd, Dallas, TX 75390-8896, USA

Daichi Hayashi
Department of Radiology, Boston University Medical Center, Boston, MA, USA

Hayden Box and Michael Huo
Department of Orthopedic Surgery, University of Texas Southwestern Medical Center, Dallas, TX, USA

Jasvinder A. Singh
Medicine Service, Birmingham VA Medical Center, Birmingham, AL, USA
Department of Medicine at School of Medicine, and Division of Epidemiology at School of Public Health, University of Alabama, Faculty Office Tower 805B, 510 20th Street S, Birmingham, AL 35294, USA
Department of Orthopedic Surgery, Mayo Clinic College of Medicine, Rochester, MN, USA

Robert S. Namba
Department of Orthopaedic Surgery, Kaiser Permanente, Irvine, CA, USA

Jason Chen, Maria C. S. Inacio and Elizabeth W. Paxton
Department of Surgical Outcomes and Analysis, Kaiser Permanente, San Diego, CA, USA

Index

www.ingramcontent.com/pod-product-compliance
Lightning Source LLC
LaVergne TN
LVHW080734210926
848485LV00003B/555
9781639274048